D0612864

The Truth About BREAST HEALTH

BREAST CANCER

Prescription for healing

Charles B. Simone, M.D.

Princeton Institute
PrincetonInstitute.com
Princeton, NJ 08654

A portion of proceeds for breast research

Manufactured in the United States of America by
Princeton Institute, LLC.
PO Box 7532 • Princeton, NJ 08540

First Printing

Cover design: Charles B. Simone, M.D.
Thermogram graciously provided by Bailes Scientific, Inc.,
Walnut Creek, CA 94595

Library of Congress Cataloging-in-Publication Data

Simone, Charles B.
The Truth About Breast Health – Breast Cancer, Prescription for Healing / Charles B. Simone, M.D.
Includes bibliographical references and index.

ISBN 0-9714574-0-9

1. Breast – Cancer – Popular works. I. Title
2. Breast – Diseases – Popular Works. I. Title
3. Antioxidants – Therapeutic use.
4. Cancer – Diet therapy.
5. Cancer – Risk factors.

RC280.B8S499 2001 01-14177
616.99'499 – dc20 CIP

Table of Contents

To my family

****
****

"It is impossible for anyone to begin to learn what he thinks that he already knows."

Epictetus

****
****

A paradigm shift occurs as exceptions, often startling changes. "Such changes, together with the controversies that almost always accompany them, are the defining characteristics of scientific revolutions."

Thomas Kuhn

Note to the Reader

This monograph does not make recommendations about breast diseases or breast cancer therapy. Neither the author nor the publisher makes warranties, expressed or implied, that this information is complete, nor do we warrant the fitness of this information for any particular purpose. This information is not intended as medical advice, and we disclaim any liability resulting from its use. Neither the author nor the publisher advocates any treatment modality. Each reader is strongly urged to consult qualified professionals for their medical problems, especially those involving cancer.

Acknowledgements: Thanks to photographers Leona Law and Sally Davidson.

Introduction

All women should strive to attain optimum breast health because the incidence of benign lumpy breast disease and breast cancer is rising at alarming rates. Eight of ten women develop benign lumpy breast disease; one in every eight women in the United States will develop breast cancer, and the odds are getting worse.

Cancer is the most feared of all diseases. People immediately associate cancer with dying. Unlike some other killer diseases, cancer usually causes a slow death involving pain, suffering, mental anguish, and a feeling of hopelessness. It now affects two of every five Americans. The number of new cancer cases has been increasing over the past nine decades; the accelerated rise in lung cancer, for example, is alarming. According to the U.S. Bureau of the Census, 47 people out of every 100,000 died of cancer in 1900, making it the sixth leading cause of death. Today, 168 people out of every 100,000 will die of cancer, ranking it second.

In 1971, the United States declared war on cancer with the following statement from President Nixon: "The time has come in America when the same kind of concentrated effort that split the atom and took man to the moon should be turned toward conquering this dread disease." In that year, 337,000 people died of cancer, and about $250 million was spent on cancer research.

Since then, billions of dollars have been invested in cancer research. Approximately $104 billion is spent on cancer treatment each year: about $35 billion for direct health care, $12 billion in lost productivity due to treatment or disability, and $57 billion in lost productivity due to premature death.[1] Each month, it seems, new therapies are trumpeted. Some show promise, others fizzle quickly. So intense is the concern to find "the cure for cancer" that more money is collected each year than can actually be spent responsibly on meaningful research. More of these funds should be directed to cancer prevention than the National Cancer Institute's current allocation of less than 5 to 7 percent.

Despite the enormous effort to combat cancer, the number of new cases of nearly every form of cancer has increased annually over the last century as shown in Table 1 and Figure 1. From 1930 to the present, despite the introduction of radiation therapy, chemotherapy, and immunotherapy with biologic response modifiers, despite CT scans, MRI scans, and all the other new medical technology, lifespans for people with almost every form of cancer except cervical cancer and lung cancer have remained constant, which means that there has been no significant progress in treatment for cancer including breast cancer.[2] See Figure 2. The incidence of stomach cancer has gone down probably due to the advent of refrigeration in the 1930s and the consequent removal of carcinogenic chemicals as food preservatives. The National Cancer Institute and American Cancer Society set an unrealistic goal of a 50 percent reduction in cancer mortality by the year 2000.[3-9] Looking at the almost vertical rise in Figure 1 in the number of new cancer cases each year, I predicted in 1994 that the goal could not be attained. It was not.

Table 1. United States Cancer Incidence

	1900	1962	1971*	2002
Total Cases	25,000	520,000	635,000	1,279,000
Leading Cancers				
Prostate	N/A	31,000	35,000	198,100
Breast	N/A	63,000	69,600	193,700
Lung	N/A	45,000	80,000	174,600
Colon/Rectum	N/A	72,000	75,000	140,000
Uterus	N/A	N/A	N/A	51,000

*President Nixon declared war on cancer. N/A = Not available. Data from US Bureau of Vital Statistics and *CA – A Cancer Journal for Clinicians*

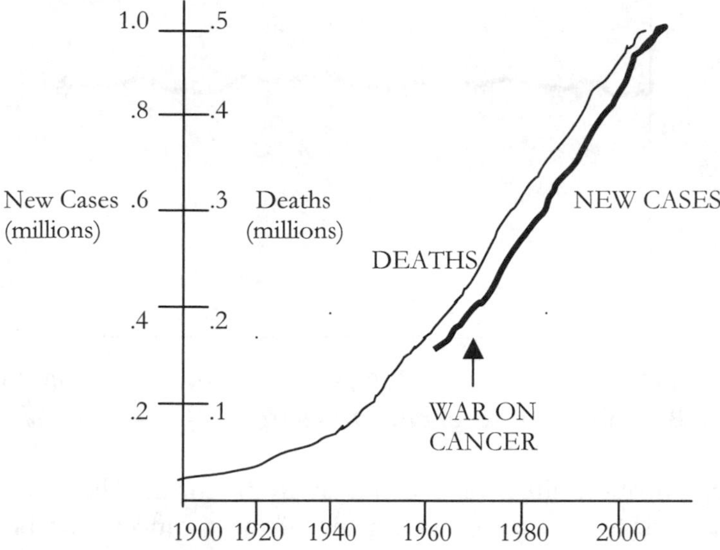

Figure 1. Cancer deaths and new cases. Note the rise in new cancer cases and cancer related deaths despite billions of dollars in research.

The chilling prospect remains: two of every five Americans will develop cancer, and the majority of them will die from it.

Cancer research and treatment are extremely complex fields of study because the exact nature of the single cancer cell is so elusive. Cancers are many diseases with many different causes. We cannot expect miracle cures just because so much money has been poured into cancer research. At the same time, we should not expect miracles from "cancer-cure" facilities that take money from cancer patients desperate to try any treatment in hope of another chance at life.

After collating the existing cancer data, I found that 80-90 percent of all cancers are produced as a result of dietary and nutritional factors, lifestyle (smoking, alcohol consumption, lack of exercise, etc.), chemicals, and other environmental factors.[10] This information has now been corroborated by major agencies: the National Academy of Sciences,[11] the U.S. Department of Health and Human Services,[12] the National Cancer Institute,[13] and the American Cancer Society.

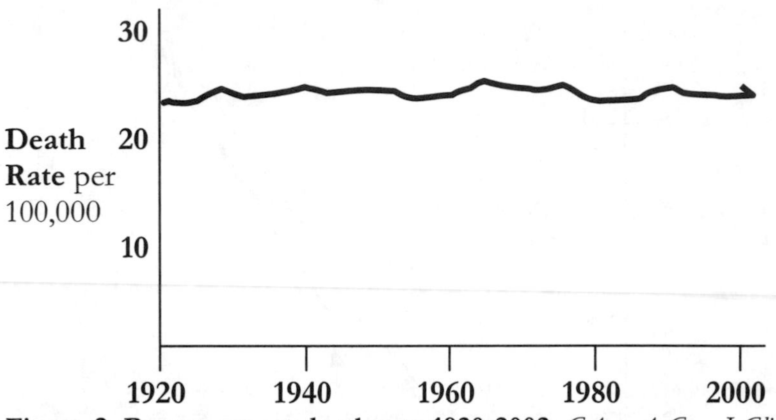

Figure 2. Breast cancer death rate 1920-2002. *CA – A Canc J Clin.*

Since nutrition, lifestyle, and the environment are the most common risk factors for cancer, many of these cancers can be eliminated or substantially reduced in number if you can identify the risk factors pertinent to you and modify them accordingly. Many people have the fatalistic attitude that anything and everything can cause cancer, and believe there is no use in trying to do anything about it. That attitude is unwarranted and fosters even more apathy. Everything does not cause cancer.

The public's perception of cancer causes and cancer "cures" comes mainly from the news media. A study finally has been done that shows serious discrepancies between media people's beliefs about what constitutes cancer risks and what scientists have actually shown to be cancer risks.[16] By reviewing over 1,100 newspaper, magazine, and television news stories between 1972 and 1992, media representatives cited the risks they believed to be the leading factors in causing cancer: manmade chemicals such as food additives and pesticides, pollution, hormone treatments, and radiation. When members of the American Association for Cancer Research were asked the same question, they cited the following as the major risk factors for causing cancer: tobacco, diet, and sunlight. Here again, it is easier for people to complain about risk factors perceived to be important and over which they have no control, rather than take on the responsibility to modify risk factors over which they have total control. People do, in fact, have total control over the leading causes of cancer.

The type of diet we eat today and its preparation are major risk factors in the development of certain cancers, risk factors that can definitely be modified. Nutrition is a very complex topic - one that is not well understood by the public or even by many physicians. Americans need to know the role that nutrition plays in major diseases.

Diet and nutrition appear to be factors in 60 percent of women's cancers and 40 percent of men's cancers as well as about 75 percent of cardiovascular disease cases. Tobacco is a factor in about 30 percent of human cancers. Other known risk factors associated with the development of cancer include alcohol, age, immune system deficiencies, chemicals, and drugs. You have total control over most of these risk factors, including the major two: diet and tobacco. The cancers most closely associated with nutritional factors are cancers of the breast, colon, rectum, prostate, and endometrium.

Having one or more of the risk factors does not mean that cancer will necessarily develop. It simply means that a person exposed to risk factors has a greater than normal chance of developing cancer.

Physicians in our country too often wind up treating the cancer rather than the whole cancer patient. Much has been learned since 1981 about the role of nutrition, the immune system, and the patient's mental state in the healing process. Because these issues are not addressed properly by the medical community, many patients with advanced tumors seek questionable treatment. At great financial and emotional cost to themselves and their families, they resort to quack remedies, get-healthy-quick schemes, and practitioners and "health" centers that claim to reverse or eliminate chronic diseases easily and quickly.

It is *your* responsibility to learn about the risk factors involved in cancer development, and specifically breast cancer, and then modify those risk factors accordingly. In order to prevent cancer, you should devise your own anticancer plan based on risk factor modification. In addition, your family, and particularly your children, should be taught about risk factor modification. If nutritional and other risk factors are modified, the benefit will be evident in all people, but especially in the young and in the succeeding generations. Obviously, there are some risk factors, like air and water that you cannot directly control; therefore, your community must devise plans to modify environmental factors.

We must eliminate or modify all known risk factors so that we will eventually be able to prevent cancer and heart disease. Nutritional factors and tobacco smoking, for example, are major risk factors, which, if modified or eliminated, can dramatically reduce the number of cancer as well as heart disease patients. Our health-care system emphasizes expensive medical technology and hospital care. It does not emphasize preventive medicine and health education. *It is your responsibility to learn about risk factors and then modify them.* Good health does not come easily, you must work for it.

You have almost total control over the destiny of your health and the health of your family! Do something about it.

PART ONE

Breast Disease Today

1

The Scope of Breast Disease

One woman in eight will develop breast cancer during her lifetime. In the United States, it is the second leading cause of death in women with cancer; 29 percent of the cancers that women develop are breast cancers. The number of new cases of breast cancer in the United States is about 193,700; 192,200 in women and 1,500 in men.[1] Total deaths from breast cancer are estimated to be 40,600; 40,200 females and 400 males. African American women are less likely to develop breast cancer than white women but they fare worse when they develop it because the cancer is more advanced at the time of diagnosis. Breast cancers also have a seasonal variation. More breast cancer cases are reported in the spring, and fewer in the autumn.[2] Physicians use the term "stage of disease" to denote the extent to which a cancer has spread. The prognosis worsens with each advancing stage. Three terms describe the stage:

Localized – cancer is in its primary site of the breast.
Regional – cancer spread to lymph nodes around breast.
Distant – cancer spread to other parts of the body.

Table 1.1 Risk of Developing Breast Cancer By Age

By age 25: 1 in 19,608	By age 60: 1 in 24
By age 30: 1 in 2,525	By age 65: 1 in 17
By age 35: 1 in 622	By age 70: 1 in 14
By age 40: 1 in 217	By age 75: 1 in 11
By age 45: 1 in 93	By age 80: 1 in 10
By age 50: 1 in 50	By age 85: 1 in 9
By age 55: 1 in 33	Ever: 1 in 8

Breast cancer is more often fatal in white men than in white women. Of all those who survive for five years after the diagnosis has been made, 65 percent are women and 53 percent are men. Because most people think that breast cancer is a woman's disease, when men get lumps in their breasts or other symptoms related to their breasts, they tend to ignore or dismiss them as not possibly being cancer. For all white breast cancer patients (both male and female) from 1960 to 1983, the length of time that most people survived after initial diagnosis was six years and seven months, compared to three years and eight months for African Americans. Since 1930 to the present, there has been little or no change in lifespan (survival rate) for breast cancer patients (Figure 2, Introduction).

For this very reason, it is important to understand the role nutrition and other risk factors play in the development of breast cancer so that you can modify them. Most risk factors for breast cancer and benign breast disease can be modified. For example, a high-fat, low-fiber diet, tobacco use, alcohol use, etc can be modified. Your genetics cannot be directly modified, but genetics play only a small role in the development of breast cancer – less than 7 percent. Age is another risk factor that cannot be modified.

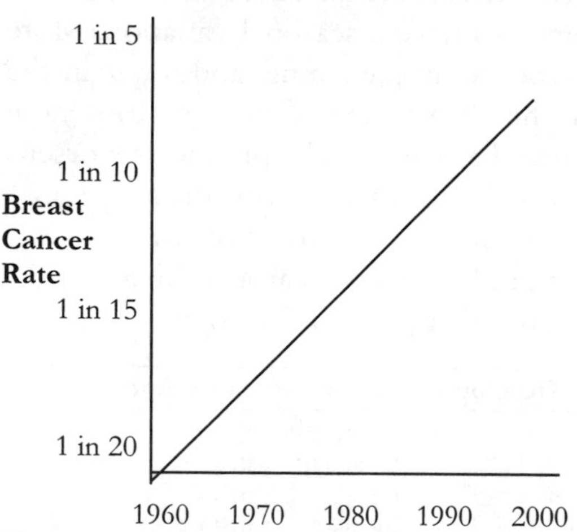

In 1960, one in twenty women developed breast cancer; in 1974, one in seventeen, and those odds have gotten worse with each succeding year. By 1990, the rate had risen to one in ten and kept zooming: in 1991, one in nine, in 1994, one in eight developed breast cancer.

Figure 1.1 Odds that a woman develops breast cancer in the US.

Breast cancer is the second most prevalent cancer in the United States. Table 1.2 shows the estimated new breast cancer cases in each state.

These statistics should be no surprise because we know that **40 percent of Americans will develop cancer**. Second only to cardiovascular disease as the leading cause of death in the United States, cancer accounts for 35 percent of all deaths These figures do not even include an estimated 450,000 patients with non-melanomas skin cancers. The leading cancers in the United States include lung cancer, breast cancer, colon-rectal cancer, prostate cancer, and cancer of the uterus; the latter four are all associated with nutritional factors. The number of new breast cancer cases increased from 82 per 100,000 women in 1973 to 195 per 100,000 in 2000. The annual percentage increase is about 2% each year.

Table 1.2 Estimated New Breast Cancer Cases by State – 2002

Alabama	2,700	Louisiana	3,200	Ohio	8,600
Alaska	200	Maine	900	Oklahoma	2,400
Arizona	2,800	Maryland	3,700	Oregon	2,200
Arkansas	1,900	Massachusetts	4,400	Pennsylvania	10,500
California	17,900	Michigan	6,700	Rhode Island	800
Colorado	2,000	Minnesota	2,800	South Carolina	2,600
Connecticut	2,300	Mississippi	2,000	South Dakota	400
Delaware	500	Missouri	3,700	Tennessee	3,800
D.C.	2,700	Montana	600	Texas	11,500
Florida	12,000	Nebraska	1,100	Utah	900
Georgia	4,600	Nevada	1,000	Vermont	400
Hawaii	500	New Hampshire	700	Virginia	4,500
Idaho	700	New Jersey	6,400	Washington	3,500
Illinois	8,900	New Mexico	1,000	West Virginia	1,400
Indiana	4,200	New York	13,700	Wisconsin	3,300
Iowa	2,100	North Carolina	5,200	Wyoming	300
Kansas	1,600	North Dakota	500	Puerto Rico	1,400
Kentucky	2,700				

When mortality figures are examined from 1930 onward, however, no change is seen in survival for women with breast cancer, which means there has been no change in the life span of women affected with breast cancer since 1930. And the number of breast cancer deaths goes up every year.

At the request of the Congress in December 1991, the Government Accounting Office released its findings concerning breast cancer – *Breast Cancer, 1971-1991: Prevention, Treatment, and Research.* The report states that there has been no progress in the prevention of breast cancer or in the reduction of breast cancer mortality. In the last two decades, the National Institutes of Health spent over $1 billion on breast cancer alone, touting spectacular progress at the research level with almost no change in reducing mortality or changing life spans. The trend of mortality rates is upward.

Treatment has improved survival only slightly. The five-year survival rate for breast cancer in 1976 was 75 percent; in 1983, 77 percent; in 1989, 78 percent; and, in 2000, 79 percent. Most scientists/physicians are convinced, however, that the slight increase in time of survival or life span is due largely to earlier detection of breast cancer by improved mammographic technology. But let us not forget what five-year survival means as defined by the oncologist. If a patient lives five years and one day, that woman is counted as a cure or survivor even though she has died. If, however, she lives one day less than five years, she is counted as a nonsurvivor.

Currently, the incidence of breast cancer is lower in developing countries than elsewhere, but almost half of all the world's breast cancer deaths will be in these developing countries.[3] The women will face all the same risk factors, and their immune systems are poor due, in part, to poor food. Breast cancer is likely to become the number one cause of death for cancer patients in the Third World. Most breast cancers in these countries will be in premenopausal women. And even if mammography were available in these countries, studies now show that screening mammography does not extend life. Breast self-examination likewise does not extend life.

The five-year mortality for patients having a 3 centimeter breast cancer lesion was studied in patients in Bombay, India, and the United States.[4] Only 25 percent of the patients in the United States die at five years compared with 41 percent of breast cancer patients who die in Bombay, India, at the end of five years. Within the first year of breast cancer detection, 21 percent of the people in Bombay, India, died, compared to only 5 percent of United States breast cancer patients in the first year. This shows that over half of the women who were going to die in the first five years, did so within the first year of diagnosis in Bombay, India.

Table 1.3 Global Incidence Rate of Breast Cancer per 100,000 – 2002

North America	86	Central America	26
Australia/New Zealand	72	Northern Africa	25
Temperate South America	69	Western Asia	24
Northern Europe	68	Melanesia	24
Western Europe	67	Southeast Asia	23
Micronesia and Polynesia	52	South Central Asia	21
Southern Europe	50	Western Africa	19
Tropical South America	39	Eastern Africa	18
Eastern Europe	36	Other East Asia	18
Caribbean	34	Middle Africa	14
Southern Africa	32	China	12
Japan	29		

As countries around the world have become more westernized especially in their dietary habits, the number of deaths from diet-related tumors has increased. For example, Table 1.3 shows the death rate of breast cancer cases per 100,000 people in various countries. When you examine the mortality from cancers in Japan, you find that tumors related to nutritional factors have increased dramatically in the last twenty-five years. Cancers of the colon and rectum, cancers of the breast, and prostate cancer all have increased dramatically. Previously, Japanese women enjoyed a very low rate of breast cancer. It affected only 3.9 women per 100,000 between the years 1955 and 1959. It rose to 6.1 women per 100,000 during the years 1985 to 1989, and is now 7.9 per 100,000. This trend is mainly seen in younger Japanese women who are more likely to have adopted Western ideas and habits, especially dietary habits.

We still hear that if more money were given for the war on cancer and specifically breast cancer, the magic bullet would be found. The major finding of the Government Accounting

Office report showed that *prevention* of cancer is paramount in the battle against cancer since there is no clear strategy for improving survival. And even though the medical management of the disease has improved, lifespan has not, and that is the primary objective of any treatment – to make the life span longer, improve survival. Two advances have come about, however: 1) minimizing pain and suffering, and 2) less mutilating surgery to achieve the same survival. Even though this information is well-known, the great majority of women still have a modified radical mastectomy rather than lumpectomy, sentinel node sampling, and radiation therapy.

The *prevention* of all cancers, including breast cancer, should be of primary importance. Less than 5 percent of the National Cancer Institute's budget currently is earmarked for prevention and of these studies, true prevention studies, unencumbered with other agenda, account for well under 2 percent. We are not winning the war against breast cancer with the current conventional approach; therefore, we must prevent the disease.

Breast diseases other than cancer also afflict many women today. It is estimated that 60 percent to 80 percent of all women develop benign breast disease. Men also develop benign breast disease. We will consider benign breast diseases at length in the next chapter.

2

Benign Breast Syndromes

The term "benign breast syndromes" embodies many benign breast disorders. Numerous terms have been used to describe these disorders including fibrocystic breasts, lumpy breasts, chronic mastitis, mammary dysplasia, cysts, and many others. Many physicians inappropriately label all the disorders that we will discuss as "fibrocystic disease."

About 60 to 80 percent of all women will develop some benign breast disorder. Most benign breast disorder symptoms occur predominantly in women who menstruate and these symptoms are relatively rare in post-menopausal women. Young women tend to have *fibroadenomas*, middle-aged women or perimenopausal women commonly have *cysts*, and only 15 percent of post-menopausal women have gross cysts.

Benign breast syndromes differ according to race. There is a decreased incidence in rural Africans, first-generation Chinese immigrants, and Native Americans. Japanese women have half as many biopsy-proven changes as American women. Lumpy breasts are more common in white women and fibroadenomas are more common in African Americans.

Many risk factors contribute to the development of benign breast symptoms and physical changes. Each of these risk factors influences all of the others.

1. High-fat diet.[1]
2. Lack of certain vitamins and minerals.[2]
3. Caffeine – coffee, tea, colas, chocolate.[3,4]
4. Nicotine, whether you smoke or inhale other's smoke.

5. Alcohol consumption.
6. Hormonal changes. Estrogen and progesterone influence different anatomical parts of the breast. Estrogen influences the cells that make up the ducts of the breasts. Progesterone influences the lobules that manufacture breast secretions.

There are two ways of classifying benign breast problems. The first and most common is based upon the clinical presentation of symptoms and physical characteristics. The second is based upon the pathologist's opinion after seeing a biopsied specimen under the microscope

SYMPTOMS AND PHYSICAL CHARACTERISTICS OF BENIGN BREAST SYNDROMES

Since the majority of lumps do not get biopsied, a clinical classification system for benign breast syndromes was developed and is based upon symptoms and physical characteristics.

Lumpiness or the feeling of grape-like structures is not the same as a single, large, dominating mass in the breast. Lumpiness is generally diffuse and located particularly in the upper outer quadrants of each breast. A dominant mass or lump does not change with the menstrual cycle, however, lumpiness does. Sometimes the difference between a dominant lump and generalized lumpiness is not very distinct.

Cyclical Swelling *Without* Tenderness starts at ovulation and continues to increase through menstruation.

Cyclical Swelling *With* Tenderness starts at ovulation (mid-cycle), and continues to increase through menstruation.

Breast Pain Both Cyclical and Non-cyclical. More than half of all women complain of breast pain at some time. Women generally seek the attention of a physician to find out if this pain is related to cancer. They simply want reassurance. Conditions that cause breast pain include:

- o Cyclical hormonal changes of menstrual cycle
- o Pain that is continuous or aching and unrelated to cycle changes (sclerosing adenosis)

o Infection of ducts
o Inflammation of the joint where the rib joins the sternum
o Cancer

Dominant Lumps – Cysts and Fibroadenomas. Dominant lumps are important because they must be distinguished from cancers. Cysts, galactoceles (milk-filled cysts), and fibroadenomas usually form dominant lumps.

- Cysts and galactoceles are fluid-filled and the fluid can be aspirated with a needle and syringe. Bile acids from the intestine, particularly lithocholic acid, a highly carcinogenic bile acid, become concentrated in breast cysts.[5] Consequently, ***palpable cysts increase the risk of developing breast cancer by 280 percent.***[6]
- Fibroadenomas, on the other hand, are solid breast tumors that are benign. Needle aspiration will yield no fluid. Fibroadenomas are usually seen in young women under the age of 25. Fibroadenomas may increase in size near the end of each menstrual cycle and are generally painless. Because they are solid masses and do not get smaller on their own, they must be removed surgically to determine with certainty that the mass is not a cancer. A ***fibroadenoma increases the risk for breast cancer by 150-200 percent.***[7]

Discharge From Nipple – Papilloma and Duct Problems. A mature woman or a newborn baby may secrete fluid from the nipple. Most hormones, including growth hormone, insulin, adrenal hormones, estrogen, progesterone, and prolactin may cause the breast to secrete fluid.

Prolactin, a hormone that is secreted from the pituitary in the brain into the blood, can cause a milky discharge from the nipple or menstrual irregularities. Many things may cause the elevation of prolactin: thyroid disorder, drugs that are used for sedation or tranquilization, oral contraceptives, breast or chest stimulation, and tumors located in the brain such as a pituitary tumor or craniopharyngiomas.

If the fluid secreted from the nipple is other than milky white, that is, if it is grossly bloody, then further investigation should be conducted. A smear may be done using the fluid put onto a slide and sent for microscopic evaluation. A mammogram should be done – and in some instances, a contrast ductographic mammogram – to determine the origin of the discharge. A bloody discharge must be evaluated. In some cases, surgical removal of the area causing the discharge is indicated. The most common causes of bloody nipple discharge:

- Intraductal papilloma (45 percent of all cases)
- "Fibrocystic" duct ectasia (35 percent - this condition affects mainly elderly females in whom the ends of the ducts are dilated and filled with debris)
- Infection (8 percent)
- Cancer (7 percent)

Infections mostly occur during lactation or shortly thereafter. Treatment is with antibiotics or surgical intervention.

A woman may have any or all of these clinical characteristics in any combination. Lumps may occur in one breast or both, but one breast is more often involved.

TISSUE BIOPSY CLASSIFICATION OF BENIGN BREAST LESIONS

The following classifications are based on biopsies. A breast lesion can only be classified in this way after a pathologist has examined tissue samples with a microscope. Some of the benign pathological categories of breast disease are precursors of future cancer and some are not. Some cause symptoms and lumps, others do not. Some grow larger, others do not.

Those benign conditions that do grow larger are termed *proliferative* lesions. Those that do not grow are termed *non-proliferative* lesions. Proliferative lesions may have either normal-looking cells or atypical cells, those that do not look normal, or typical. Any benign-looking lesion that has atypical cells brings with it a much higher risk of developing cancer. The more abnormal the cells look, the higher the risk. The lesions and categories below represent the majority of benign breast conditions that are typically seen. By no means, however, are all of them represented.

Non-Proliferative Lesions (Non-Growers)

- **Cyst.** Once the walls of a cyst are formed, they do not increase but they can stretch like a balloon being filled with water. The size varies during the menstrual cycle. Small cysts, less than 3 mm in diameter, pose little or no risk for cancer development. Large cysts can be palpated clinically when they reach 10 mm or more. The larger the cyst, the higher is the risk for cancer. The more atypical the cells that line the chamber of the cyst, the higher the risk for cancer.
- **Radial Scars** have a fibroelastotic core from which ducts and lobules radiate and can include cysts and proliferative lesions.[8]
- **Apocrine Cells** generally make up all sweat glands – the breast is classified as a sweat gland. In some patients, these cells may become abnormal. Generally, this poses little or no risk for the subsequent development of cancer.
- **Fibroadenoma** is a solid non-cancer mass and generally occurs in young women. It must be removed to differentiate it from a cancer.
- **Hyperplastic Cells** are normal in appearance under the microscope but there are many more of them than usual.

Proliferative Lesions With Normal Cells

- **Sclerosing adenosis** is not a cancer but may look like one under the microscope. It can be small or large and palpable and is usually located in one area of the breast. Microcalcifications on a mammogram are typical for an adenosis, which must then be distinguished from a cancer since some cancers also present with microcalcifications on a mammogram.

Proliferative Lesions With Abnormal or Atypical Cells

- **Hyperplasia – high degree.** A much larger number of cells are seen. Some may appear abnormal and thereby have a higher malignant potential.

- **Lobular Neoplasia.** An abnormal growth of cells that line the ducts and lobules, lobular neoplasia, misnamed lobular carcinoma *in situ*, usually does not form a palpable tumor. It does predispose to cancer.
- **Intraductal Papilloma.** Multiple intraductal papillomas involve a number of ducts, and generally form palpable masses. These also predispose to the development of cancer.

CERTAIN BENIGN ENTITIES INCREASE CANCER RISK

Numerous studies have examined the relationship between the above benign conditions and future risk of cancer. The bottom line with all these is a single important factor: the more abnormal the cells look under the microscope, i.e., the more atypical they are, the higher the chance for developing cancer. The less atypical or abnormal, the less is the risk for future cancer. Hence, any pathologically benign disorder of the breast should be treated aggressively because all cells are on a continuum starting with normal cells that can transform to various degrees of abnormality or atypia, and proceeding onward to a cancer cell. Once a benign condition is diagnosed, tremendous effort should be made to change the lifestyle factors that produced this condition. If those lifestyle factors are not changed, that benign condition may transform ultimately into a higher form of atypical cells or abnormal cells, and then into a cancer.

Table 2.1 represents a consensus statement issued by the Cancer Committee, College of American Pathologists, Relative Risk of Invasive Breast Cancer based on pathological examination of benign breast tissue.[9] About 25 percent of all women with benign breast conditions have pathology that puts them into the "slightly increased risk" category. However, for women with atypical or abnormal hyperplasia (borderline lesions) who also have a first-degree relative with breast cancer, the risk for developing breast cancer is 20 percent in the next 10 to 15 years.

Table 2.1. Risk of Developing Cancer Based on Pathological Examination of Benign Breast Tissue

No Increased Risk
Adenosis
Apocrine cellular changes
Small cysts
Mild Hyperplasia
Duct Ectasia
Fibrosis
Inflammation/ Infection (mastitis)
Squamous cellular changes
Slightly Increased Risk (1.5 to 2 times)
Large cysts and a first degree relative with breast cancer
Fibroadenoma – moderate to extensive hyperplasia
Papilloma
Sclerosing Adenosis, well developed
Radial Scars
Moderately Increased Risk (4 to 5 times)
Hyperplasia with abnormal or atypical cells
High Risk
Comedo (a pathological cell type) or non-comedo carcinoma *in situ*

GYNECOMASTIA

Gynecomastia is the condition in which the male breast enlarges. This male breast condition occurs when the influence of estrogen or estrogen-like chemicals is greater than the influence of testosterone. Gynecomastia generally affects the left breast more often than the right.[10] This condition may affect as much as one-third of the male population of all ages from puberty to old age and is seen in 57% of men over age 44.[11,12] Gynecomastia is associated with four causes:

1. Hormonal Changes

- Normal changes in the Neonatal period, Puberty, or Elderly
- Abnormal disease conditions:
  - Testicle fails to work
  - Puberty or Postpuberty abnormalities
  - Klinefelter's syndrome
- Testicle fails to work secondary to:
  - Radiation, or Trauma
  - Infection: orchitis, tuberculosis, leprosy
  - Cryptochidism
  - Hydrocele, or Varicocele, or Spermatocele

- Thyroid underactivity or overactivity
- Hormone produced from cancers of:
  - Testicle – Seminoma, Teratoma, Embryonal cell carcinoma, Androblastoma, Choriocarcinoma, Interstitial (Leydig) cell
  - Adrenal – Hyperplasia, carcinoma
  - Pituitary – Adenoma
  - Bronchogenic carcinoma
  - Hepatoma

2. Drugs

Amiloride	D-penicillamine	Marijuana	Reserpine
Amphetamines	Ergotamine tartrate	Methadone	Spironolactone
Anabolic steroids	Estramustine	Methyldopa	Sulindac
Busulfan	Estrogen	Metronidazole	Tamoxifen
Chlorpromazine	Fluphenazine	Neuroleptics	Theophylline
Cimetidine	Flutamide	Perphenazine	Thiazide
Clomiphene	Guanabenz	Phenothiazines	Thiethylperazine
Diazepam	Heroin	Procarbazine	Thioridazine
Diethylstilbestrol	Isoniazid	Prochlorperazine	Trifluoperazine
Digoxin	Ketoconizole	Propanolol	Tricyclics
Diphenylhydantoin	Leuprolide	Ranitidine	Vincristine

3. Systemic Disorders

Chronic disease of: liver, kidney, lung, brain
Malnutrition or starvation
Cancer of the colon, prostate, or lymphoma
Ulcerative colitis, Rheumatic fever

4. Idiopathic – Cause unknown

EXAMINATION AND FOLLOW-UP OF BENIGN BREAST SYNDROMES

Patients who have benign breast syndromes are difficult to physically examine. No matter how thorough a physician is in examining lumpy breasts, he/she can never be absolutely sure that there is not something evil like a cancer lurking within the nodularity or lumpiness or, in fact, behind them. The same caveat holds true for mammogram interpretation because the nodularity and fibrous tissue may mask areas that can also harbor a cancer. In addition, there are no good blood tests that can detect an early breast cancer. So the best course is to practice self-examination and "memorize" your breasts as much as possible, noting the location of the nodularities. Notify your physician if any *new* nodules develop, persist, or become hard.

Before a physician examines your breasts, he/she should know your risk factors for developing breast cancer. These risk factors should include those from Chapter 1 and, if you had a previous breast biopsy, the assigned risk from Table 2.1. This overall risk assessment will enable the physician to assign a certain degree of suspicion of possible cancer to your breast examination. If you have a high potential for malignancy as determined by your overall risk assessment, then minor changes in your breast should be viewed as highly suspicious. If your risk assessment is low, then minor breast changes would not be as suspicious.

For instance, if you are in a high risk category on the self-assessment test in Chapter 3 and also had a breast biopsy that was "hyperplasia with abnormal or atypical cells" (Table 2.1), I would examine you with a high degree of suspicion, looking for even subtle changes. If, on the other hand, you are in a low-risk category and had a biopsy that also conferred low-risk, like adenosis (Table 2.1), I would feel more relaxed about any minor breast changes. If you never had a breast biopsy, then the examiner's degree of suspicion should be linked to the level of risk as determined by the self-assessment test alone.

How Often Should You Be Examined?

If you have lumpy breasts, you should be examined three to four times a year by a physician who has extensive clinical experience in breast diseases. Gynecologists do the majority of all breast examinations but, in one study, did not find as many breast masses when compared to the number of breast masses detected by internists or family physicians, who spend the most amount of time doing a breast examination and found the most abnormalities.[13]

TREATMENT OF BENIGN BREAST DISORDERS

The most important thing a physician can do for a patient who comes into the office complaining of a lump is to make sure that the lump is not a cancer. A full discussion of the proper work-up of a lump begins in Chapter 21. Needle aspiration, ultrasound, and mammogram are all part of the evaluation process if indicated. Cyclical pain and generalized lumps have been handled in many different ways:

- Hormonal manipulation using progesterone, thyroid hormones, gonadotropins, tamoxifen, danazol, bromocriptine.
- Diuretics and/or Oral Contraceptives
- Steroids injected directly into the breast
- Surgical maneuvers
- Caffeine restriction
- Vitamin E, Evening Primrose Oil

Although some of these have provided relief for women, many of these drugs are too expensive or have too many side effects, including cancer that most women are not willing to tolerate. For instance, there is a 200 percent increased risk of developing breast cancer for women who used oral contraceptives for four years or more before the age of twenty-five.

PREMENSTRUAL SYNDROME

Premenstrual syndrome, or PMS, is a syndrome caused by the changes of estrogen and progesterone and other hormones during ovulation and, ultimately, premenstrually and menstrually. These hormonal changes are necessary if ovulation (the release of an egg from the ovary into the uterus) is to proceed. However, the hormonal changes lead to a combination of cyclical and distressing physical, psychological, and/or behavioral changes in many women. Some of these changes include acne, cravings for sweets, bloating, breast tenderness as already discussed, constipation, depression, anxiety, irritability, fatigue, insomnia, and headaches. Premenstrual syndrome even has legal implications. It has been used as a defense to mitigate women's responsibility for criminal acts.

SIMONE TEN-POINT PLAN FOR TREATING BENIGN BREAST SYMPTOMS

The Simone Ten-Point Plan has been effective for decreasing breast pain, nodularity, lumpiness, the size of many cysts, and many PMS symptoms. After adherence to the Simone Ten-

Point Plan for two full menstrual cycles, virtually 90 percent of all women have decreased breast tenderness, decreased swelling, little or no breast pain, softer breasts, and improvement in many PMS symptoms. After approximately six months, the majority of women experience a decrease in nodularity as well. The plan is fully discussed in Chapter 27.

Point 1. Nutrition.

- Maintain an ideal weight – decrease calories.
- No four-legged animals, shellfish, or dairy products unless they are skim products, not whole, 1%, or 2%. Poultry cooked without the skin.
- Consume *soluble* and *insoluble* fiber (25-35 grams/day). Fruits, vegetables, cereals are mainly *insoluble* fibers. Pectins, gums, and mucilages have *soluble* fibers that can decrease cholesterol, trigylcerides, sugars, and carcinogens. Use a supplement of *soluble* fiber to insure a consistent amount each day.
- Supplement your diet with certain nutrients in the proper doses, form, and combination based on your lifestyle. Take high doses of all antioxidants (the carotenoids, vitamins C and E, selenium, cysteine, bioflavonoids, copper, zinc), and the B vitamins with food. Calcium and its enhancing agents should be taken at bedtime.
- Eliminate salt, food additives, smoked and pickled foods. Limit barbecues.
- Take 325 mg aspirin every other day if you are able.

Point 2. Tobacco. Do not smoke, chew, snuff, or inhale other people's smoke.

Point 3. Alcohol and Caffeine. No alcohol or less than 2 drinks a week. Avoid caffeine (coffee, tea, chocolate).

Point 4. Radiation. X-rays only when needed. Use sun screens, and wear sunglasses. Avoid electromagnetic fields.

Point 5. Environment. Keep air, water, workplace clean.

Point 6. Sexual-Social Factors, Hormones, Drugs. Avoid promiscuity, hormones, and any unnecessary drugs.

Point 7. Learn the Seven Early Warning Signs

- Lump in breast
- Nonhealing sore
- Change in wart/mole
- Unusual bleeding
- Persistent cough/hoarseness
- Change in bowel/bladder habits
- Indigestion/trouble swallowing

Point 8. Exercise

Point 9. Modify Stress, Spirituality, Sexuality

Point 10. Comprehensive Physical Exam Yearly. Early diagnosis is important. Prevention is the key to wellness.

You will feel the difference and stay well by following this Simone Ten Point Plan. If you adhere to this Ten-Point Plan and still have not had significant relief from your breast pain or have not had improvement in other symptoms, then the various nutrients can be modified by an experienced clinician to attain a clinical response.

CAN TAMOXIFEN PREVENT BREAST CANCER ?

In April 1992, the US National Cancer Institute announced the beginning of the Breast Cancer Prevention Trial that would "last for only five years" and involve 16,000 women deemed to be at increased risk for developing breast cancer. The objective was to determine whether tamoxifen could significantly reduce the incidence of breast cancer in these high-risk individuals. Any woman over the age of 60 was eligible automatically. Women between the ages of 35 and 59 were eligible only if they had the following six risk factors: (a) Previous diagnosis of lobular carcinoma *in situ*; (b) First-degree relatives (mother, daughters, sisters) who have breast cancer; (c) Early age at menarche (first occurrence of menstruation); (d) Late age at delivery of first child; (e) No pregnancies; and, (f) History of having had breast biopsies.

On February 22, 1996 the International Agency for Research on Cancer ruled that tamoxifen was a carcinogen and causes human endometrial cancer

Because of improprieties, the US government halted the Breast Cancer Prevention Trial for over a year. But in April 1998, 14 months earlier than the scheduled five-year study period, the Breast Cancer Prevention Trial (13,338 women, 58 months) reported, via the news media, that tamoxifen reduced the risk of breast cancer by 45 percent.[14] Cancers were reported in 85 women taking tamoxifen, and 154 women taking the placebo. These data were not peer-reviewed, but nonetheless, on October 29, 1998 the Food and Drug Administration gave approval for tamoxifen's use to reduce the risk of breast cancer in high-risk women.

Two other studies, the British trial (2471 women, 70 months) and the Italian trial (5408 women, 46 months) showed that tamoxifen did not reduce the rate of breast cancer in women at high risk.[15,16] Why the discrepancy? Possibly because the preventive effect seen in the large Breast Cancer Prevention Trial with its short follow-up time is not prevention at all, but rather treatment of early breast cancers that were not detected – a finding that may disappear with longer follow-up time. This is precisely what the principal architect of this Trial explained as the rationale for its use. He said, "breast cancers that are diagnosed today did not begin to develop yesterday. A number of women who have what appeared to be normal breasts without detectable cancers already have the biological changes that will cause the disease. For any of these early changes an intervention such as tamoxifen may be able to halt the development or progression of breast cancer."[17]

Tamoxifen increases a woman's risk of developing four life-threatening conditions: endometrial cancer, deep vein thrombosis, pulmonary blood clots, and stroke.

According to the architects of the Breast Cancer Prevention Trial, tamoxifen was supposed to also protect against osteoporosis and heart disease. However, in two retrospective series[18,19] and in three prospective investigations[20-22] tamoxifen had no protective effect on bone density at all. Similarly, tamoxifen did not protect against heart disease – "the difference was not statistically significant."[23]

Tamoxifen has been around since 1980 to treat patients who have advanced breast cancer. It is the most widely prescribed cancer drug in the world. Tamoxifen is extremely helpful in a breast cancer patient's care. However, it is a drug used in patients who already have cancer, and it has side effects and risks, including endometrial cancer, liver cancer, lung clots, blood clots, hot flushes, and vaginal discharge. As toxic drugs go, it is one of the least toxic drugs. But when you have a cancer, you accept risks of drugs because you are trying to kill the cancer that can otherwise kill you.

The British Trial and the Italian Trial cast doubt on the results of the Breast Cancer Prevention Trial. None of these trials even assessed the length of life – the most important endpoint of any such study. There is no quick fix that most Americans want, a single pill like tamoxifen to get rid of all their woes.

If you have an illness, then take medicine for it. If you don't have an illness but are at high risk for it, change your lifestyle. It is your responsibility to keep yourself healthy. No single pill is a green light for you to continue to eat the wrong foods, to smoke, to drink alcohol, and otherwise not follow a healthful lifestyle.

3

An Overview of Risk Factors

Numerous risk factors are associated with cancer. Many of them are also risk factors for cardiovascular and other chronic diseases. Learn and modify these risk factors and your risk for all illnesses will be reduced.

DIET AND NUTRITIONAL RISK FACTORS

There is a strong correlation between nutritional factors and many cancers (Table 3.1). The National Academy of Sciences and others estimate that nutritional factors account for 60 percent of cancer cases in women and 40 percent in men.[1-3] Cancers of the breast, colon, rectum, uterus, prostate, and kidney are closely associated with consumption of total fat and protein, particularly meat and animal fat. Other cancers that are directly correlated with dietary factors are cancers of the stomach, small intestine, mouth, pharynx, esophagus, pancreas, liver, ovary, endometrium, thyroid, and bladder.[4-9] Aflatoxin, a fungus product that is found on certain edible plants (especially peanuts), is related to human liver cancer.[10] Obesity is also an independent risk factor for cancer, especially breast cancer.

Japanese men and women who leave Japan and settle in Hawaii or the continental United States have a lower risk of stomach cancer than those who remain in Japan. Stomach cancer in the United States has been steadily decreasing with the advent of refrigeration and the consequent removal of carcinogenic chemicals as food preservatives. Also, the Japanese generally have lower rates of breast and colon cancer, but when

Table 3.1 Risk Factors and Associated Cancers

Risk Factor	Associated Human Cancer
Nutritional Factors	
High-fat, low-fiber	**Breast**, colon, rectum, prostate, stomach, mouth, pharynx, esophagus, pancreas, liver, ovary, endometrium, thyroid, kidney, bladder
Iodine deficiency	**Breast**, thyroid
Aflatoxin (fungus)	Liver
Obesity	**Breast**, endometrium, colon, prostate
Tobacco Smoking, Chewing, Snuffing	**Breast,** lung, larynx, mouth, pharynx, head and neck, esophagus, pancreas, bladder, kidney
Involuntary Inhalation	**Breast,** lung, cervix, mouth
Alcohol	**Breast**, mouth, pharynx, esophagus, gastrointestine, liver, pancreas, head and neck, larynx, bladder
Radiation	
X-rays, etc. (ionizing)	**Breast**, skin, myelogenous leukemia, thyroid, bone
Sunlight (UV)	Skin
Hormonal Factors	
Late/never pregnant	**Breast**
Lumpy Breast disease	**Breast**
DES-diethylstilbestrol	**Breast**, vagina, cervix, endometrium, testicle
Conjugated Estrogen	**Breast**, liver
Androgen-17 methyl	Liver
Undescended Testicle	Testicle
Sexual-Social Factors	
Female promiscuity	Cervix
Male homosexual promiscuity	Kaposi's sarcoma, anus, tongue
Poor male hygiene	Penis
Sedentary Lifestyle	**Breast**, colon, other sites
Stress	Implicated in multiple sites
Immune Abnormality	Lymphomas, carcinomas
Age greater than 55	Multiple sites
High Blood Pressure	**Breast**, colon
Environment	Leukemia, lung, skin, other sites
Pesticides	Breast, lung, prostate, liver, skin, other sites
Hair dye	Lymphoma, multiple myeloma
Occupation or Workers in:	
Chemists	Brain, lymphoma, leukemia, pancreas
Flight personnel	**Breast**, skin, melanoma, leukemia
Furniture/Shoe/Textile	Nasal sinus
Painters	Leukemia

Table 3.1 (continued) Risk Factors and Associated Cancers

Risk Factor	Associated Human Cancer
Petroleum, tar	Lung, skin, scrotum
Printers / Foundry	Lung, mouth, pharynx
Rubber workers	Lung, bladder, leukemia, pancreas
Infections – specific	Stomach, lymphoma, leukemia, cervix, anus

they immigrate to the United States, after only twenty years, they have the same rate of colon cancer as Americans. After only two generations, they have the same rate of breast cancer. Cancers and their relationship to diet and nutritional factors are discussed in depth in Chapters 7 through 10.

CHEMICAL RISK FACTORS

Chemical and environmental factors, including diet and lifestyle, may be responsible for causing 80 to 90 percent of all cancers. Most cancers could be prevented if the factors that cause them were first identified and then controlled or eliminated. People are exposed to many chemicals and some drugs in small amounts and in many combinations unique to their culture and environment. Many drugs and chemicals are now known to cause human cancer, and many more are suspected carcinogens.[11] The drugs include: calcium channel blockers,[12,13] chlorambucil, chloramphenicol, cyclophosphamide, dilantin, hair dyes,[14] melphalan, phenacetin, and thiotepa. The chemicals include: acrylonitrile, aminobiphenyl, aniline, arsenic, asbestos, auramine, benzene, benzidine, beryllium, cadmium chemicals, carbon tetrachloride, chlormethyl ether, chloroprene, chromate, isopropyl alcohol, mustard gas, nickel, radon, and vinyl chloride.

Due to differences in their genetic make-up, individuals exposed to a carcinogen (a chemical substance that causes cancer) will not all have the same probability of getting cancer. Enzymes can break down or activate the carcinogen at different speeds in different people to either render it harmless or promote it to cause cancer. Food sources that induce these enzymes are vegetables of the *Brassicaceae* family – Brussels sprouts, cabbage, broccoli.[15]

ENVIRONMENTAL RISK FACTORS

Environmental factors are just as important. Those living in cities encounter many sources of pollution. More people in cities than in rural areas smoke cigarettes. Air pollution is a risk factor for cancer, especially lung cancer. Carcinogens derived from car emissions, industrial activity, burning of solid wastes and fuels remain in the air from four to forty days and thereby travel long distances.[16] Asbestos, a potent carcinogen, can also be found airborne in cities.

Our drinking water contains a number of carcinogens, including asbestos, arsenic, metals, and synthetic organic compounds that are associated with gastrointestinal cancers, skin cancers, and urinary bladder cancers.[17,18]

With many carcinogens, the time between exposure to the carcinogen and actual development of cancer may be quite long. Hence, a cancer initiated by trace amounts of either airborne or waterborne carcinogens years before the cancer appears may be attributed to an unrelated or unknown cause at the time of diagnosis.

We are able to detect many carcinogens in our environment, but many others exist in low concentrations. These environmental carcinogens may themselves cause cancer in certain individuals, or they may interact with other risk factors to initiate or promote cancers. Therefore, we must avoid introducing harmful substances into the environment.

RADIATION RISK FACTORS

The more radiation to which a person is exposed, the higher is the risk of developing cancer, especially if the radiation exposure is to bone marrow, where the blood cells are made. Almost 85 percent of the radiation to which we are exposed in developed countries is from natural sources, but 15 percent is from human-made sources. Of these, about 97 percent is from diagnostic radiology – mainly CT scans.[19]

Women who received many chest X-rays to follow the progress of treatment for tuberculosis had an increased incidence of breast cancer with as little as 17 cGy total dose. A cGy, or centiGray, is a defined amount of energy absorbed by a certain amount of body tissue. One chest X-ray using modern equipment delivers about 0.14 cGy. Riding in an airplane at 35,000 feet for six hours exposes a person to 0.01 cGy.

People who received radiation to shrink enlarged tonsils or to treat acne have a higher risk of developing cancer of the thyroid and parathyroid glands located in the neck. Survivors of the bombings of Hiroshima and Nagasaki had an increased incidence of leukemia, lymphoma, Hodgkin's disease, multiple myeloma, and other cancers. Female radiology technologists may have only a small increased risk for developing breast cancer.[20] People who painted radium on wrist-watch dials have a high incidence of osteogenic sarcoma, a bone cancer. Chronic exposure of fair-skinned, easily sunburned people to sunlight (ultraviolet light) will lead to a higher rate of skin cancer.

People who work in or live near nuclear power plants have a higher risk of cancer. A higher incidence of childhood leukemia has been reported in children living near several nuclear facilities, most notably a fuel reprocessing plant located at Sellafield in England.[21] The results of another study involving over 8,000 men who worked in the Oak Ridge National Laboratory in Tennessee between 1943 and 1972 show that they had a higher risk of developing cancers, especially leukemia.[22] Another study shows no such increase in cancer incidence.[23]

Female flight attendants have a two-fold increased risk of developing breast cancer because they have chronic disturbances in sleep-wake cycles (circadian rhythms) with a resultant deficiency of melatonin.[24,25] Male cockpit flight members flying 5000 hours or more in jets have a higher risk of acute myeloid leukemia.[26]

Workers in many industries are chronically exposed to low-dose radiation and, hence, may be at risk for cancer and heart disease. We therefore have to reexamine standards for acceptable radiation levels in industry.

OCCUPATIONAL RISK FACTORS

About 10 percent of all cancers are related to exposure to carcinogens on the job. The relationship between a person's job and cancer was noted in the eighteenth century when it was observed that the incidence of cancer of the scrotum was very high in chimney sweeps. Occupations and their associated human cancers are listed in Table 3.1.[27]

AGE AS A RISK FACTOR

Breast cancer is related to age. Between ages 30 and 40, there is a steep rise in the number of breast cancer cases, then a plateau between 40 and 55, and then another steep rise thereafter. The incidence of breast cancer in the elderly is more than double that for younger women.

The older you are, the higher the risk of developing any cancer. The Biometry Section of the National Cancer Institute show that with every five-year increase of age there is a doubling in the incidence of cancer[28] because of the amount of time you have been exposed to risk factors. The elderly often suffer from nutritional deficiencies, and they have an increased number of infections, autoimmune diseases, as well as cancer. Werner's syndrome, which prematurely ages very young children so that they die in early adolescence, is characterized by an impaired immune system. These facts suggest that the immune system in the elderly is working inefficiently, partly due to poor nutrition.[29] Because the gastrointestinal tract absorbs nutrients less efficiently with age, the elderly need more nutrients in their diets. The number of elderly aged 65 or older in the US for the year 2000 is about 35 million and in 2030 will be 66 million.

GENETIC RISK FACTORS

People with certain inherited diseases are more prone to getting cancer. There are over 200 genetic conditions that have an increased incidence of cancer,[30] including mongolism or trisomy 21 syndrome, the immunodeficiency syndromes, Gardner's syndrome, and many more. These genetic abnormalities, although important for the physician to recognize, make a minor contribution to the causation of cancer. ***Inherited genetic factors account for only a small fraction of all human cancers – less than 7 percent.*** [31,32]

ATHEROSCLEROSIS AND CANCER Atherosclerosis is a major cause of death. Commonly called "hardening of the arteries," it is a disease that narrows the inside diameter of the artery and thereby restricts the blood flow and oxygen beyond the narrowed portion causing tissue death. Pain is a symptom of either very low oxygen or outright death of tissues. When a person has a "heart attack," pain occurs because some tissues die and others don't receive enough oxygen.

What does atherosclerosis have to do with breast cancer? Well, a cancer-like growth of cells may be responsible for the development of heart and vessel disease. The first step in the formation of a narrowed artery is the manufacture of cells (endothelial cells) that line the inside of the artery. Then cholesterol gets deposited in these cells after they have increased in number – called a plaque. There is good evidence that these cells come from a single cell, that is, they are cloned from one common cell. Cloning is a form of cancer [33] and can be initiated by carcinogens, like hydrocarbons. If we eat food contaminated with these hydrocarbons or are otherwise exposed to them so that they get into our bloodstream, atherosclerosis may begin to develop. Of course this is just one of many factors involved in the development of atherosclerosis.

There is a relationship between high blood pressure and certain cancers, like breast, colon, lung, and others.[34-36] The higher the blood pressure and the older the person, the more alterations of DNA occur in cells. The more abnormal the DNA of a cell, the more often it will lose control and form a cancer.

HORMONAL RISK FACTORS

Hormones influence a cell's growth and development, so if there is an excess or deficit of hormones in the body, cells will not function properly and may grow abnormally or aberrantly and become cancer cells.

The longer a woman's body is bathed with estrogen, the higher is her risk for breast cancer. Women who start menstruating early (age 11), or stop menstruating late (after age 55), or who have never been pregnant, or who have become pregnant after the age of 35, all have a greater risk for developing breast cancer. Women who become pregnant before age 20 have a reduced risk. Women whose mothers or other close relatives have breast cancer have three times the normal risk of getting breast cancer. Women who do not menstruate during their lifetime have a three to four times higher risk of developing breast cancer after the age of 55. A lower risk of breast cancer is seen in women whose ovaries cease to function or are removed surgically before age 35. Women who use oral contraceptives before age 25 for four years or more, or women who use hormone replacement therapy for 5 years or more have a two-fold higher risk for developing breast cancer.

Daughters of women who received DES (diethylstilbestrol) therapy during pregnancy have developed cancer of the cervix and vagina.[37] Sons of women who took DES have a higher risk of developing cancer of the testicles because DES causes urinary tract abnormalities including undescended testicles, which, if not corrected surgically before age 6, can develop into cancer of the testicles.[38] Furthermore, women exposed to these same synthetic estrogens in adult life have a higher risk of developing cancer of the cells that line the inside of the uterus (endometrial cancer). Male hormones can predispose to both benign and malignant liver tumors.

Benign lumpy breast disease, a disease that affects about 80 percent of all women sometime during their lives, probably represents a hormone imbalance. If a woman has had the disease over many years, she is at an increased risk of developing breast cancer. We have shown that benign lumpy breast disease can respond to certain nutrients and dietary modification.

SEXUAL-SOCIAL RISK FACTORS

Cancer of the cervix is associated with having sexual intercourse at an early age and with having multiple male sex partners, especially uncircumcised male partners. The human papilloma virus is usually responsible.

Cancer of the penis is a very rare disease in the United States. The primary risk factor is poor hygiene, especially in the uncircumcised male. Secretion and different organisms retained under the foreskin produce irritation and infection that predispose to cancer's cellular changes.

Promiscuous male homosexuals have a higher risk of Kaposi's sarcoma, cancer of the anus, cancer of the tongue, AIDS, and an abnormal immune system.

INFECTIOUS DISEASES AS RISK FACTORS

The International Agency for Research on Cancer concludes that certain infectious diseases cause human cancer[39,40] (Table 3.3).

Table 3.3 Infectious Disease Pathogen – Cancer Associations

Pathogen	Cancer
Helicobacter pylori	Stomach Cancer
	Mucosa-Associated Lymphoma Tissue
Schistosoma haematobium	Bladder Cancer
T-cell Lymphoma/Leukemia Virus I	Adult T-cell Lymphoma/Leukemia
T-cell Lymphoma/Leukemia Virus II	Hairy Cell Leukemia
Hepatitis B and C virus	Liver Cancer
Human Herpes Virus 8	Kaposi's Sarcoma
Epstein Barr Virus	Lymphoproliferative disorders
	Nasopharyngeal cancer
	Burkitt's Lymphoma
Human Papilloma Virus	Cervix Cancer, Anal-Genital Cancer
Chlamydia trachomatis	Cervix Cancer

Some pathogens cause cancer in animals, like feline leukemia virus that causes leukemia in cats. However, human cell lines can be infected by feline leukemia virus.[41] It has now been documented that fatal viral infections can be transmitted from one species to another – like a cow to human.[42,43]

Therefore, cats infected with feline leukemia virus should be kept away from pregnant women (developing human fetus), children, and immunosuppressed people.

RISK FACTOR ASSESSMENT

My Cancer Risk Factor Assessment test that follows has been designed to assess your own risk factors based upon diet, weight, age, lifestyle, and other variables covered in this chapter. Take the test to evaluate your risk. We define risk for potentially developing cancer based upon the following letter combination totals:

Risk Level	Number A's	Number B's	Number C's
High Risk	2+	Any	Any
	1	4 or more	Any
	1	3 or less	Any
Moderate Risk	0	4 or more	Any
	0	2 to 3	2 or more
	0	0	0
Low Risk	0	1	2 or less
	0	0	2 or less

A person in a high-risk category will not necessarily develop cancer, but simply he/she is more at risk than a person in another category. Following are a few examples of persons with various risk factors, their relative degrees of risk for developing cancer, and what they should do to modify those risks, thereby reducing their chance of developing cancer (and/or cardiovascular disease). After each risk factor, the score is indicated in parentheses.

Consider Linda, a 56-year-old (C) New Jersey (B) housewife (0). She is 5 feet 5 inches tall, weighs 160 pounds (B), eats red meat daily, eats several eggs per week, drinks milk daily, consumes very little fiber-containing foods, and does not eat a balanced diet (A). She also smokes two packs of cigarettes a day, and has done so for over fifteen years (A). Linda drinks socially (0) and has never had cancer (0), but her mother had breast cancer (B). She started having sexual intercourse at age 20 (0), first got pregnant, at age 24 (0), has a history of lumpy breast disease (C), never had any radiation (0), and is usually calm (0).

Linda's total score is two A's, three B's, and two C's. She is in the high-risk group. What can she do to modify her risk factors? She directly controls the most serious ones. I would advise her to terminate cigarette smoking abruptly and completely. Then I would suggest that she permanently modify her diet in order to reduce two other serious risk factors: her high-animal-fat, high cholesterol, low-fiber diet, and her overweight problem. This would serve also to counter any weight gain that may occur when she stops smoking. Linda has no control over her age, the state in which she has lived, or her history of fibrocystic breast disease; but these are minor risk factors. By modifying the risk factors that she directly controls, she will, over the course of time, lessen her overall risk category and reduce her risk of developing cancer or cardiovascular disease.

The second example is Dave, a 24-year-old sexually active male homosexual who has many male partners and uses a drug called amyl nitrite (C). He smoked two packs of cigarettes a day for eleven years but quit one year ago (A). Up until a few months ago, he ate red meat daily, ate cheese daily, ate very few fiber-containing foods, and took no vitamins (A). His weight is normal (0), and he has never had cancer (0) nor have any of his family members (0). Until Dave was 21 years old, he lived in Alaska (0), but he has since lived in New York City.

Dave's total score is two A's, zero B's and one C. He is in the high-risk group, but by continuing not to smoke and by modifying his diet, he can dramatically lessen his overall risk.

Next is Nancy, a 27-year-old woman who smoked two packs of cigarettes a day until she quit eight years ago (B). She eats a well-balanced diet consisting of red meat five times a week, low-fat dairy products, and an average intake of fiber (B), and she is twenty pounds overweight (C). As a lifelong resident of Vermont (C), Nancy has been working in the furniture industry for the past seven years (B). She is taking birth control pills (B) and has been doing so for the past ten years. She is fair-skinned, sunburns easily, and enjoys sunbathing and using a suntanning booth year-round (B).

On the surface of things it looks as though Nancy's overall risk is not so bad, but when you examine the whole picture, you find she is in the moderate-risk category. Her total score is five B's and two C's. However, she is on the right track. She should do the following to reduce her overall risk: continue not to smoke, lose twenty pounds, modify her nutritional status, seek another means of birth control, use sun screens when sunbathing, and avoid suntanning booths.

The last example is Bob, a 50-year-old (0) male chemist (B) who is twenty-five pounds overweight (B) and a meat-and-potatoes man all the way (A). He has smoked two packs of cigarettes a day for the past thirty years (A), drinks four ounces of whiskey every day (A), has lived in Illinois most of his life (B), and is easily angered (C). His father died of lung cancer (B).

You know that Bob is in the high-risk category: three A's, four B's, and one C. As you can see, he does have risk factors that he can directly control. He should: stop smoking, modify his diet and lose weight, stop drinking alcohol or less than 2 drinks per week, and learn how to relax. All these modifications will greatly reduce his overall risk.

What can *you* do to reduce *your* risk for cancer? You have now identified the problem areas that need modification. Simple preventive measures can be taken to help you reduce your chances of developing cancer or cardiovascular disease. This book will show you how you can make relatively minor adjustments in your lifestyle to lessen your risk. In the following chapters, I will review nutritional risk factors and other risk factors that can lead to the development of breast cancer. I will also tell you how the risk factors can be modified. Maintaining a good weight, eating a healthful diet (one that is low in animal fat, low in cholesterol, and high in fiber), choosing not to smoke or drink alcoholic beverages, avoiding or limiting exposure to the sun – all of these are just a few of the ways you can protect yourself from cancer. You must strive to maintain good health. Good health is no accident!

SELF-TEST

What is your risk of developing cancer? Take my **Cancer Risk Factor Assessment Test** to determine your risk for developing cancer according to your lifestyle factors. You will be able to determine which factors pose a risk, and then how to modify them according to my recommendations. Repeat the test in the future to see if your risk has been reduced.

Choose the statement that most applies to you and mark the score accordingly. After completely the questionnaire, add up your scores. The zero scores won't count in the total.

Cancer Risk Factor Assessment Test

Risk Factor	Score
1. Nutrition	
• If during 50% or more of your life two or more apply to you:	
(1) one serving of red meat daily (including luncheon meat)	
(2) 6 eggs per week	

(3) butter, milk, or cheese daily
(4) little or no fiber foods (3 gm or less daily)
(5) frequent barbecued meats
(6) below average intake of vitamins and minerals Score A__

- If during 50% or more of your life two or more apply to you:
(1) red meat 4-5 times a week (including luncheon meat)
(2) 3-5 eggs per week
(3) margarine, low-fat dairy products, some cheese
(4) 4-15 gm fiber daily
(5) frequent barbecued meats
(6) average intake of vitamins and minerals Score B__
- If during 50% or more of your life two or more apply to you:
(1) red meat and one egg once a week or none at all
(2) poultry or fish daily or very frequently
(3) margarine, skim milk, or skim milk products
(4) 15-20 gm fiber daily
(5) above average intake of vitamins and minerals Score C__

2. Weight

Ideal weight for men is 110 lbs + 5 lbs per inch over 5 feet.
Ideal weight for women is 100 lbs + 5 lbs per inch over 5 feet.

- If you are 25 pounds overweight Score B __
- If you are 10-24 pounds overweight Score C __
- If you are less than 10 pounds overweight Score 0 __

3. Tobacco

- Smoke 2 packs or more per day for 10 years or more Score A __
- Smoke 1-2 packs for 10 yrs or more, or quit less than 1 yr Score A __
- Smoke less than 1 pack for 10 yrs or more, or pipe or cigar Score B __
- Smoked 1-2 pks/d, a pipe or cigar, but stopped 7-14 yrs agoScore B __
- Chew or snuff tobacco Score B __
- Inhaled others' smoke for 1 or more hrs/day up to age 25 Score B __
- Inhaled others' smoke for 1 or more hrs/day from age 25 Score C __
- Never smoked, quit 15 years ago, never inhaled others' Score 0 __

4. Alcohol

- If you drink 4 oz whiskey, and/or 8 oz wine, and/or
24 oz beer daily or more Score A __
- If you drink 2-4 drinks per week Score B __
- If you drink less than that indicated above Score 0 __
- If you drink 4 oz whiskey, 8 oz wine, 24 oz beer daily, and also
Smoke less than 1 pack /day, or chew or snuff tobacco Score B __
Smoke 1-2 packs per day, pipe or cigar Score A __
Smoke 2 or more packs per day Score A __
- If you do not drink at all Score 0 __

5. Hormonal

- If you started menstruating between ages 8 and 12 Score C __
- If you stopped menstruating at age 50 or older Score C __
- If you never had menses at all Score C __
- If your mother took DES, or if you took DES or estrogens Score C __
- If you took oral contraceptives for 4 years + before age 25, or 10 or more during your lifetime Score B __
- If had miscarriage or abortion in 1st trimester, 1st pregnancy Score C __
- If 1st pregnant after age 35, or never, or had lumpy breasts Score C __
- If your bra cup size is D or greater Score C __

6. Breast Biopsy Report

- If your biopsy showed fibroadenoma, papilloma, sclerosing adenosis, or large cyst Score C __
- If your biopsy showed hyperplasia with atypia Score B __
- If your biopsy showed comedo or non-comedo *in situ* Score A __

7. Radiation Exposure

- If you received multiple X-rays or radiation treatments, or if you were exposed to radioactive isotopes, radioactive weapons Score C __
- If you are fair-skinned and sunburn easily Score B __
- If neither applies Score 0 __

8. Occupation

- If you are a radiologist, chemist, painter, luminous dial painter, or worker in: leather, foundry, flight, dye, printing, rubber, petroleum, furniture, textile, nuclear, slaughterhouse, plutonium/uranium Score A __
- Never was one of the above workers Score 0 __

9. Chemicals

- If you worked with: acrylonitrile, aminobiphenyl, aniline, arsenic, asbestos, auramine, benzene, benzidine, beryllium, cadmium chemicals, carbon tetrachloride, chlormethyl ether, chloroprene, chromate, isopropyl alcohol, mustard gas, nickel, radon, and vinyl chloride Score A __
- If you worked indirectly with one of the above Score C __
- Never worked with one of the above Score 0 __

10. Sexual-Social History

- If you are a female who started having intercourse before age 16 with multiple male partners, particularly uncircumcised Score C __
- If you are a promiscuous male homosexual Score C __
- If neither applies Score 0 __

11. Immunity, Drugs, Hormones

- If your doctor said you have an immune deficiency Score A __
- If you had an organ transplant Score A __

- If you've taken for prolonged time: calcium channel blockers, chlorambucil, chloramphenicol, cyclophosphamide, dilantin, hair dyes, melphalan, steroids Score A __
- If you've taken for prolonged time: phenacetin, thiotepa Score A __
- If none of the above applies Score 0 __

12. Geography

- If during most of your life you've live in the Northeast Score A __
- If during most of your life you've lived in the Midwest Score C __
- If during most of your life you've lived in elsewhere in US Score 0 __

13. Age

- If your age is 70 or more Score B __
- If your age is 55 to 60 Score C __
- If your age is 54 or less Score 0 __

14. Personal History

- If you had cancer Score B __
- If you never had cancer Score 0 __

15. Family History

- If your parents or grandparents had cancer Score B __
- No family history of cancer Score 0 __

16. Exercise

- If you exercise very little or not at all Score C __
- If you exercise 3 or more times per week and get your heart rate 50% higher than normal for 20 minutes Score 0 __

17. Stress

- If you easily get frustrated or angered, or can't control stress Score C __
- If you are comfortable while waiting, and can control stress Score 0 __

TOTAL SCORE: ____A's; ____B's; ____C's

PART TWO

The Body's Defenses

4
Nutrition, Immunity, and Cancer

Nutrition affects immunity [1,2] and also affects the development of cancer [3,4] either directly or indirectly via the immune system. The immune system is a complex interaction of blood cells, proteins, and processes that protect you from infections, foreign substances, and cancer cells that spontaneously develop.

White blood cells and antibodies are two major armies of the immune system. A lymphocyte is a type of white cell involved in cellular immunity. Lymphocytes are divided into two groups, T cells and B cells. T lymphocytes, or T cells, are derived from or are under the influence of the *thymus*, an organ in the neck and front part of the chest that is functionally active in early childhood. T cells fight cancer, fungi, certain bacteria (intracellular), some viruses, transplant rejections, and delayed skin reactions (tuberculosis skin test). T cells can be divided into helper T cells and suppressor T cells, those that either help or hinder normal immune cellular function. B cell lymphocytes produce proteins called antibodies or immunoglobulins. B cells originate in the *bone* marrow, from which they derive their designation. Antibodies are formed by the B cells in response to a foreign substance introduced into the body.

In 1980, I showed how a white blood cell and complement proteins kill abnormal cells. They do so by making holes in the abnormal cell's membrane, thereby allowing water to rush in and explode the cell. White blood cell extends feet-like processes that kill the targets. [5]

Phagocytes are another group of white cells that reside in the blood and body tissues to recognize and dispose of abnormal cancer cells and other foreign substances. Phagocytes can perform this task alone or can recruit antibodies and complement proteins to aid in the disposal.

IMMUNOLOGY AND CANCER

The immune system is extremely intricate and finely tuned. If any one aspect of the system malfunctions because of poor nutrition, or if it is destroyed, you may become susceptible to cancer and foreign microbial invaders. The white blood cell army and the antibody army must be functioning perfectly to destroy any cancer cell or foreign invader and prevent either one from gaining a foothold in your body.

The major histocompatibility complex is part of your genetic make-up and is another component of the immune system, acting as a commander of the white blood cell and antibody armies. This complex allows the immune system to recognize the parts of your body so that it does not destroy them as it would destroy foreign substances. At the same time, it can recognize a substance or tissue (histo-) that does not belong to its body and subsequently take the necessary steps to destroy it.

Killer cells of the immune system watch, or keep a surveillance on, all cells in the body and immediately destroy any cells that start to have a malignant or cancerous potential.[6] The most convincing evidence for this comes from observations of patients with suppressed immune systems caused by drugs or radiation or an inherited disorder. Patients with inherited immunodeficiencies, whose immune systems do not function normally from birth, or patients whose immune systems acquire a malfunction later in life have 100 times more deaths due to cancer than the expected cancer death rate in the normal population.[7,8] Kidney transplant patients, who receive drugs to suppress the immune system's ability to reject the new kidney, also have a higher rate of cancer than expected.[9,10] The cancers most frequently seen in these cases are the lymphomas and epithelial cancers; however, all other types of cancers have been reported.

The immune system is relatively immature in infancy, and then becomes weak with advancing age. These two times of life have the highest incidence of lymphocytic leukemia. Other immune-deficiency states that can lead to cancer are seen with malaria, acute viral infections, and malnutrition.

NUTRITION AND THE IMMUNE SYSTEM

Nutritional deficiencies decrease a person's capacity to resist infection, and decrease the capability of the immune system.[11] In old age, the immune system is impaired mainly because of nutritional deficiencies.[12] Poor nutrition adversely affects all components of the immune system, including T cell function, other cellular-related killing, the ability of B cells to make antibodies, the functioning of the complement proteins, and phagocytic function. When several of these functions or processes are impaired, the ability of the entire immune system to keep a watchful eye for cancer cells, abnormal cells, or foreign substances and to dispose of them is also markedly impaired. Table 4.1 summarizes the factors that affect the functioning of the immune system.

Table 4.1 Factors That Influence the Immune System

Enhance	Suppress
Nutrition	Nutrition
Low-fat, high-fiber diet	High-fat diet
Antioxidants	High sugar level
Carotene, vitamins E & C,	Obesity
Selenium, cysteine, copper	Soy and Corn oil
flavonoids, zinc	Tobacco
B vitamins, pantothenic acid	Alcohol
Calcium	Radiation
Exercise	Lead, cadmium, mercury
Stress Modified; Loving	Certain Drugs
Clean air and pure water	Environmental pollutants
	Ozone depletion [13-16]
	Stress
	Sedentary Lifestyle
	Exhaustive Exercise [17,18]

Protein deficiency impairs the ability of phagocytes and T cells to kill.[19,20] Antibody production is reduced as is the speed with which it attaches to an "enemy."[21] Complement proteins also are impaired.

Sugar levels – high or low – adversely affects the immune system. The function of phagocytes, and T and B cells are impaired if the sugar is too high (diabetes) or too low (hypoglycemia).[22-24] The degree of impairment correlates well with the fasting blood sugar level and improves as the sugar level becomes normal.

Lipids have a significant effect on the functioning of the immune system. Cholesterol and fats inhibits antibody production[25] and the functioning of T cells and phagocytes.[26,27]

The Epstein-Barr virus may manifest itself by causing entirely different diseases in different people as a result of varying degrees of impairment of the immune system. The extent to which the immune system is weakened or damaged is partly determined by the nutritional status of the individual prior to infection. Epstein-Barr virus is implicated in many diseases: a relatively benign disease, infectious mononucleosis; a slow-growing cancer, nasopharyngeal cancer; and a rapidly growing, usually fatal cancer, Burkitt's lymphoma; as well as other diseases. Why does one person's immune system permit infectious mononucleosis to develop and another person's immune system permit a fatal cancer to develop? The answer is very complex and not well defined at all, but nutritional status is a factor.

Your nutritional status is determined by how well your diet and supplementation program is meeting your nutritional needs. The better your nutritional status, the better your immune system, and the better off you will be.

5

Antioxidants and Other Cancer-Fighting Nutrients

Living cells contain proteins, nucleic acids, carbohydrates, lipids, and certain organic substances that function in very small amounts, called vitamins. Vitamins are essential to life and the immune system, and play a crucial role as helper enzymes in important chemical functions of the body. Vitamins interact with each other, and some can be stored for long periods of time, while others have to be supplied on a daily basis. Certain drugs and hormones can produce a gradual vitamin deficiency.

A person who is grossly deficient in vitamins demonstrates specific symptoms and complaints. But a person with only marginal deficiencies demonstrates no such signs or symptoms and does not appear to be ill.

Do you consider your diet to be well balanced? Do you think it is meeting your nutritional needs? Although you may believe it is fulfilling your requirements, you will most likely find that your diet is deficient in at least one nutrient. Consider the following sections.

MARGINAL DEFICIENCIES

Marginal deficiency is a gradual vitamin depletion in which there is evidence of personal lack of well-being associated with impairment of certain biochemical reactions.[1,2] The person may complain of non-specific symptoms such as fatigue, decreased mental acuity, loss of appetite, irritability, inability to sleep, and decreased resistance to disease, infection, as well as poor wound healing. Comprehensive studies confirm marginal deficiencies by measuring blood levels or assessing dietary ingestion.[3-6] **About 50 percent of all people examined and surveyed, whether rich or poor, educated or not, had at least one, and usually two or three marginal nutrient deficiencies.**

LIFESTYLE AND EATING PATTERNS

Lifestyle and eating patterns can lead to nutrient deficiencies. There is an increased demand for convenience foods and fast-food. Eating patterns have changed. About 25% of Americans skip breakfast, 25% skip lunch, almost 50% snack, and most eat one meal a day away from home. In 1965 affluent whites ate less healthy compared to poor African-Americans; by 1991, the diets of both were similar.[7]

In the federally sponsored HANES II study, people were asked to choose a food that they liked and considered "balanced." For a "balanced" vegetable, the majority chose French fries over broccoli; for meat/legume, hot dogs over split peas; and for grain, white bread over whole wheat. In the same study, favorite foods included coffee, doughnuts, soft drinks, and hamburgers. The percentage of calories in the American diet derived from fat is 42; from sugar, 24.

When caloric intakes fall below 1,600 calories, most nutritional guidelines cannot be met.[8] And below 1,800 per day, which about 50 percent of the population consumes at times, trained nutritionists have trouble designing meals to provide the minimum RDIs.[9] The Nationwide Food Consumption Survey [10] found that over 50 percent of people who thought they ate the "well-balanced" diet had deficiencies in vitamins A, C, B1, B2, B6, B12, calcium, magnesium, and iron. Women of all economic levels had low intakes of vitamins A, C, B6, calcium, iron, and zinc. [11]

Outright vitamin deficiencies occur in two groups of people. In the first group, people are unable to buy the right kinds of food either because of the expense or because they are not knowledgeable about the proper foods. The second group consists of people whose nutrient deficiency occurs as the result of a specific disease or a drug or other treatment therapy.

Americans unknowingly eat foods that are sprayed with chemicals, refined, processed, over-cooked, frozen, canned, stored, and trucked around the country. Many of our meats contain the hormones and chemicals that have been fed to animals. All of these foods have been depleted of nutrients to varying degrees. Some methods of cooking can totally destroy nutrients or decrease their concentration, and some nutrients are not stable in heat or boiling water. As a result, Americans do not or cannot eat a healthful balanced diet.

We get about one-third of our calories from sources of little or no nutrient value. The average American consumes about 60 pounds of sugar each year and four to five times the amount of salt necessary, favors carbonated drinks to others when not consuming 2.6 gallons of alcoholic beverages each year (if of drinking age). In short, it is very difficult to find an individual who consistently, on a daily basis, eats a "well-balanced diet" – that is, one containing foods that are freshly prepared, varied, and nutritionally adequate.

GROUPS AT RISK FOR NUTRIENT DEFICIENCIES

There are multiple groups of our population that may not be "healthy" and that may be considered to be "at risk" for inadequate nutrient intake. The RDIs do not take into account the special needs of these people. The greater requirements of the groups listed in Table 5.1 need to be recognized and addressed.

ANTIOXIDANTS REDUCE CANCER RISK

Since the 1950s a huge volume of evidence has demonstrated that antioxidants reduce the risk of cancer. The evidence is so overwhelming that I will cite only the main references and review articles.

Oxidation causes cancer, and inflammation causes cancer because of free radical production.[91-103] Antioxidants reduce the risk of cancer because they neutralize free radicals (Chapter 7) and the oxidative reaction that is caused by free radicals, thus interfering with the initiation and promotion phases of cancer

Table 5.1 Candidates for Nutrient Supplementation

Risk Group	Million	Nutrient Deficiencies
Alcohol drinker (3+ drinks/week)	90	Carotene, vitamins A, B6, D, folate, thiamine [12-22]
People with Alleriges or Food Intolerance	80	Any or all
Cigarette Smokers	50	Carotene, vitamins C, E, B6, Folate [23-32]
Dieters	45	Any or all [33-37]
Hospitalized Patients	36	Any or all [38]
Osteoporosis Patients	34	Calcium, vitamin D, others
People with Chronic Diseases	31	Any or all [39-44]
Elderly Patients	25	Folate, vitamins C and D [45-51]
Surgical Patients	24	Any or all
Oral Contraceptive Users	18	Carotene, folate, B6 [52-57]
Teenagers	17	Vitamin A, folate [58,59]
Diabetics	11	Vitamins C, D, B6, Magnesium [60,61]
Pregnant Women	7	All [62]
People with Infections	5	Any or all
Strict Vegetarians	1	Vitamins B12 and D
Stressed People	*	B vitamins, any and all
Athletes, Exercisers	*	B vitamins, any and all
Consumers of High-Fat Foods	*	Any and all
Low income people	*	Vitamin A and C, B vitamins, iron [63]
Premature Infants/Toddlers	*	Vitamins A,C,E, iron [64-68]
Children with low IQs	*	Any and all [69-83]
Psychiatric Patients	*	Any and all [84]
People with Aggressive / Criminal Behavior	*	Any and all [85-90]

*Unknown Millions

formation.[104,105] Antioxidant nutrients include beta-carotene, vitamin C, vitamin E, selenium, alpha-lipoic acid, copper, zinc, bioflavonoids, and cysteine.

CELLULAR AND ANIMAL STUDIES [106-114]

Hundreds of studies demonstrate that antioxidants protect normal cells from transforming to cancer and animals from developing cancer. Antioxidants like the carotenes, vitamins E and C as well as selenium protect the cell membrane from carcinogens by allowing it to communicate efficiently and by preventing uncontrolled growth characteristic of cancer. Antioxidants can even reverse the transformation process.

HUMAN EVIDENCE

Epidemiological and Cohort Studies

An **extensive review** of the evidence **shows that vitamin E and C reduce the risk for cancer**, and neither antioxidant cause any harm.[115,116] Multiple observational studies, including the Iowa Women's Health Study, demonstrate protection against colorectal cancer with vitamin E, some protection with vitamin A, but none with vitamin C. [117,118]

A cohort study is one that investigates a specific group of people prospectively. **A review of 24 cohort studies demonstrate that supplemental vitamins C, E, A, carotene, selenium, multivitamins, or any combination of these confer protection against cancer or had no effect, but none report harm.** [117] This is a massive amount of data. Below are some additional studies.

- *Breast Cancer* [118-124] Antioxidants, including beta-carotene, vitamins C and E, or vitamin A, other nutrients, and/or fiber alone or in combination decrease the risk for breast cancer by as much as 20 percent. In one of these studies, vitamin E was shown to reduce the risk for cardiovascular disease.
- *Endometrial Cancer* [125] occurs mainly in older women who are obese and eat a high-fat diet. Antioxidants help protect against it. The antioxidant enzymes glutathione S-transferase and superoxide dismutase were significantly lower in patients who had cancer of the endometrium compared to patients undergoing hysterectomy without cancer.
- *Cervical Cancer* [126] Patients who had cervical cancer or cervical dysplasia had significantly lower levels of beta-carotene than women who had normal cervices.
- *Oral And Pharyngeal Cancer* [127-129] People who took supplements containing vitamins A, C, E, and B complex had a much lower risk for oral and pharyngeal cancer after controlling for the effects of tobacco, alcohol, and other risk factors. This was confirmed by a US National Cancer Institute study. Another study showed people with high levels of carotenoids

including beta-carotene, alpha-carotene, cryptoxanthin, leutin, and lyocopene – but particularly beta-carotene – had a much lower rate of getting oral cancer than the control population. High blood levels of vitamin E and beta-carotene together provided the most protection against oral cancer.

- *California Study* [130] investigated over 11,600 people during 8 years. Women with higher dietary intakes of vitamin C, vegetables and fruits or fruits alone, had a lower risk for developing cancer at all sites, especially colon cancer. Taking supplements of beta-carotene, vitamin A as well as vitamin C and E were associated with a lower risk of getting lung cancer, colon cancer, and bladder cancer.
- *Hawaiian Study* [131] Beta-carotene, alpha-carotene, and lutein all conferred protection against lung cancer. Lycopene and beta-cryptoxanthin showed no such protective effects. It was found that beta-carotene conferred the most protection.
- *Finland Study* [132] Over 4,500 men entered a 20 year study. The nonsmokers who had low intakes of carotenes, vitamin E, and vitamin C had high risk of developing lung cancer. Those who had the least intake of these antioxidant nutrients were twice as likely to develop lung cancer.
- *Switzerland Study* [133] Serum levels of vitamins A, C, and E as well as beta-carotene were measured in almost 3,000 men. Men with low levels of beta-carotene and vitamin C had a higher risk of dying from lung and stomach cancer. Men who had low levels of both vitamin A and beta-carotene had an increased risk of all cancers.

Case Control Studies

Over 45 case control studies have been done and several reviews of them have been written.[117,134] **The overwhelming conclusions are that antioxidants reduce the risk of cancer and no harm is caused by them.** Additional studies below:

- *Pediatric Brain Cancer Study* [135] The risk of a child developing brain cancer decreased by 30% if the mother took antioxidants for 2 trimesters of the pregnancy.

- *Basel Study* [136] showed that high plasma levels of vitamins C, E, retinol, and carotene reduced the risk of death overall and reduced the risk for lung cancer and prostate cancer.
- *Physicians' Health* Study [137,138] found that higher levels of lycopene and vitamin C reduced the risk for prostate cancer.

Intervention Studies involve a specific treatment, like nutrients, over a course of time to determine an outcome. The best known are: Linxian study, ATBC study, Physician's Health study, Carotene and Retinol Efficacy Trial (CARET), Clark's study of selenium. The authors who reviewed all of these state: **"Overall there is evidence for protective effects of nutrients from supplements against several cancers."**[117]

- *Linxian, China Study* [139-141] In north central China in the county of Linxian, Henan Province, are people who have the world's highest rates of esophageal cancer and a high rate of stomach cancer. The people of Linxian also have a very high rate of marginal nutritional deficiencies. In Linxian, esophageal cancer deaths are one hundred times higher than the rate for Caucasian Americans and ten times higher than the rate for China in general. Since poor nutrition is linked to these two cancers and since marginal deficiencies are very common in the people of Linxian, an intervention trial was conducted.

  Researchers from the Cancer Institute of the Chinese Academy of Medical Sciences and the US National Cancer Institute studied almost 30,000 adults, randomizing them over five years. The findings were spectacular.

  - Three antioxidant nutrients taken together daily – beta-carotene (15 mg), vitamin E (60 IU), and selenium (50 mcg organic) – significantly reduced total mortality (9 percent) especially from all cancers (13 percent) and particularly stomach cancer (21 percent).
  - These antioxidants also reduced the risk of cancer.
  - These antioxidants substantially reduced the prevalence of cataracts in the oldest patients (aged 65-74 years).
  - These antioxidants reduced the mortality from stroke.

The doses used in the study are relatively low; I recommend much higher doses. Five years is a short time; imagine what the results would be in a population taking these antioxidants as well as other nutrients in higher doses for a lifetime.

- *Small Cell Lung Cancer Study* [142] Patients who received conventional therapy and also antioxidants lived longer than those who just received conventional treatment. The patients receiving the antioxidants were able to tolerate chemotherapy and radiation therapy better. And when antioxidant treatment was started earlier, survival was longer.

ANTIOXIDANTS AND PRE-CANCER CONDITIONS

- *Esophageal Dysplasia Intervention Study* in Linxian, China [143]

More than 3,300 patients with esophageal dysplasia, a precursor to esophageal cancer, were studied by the same team of researchers from China and the United States as above. One group received a placebo. The other group received a multiple vitamin-mineral supplement daily for six years that contained doses two to three times higher than the U.S. Recommended Dietary Intake: beta carotene 15 mg, vitamin A 10,000 IU, vitamin E 60 IU, vitamin C 180 mg, folic acid 800 mcg, thiamin 5 mg, riboflavin 5.2 mg, niacinamide 40 mg, vitamin B6 6 mg, vitamin B12 18 mcg, vitamin D 800 IU, biotin 90 mcg, pantothenic acid 20 mg, calcium 324 mg, phosphorus 250 mg, iodine 300 mcg, iron 54 mg, magnesium 200 mg, copper 6 mg, manganese 15 mg, potassium 15.4 mg, chloride 14 mg, chromium 30 mcg, molybdenum 30 mcg, selenium 50 mcg, and zinc 45 mg. The group that took the supplement:

- 8% lower mortality from esophageal and stomach cancers.
- 7% lower overall mortality.
- 4% lower rate of death from cancer in any site.
- 38% lower risk of dying from stroke.

Here again the results are spectacular despite the short duration of time and the low doses. Other trials with positive results used 30 to 90 mg of beta-carotene[144,145] and 800 IU of vitamin E to treat precancerous oral lesions.[146,147]

• *Colorectal Polyp Adenomas*

Most colon cancers arise from adenomas. Patients with colorectal adenomas[148] were given vitamins A, C, and E for six months after complete polypectomy. After thorough analysis, those who received the vitamins were less likely to develop future adenomas compared to the placebo group.

ANTIOXIDANTS AND OTHER DISEASES

Free radicals are now considered to be the cause of many chronic illnesses (Table 7.1 in Chapter 7). It is therefore crucial that we be aware of the protection offered by antioxidants. Only the major studies or reviews will be cited in Table 5.2.

Table 5.2 Antioxidant Supplementation

Decreases Risk for	Enhances
Aggressive Behavior [85-90]	I.Q. [69-83]
Angina [149]	Memory [218]
Arthritis and Inflammation [150]	
Cardiovascular Disease [151-181]	
Cataracts [139-141, 181-199]	
Hepatitis C [200]	
Hypertension [201]	
Macular Degeneration [202-206]	
Neurological Diseases	
Alzheimer's [207,208]	
Dementia [209]	
Epilepsy [210]	
Lou Gehrig's Disease [211]	
Parkinson's Disease [212-214]	
Tardive Dyskinesia [215-217]	

INDIVIDUAL ANTIOXIDANTS

Many nutrients have been identified as antioxidants. You should be aware of the beneficial effects, recommended doses, and the possible toxicity of:

Beta-carotene

• Most powerful antioxidant of free radicals and singlet oxygen.
• Cancer and Cardiovascular Disease risk – reduced. [219-221]

- Immune System – enhanced. [222]
- Cataracts and other eye disease risk – reduced. [223]
- Toxicity: None in any amount. [224]

The ATBC and CARET studies erroneously suggested that beta-carotene increased the risk of lung cancer in heavy smokers who drank alcohol and had asbestos exposure. Multiple reasons cast doubt that carotene increases cancer risk: [225,226]

1. Cancers start between 10 and 20 years before symptoms occur or our technology can detect them. These heavy smokers and drinkers already had developed their cancers that were simply not detected with the methodology used.
2. The smokers who had high carotene serum levels at the start of the study had the lowest incidence of lung cancer.
3. Most of the study participants were alcoholics, and all ate a high fat diet – both risk factors independently increase cancer risk. Other risk factors were not indicated.
4. Beta-carotene did not increase the risk of lung cancer for those who smoked less than 20 cigarettes a day and drank little or no alcohol.
5. Beta-carotene works most efficiently at the early stages of carcinogenesis, not at the later stages when a cancer is already formed.
6. Over 200 studies have demonstrated that beta-carotene is safe and can lower the risk of developing cancer and cardiovascular disease, or has no effect, including harm.
7. All intervention studies show that beta-carotene and other nutrients can decrease cancer rates and cancer progression.
8. A total of 22 epidemiological studies that included 400,000 smokers and nonsmokers have shown those who had a high blood level of beta-carotene had a lower incidence and mortality of lung cancer.
9. None of these studies reported any association with an increased incidence of lung cancer, including the Physician's Health Study which was the longest and largest trial of beta-carotene in which 11% of the physicians remained smokers. In fact, the reduction in risk was more pronounced in smokers than in nonsmokers.

It is important to rely on the synergism of all the antioxidants, including the carotenoids, vitamins C and E, selenium, and also the B's, etc., as well as lifestyle changes to decrease one's risk of cancer and heart disease. It is foolish to expect that a single nutrient can give the "green light" to continue lifestyle behavior that will cause disease.

- Simone recommended dose: 30-40 mg per day.

Vitamin E

One vitamin E molecule fits snugly between polyunsaturated fat molecules. This location and closeness to the polyunsaturated fats is extremely important because vitamin E competes with the polyunsaturated fat for free radicals that are formed when polyunsaturated fats react with oxygen. This means that if there are more vitamin E molecules than polyunsaturated fat molecules, the radicals will be taken out of the system and neutralized by vitamin E. The more polyunsaturated fats you eat, the more vitamin E you require.

- Potent antioxidant.
- Cancer risk – reduced, [227-257] especially bladder, breast, cervix, colon polyps, colon, lung, oral cavity, prostate, skin, stomach – as shown in intervention, prospective, retrospective studies.
- Cardiovascular Disease risk – reduced and reduces progression of coronary artery blockages. [258-262]
- Smog – protects you from free radicals of smog. [263]
- Lumpy Breast Disease (fibrocystic) – reduced. 85% of women who took 600 IU of vitamin E daily for eight weeks had relief of their breast pain pre-menstrually, and some had demonstrable regression of disease. [264]
- Diabetes complications – reduced when taking 600 to 1200 IU of vitamin E daily. [265]
- Allergy Reactions – reduced. [266]
- Toxicity: There is no case on record of vitamin E toxicity or any indication of vitamin E toxicity. A daily intake of 800 IU of vitamin E per 2.2 pounds of body weight for five months has not been toxic. This equals 56,000 IU for an average man weighing 140 pounds, or about 5,600 times the RDI.

As ridiculous as it may sound, some people, including some physicians, "believe" that vitamin E causes cancer. They reason that since the molecule of vitamin E looks similar to estrogen, it can cause breast cancer. This is absolutely absurd! There are hundreds of molecules in the body that are formed from the same basic cholesterol ring structure. The body is able to discriminate one molecule from another even if there is only a slight difference between their structures. For instance, what differentiates men from women is a mere methyl group, CH_3, on a cholesterol-steroid chemical compound. Obviously, Mother Nature has this under control.

- Toxicity – None. Vitamin E has never been shown to cause cancer or changes in the DNA or RNA, nor has it ever been shown to cause changes in fetal development – even at very high doses of 3,200 IU per day. [267-269]
- Simone recommended dose: 400-1600 IU per day.

Vitamin C

Vitamin C is a major factor in controlling and potentiating multiple aspects of human resistance to many diseases including cancer. Unlike most animals, humans do not manufacture their own vitamin C.

- Potent antioxidant. Deficiency of vitamin C leads to deficiency of other antioxidants. [270]
- Cancer risk – reduced [228, 237, 271-307] especially bladder, breast, cervix, colon, colon polyp, lung, upper digestive tract, pancreas, prostate, stomach – as shown in intervention, prospective and retrospective studies. It also inhibits the spread of cancer by neutralizing an enzyme (hyaluronidase) made by cancer cells.[308,309]
- Hypertension – decreased. [310]
- Bone density – increased. [311]
- Gall Stones – reduces formation. [312]
- Immune System – enhanced. [313]
- Viral infection – reduced.
- Smoking reduces vitamin C in blood.
- Ultraviolet light harm – reduced.

- Toxicity: Doses of 3 to 30 grams of vitamin C in more than 1,000 patients since 1953 has not caused one miscarriage, kidney-stone formation, or any other serious side effect. [314] Klenner has given patients 10 grams of vitamin C daily for over thirty years without any serious toxic side effects. [315]
- Simone recommended dose: 350-6,000 mg per day or more, depending upon circumstances.

Bioflavonoids

- An antioxidant.
- Cancer and Cardiovascular Disease risk – reduced. [316,317]
- Helps vitamin C to work efficiently.
- Toxicity: None reported.
- Simone recommended dose: 10-20 mg per day.

Selenium [318]

- A powerful antioxidant.
- Cancer and Cardiovascular Disease risk – reduced.
- Immune System – enhanced.
- HIV progression to AIDS – inhibited.
- Arthritis inflammation – reduced.
- Brain function and mood – enhanced.
- Miscarriage risk – reduced.
- Thyroid function – enhanced.
- Neutralizes toxic metals (mercury, cadmium, arsenic).
- Vision – enhanced.
- Toxicity: Occurs after prolonged ingestion of 2,400 to 3,000 micrograms of selenium per day.[319] Approximately 500 micrograms of selenium per day is safely tolerated by people in Japan.[320] "Organic" selenium, as found in certain yeasts, is better than inorganic selenium for supplementation because it has less systemic toxicity at high concentrations, it resists chemical changes, and it is stable during food processing.
- Simone recommended dose: 200-300 mcg per day.

Zinc

- An antioxidant.
- Cancer risk – reduced. [321]
- Immune System – enhanced. [322]
- Toxicity: 80-150 mg/day or more.
- Simone recommended dose: 15-20 mg per day.

Copper

- An antioxidant.
- Cancer and Cardiovascular Disease risk – reduced.
- Immune system – enhanced.
- Cholesterol and Glucose levels – helps to control.
- Toxicity: 10 mg/day for prolonged periods.
- Simone recommended dose: 3-5 mg per day.

alpha-Lipoic Acid

- Powerful antioxidant.
- Recycles vitamins C and E, regenerates glutathione, removes heavy metals, generates energy.
- Liver damage is repaired.
- Diabetes – improved. [323-327] Makes cells more sensitive to insulin. Improves peripheral neuropathy (painful feet/hands).
- Cataracts – decreases formation. [328]
- Glaucoma – improves pressures (150 mg per day). [329]
- Ischemia-Reperfusion Injury. A stroke or heart attack deprives that area of the body of blood for a while. When blood gains access to the deprived tissue, a burst occurs of free radicals that can be neutralized by alpha-Lipoic acid. [330]
- Other uses: Prevents HIV replication in animals, protects against radiation injury, prevents neurological disorders.
- Toxicity: None reported for doses between 2,000-3,000 mg per day. Some people have reported allergic skin reactions.
- Simone Recommended Dose: 300-600 mg per day

Cysteine (an amino acid)

- An antioxidant.

- Cardiac toxicity of adriamycin – reduced
- Immune System – enhanced.
- Toxicity: None.
- Simone recommended dose: 20-500 mg per day.

OTHER NUTRIENTS

Antioxidants are not the only nutrients that provide protection against cancer. You should also include the following:

Vitamin A

- Cancer risk – reduced. [331-335]
- Immune System – enhanced. [336]
- Cataract risk – reduced. [337]
- Hearing – enhanced. [338]
- Toxicity: Daily doses of 100,000 IU (30 milligrams of retinol) have been given to adults for many months without serious side effects. [339] Children who ingest 50,000 to 500,000 IU (15 to 150 milligrams of retinol) per day do exhibit toxicity. [340] The safety of vitamin A has been extensively reviewed. [341]
- Simone recommended dose: 5,000-7,500 IU per day.

Vitamin D

- Cancer risk – reduced, especially breast, colon cancer. [342-344]
- Oncogene c-myc - inhibited. [345]
- Immune System – enhanced [346]
- Osteoporosis risk – reduced.
- Toxicity: A daily dose of 100,000 to 150,000 IU of vitamin D (250 to 375 micrograms of cholecalciferol) for many months can be tolerated by a healthy adult.[337]
- Simone recommended dose: 400-600 IU per day.

Vitamin K

- Cancer risk – reduced. [347]
- Immune System – enhanced.
- Toxicity: Not toxic in large doses.
- No supplement is needed.

Thiamine (B1)

- Cancer and Cardiovascular Disease risk – reduced. [348]
- Immune System – enhanced.
- Toxicity: None recorded.
- Simone recommended dose: 10-15 mg per day.

Riboflavin (B2)

- Immune System – enhanced.
- Toxicity: None.
- Simone recommended dose: 10-15 mg per day.

Niacin

- Cancer and Cardiovascular Disease risk – reduced. [349]
- Cholesterol and Triglycerides – reduced. [350]
- Toxicity: Those using niacin should take only the immediate-release form. The timed-release form can damage your liver. Do not exceed 1,500 milligrams of niacin per day. Take it with food to decrease the red flush to skin. Niacin may aggravate gout, and stomach problems.
- Simone recommended dose: 40-80 mg per day; 1000-1500 mg per day to lower cholesterol and triglycerides.

Pantothenic Acid

- Energy - boosted.
- Diabetes – controls sugar.
- Toxicity: None.
- Simone recommended dose: 20-30 mg per day.

Pyridoxine (B6)

- Cancer risk – reduced. [351]
- Immune System – enhanced.
- Toxicity: Taking 500 mg/d for months will damage nerves.
- Simone recommended dose: 10-15 mg per day.

Vitamin B12

- Immune system – enhanced.
- Toxicity: None.

- Simone recommended dose: 18-30 mcg per day.

Folic Acid

- Cancer risk – reduced, breast, colon, and colon polyps. [352,353]
- Immune system – enhanced; Neural tube defects – reduced.
- Toxicity: None.
- Simone recommended dose: 400-800 mcg per day.

Biotin

- Its deficiency results in depression, anemia, sleepiness, muscle pain, hair loss, and increased cholesterol levels.
- Immune system – enhanced.
- Toxicity: None.
- Simone recommended dose: 150-250 mcg/day.

Calcium

The average daily calcium intake for Americans is 450-500 mg, an amount well below even the US RDI of 1000 mg per day for those under age 50 or menstruating, and 1500 mg per day for those over 50 or menopausal.

- Cancer risk – reduced, especially breast, colon, and pre-colon cancer (adenomas). [354-358]
- Cardiovascular Disease risk – reduced.
- Osteoporosis risk – reduced. Adolescent girls have evidence of osteoporosis.[359,360] Even eight year old girls and women of all ages benefit from calcium supplemenation.[361,362] Based on 3 studies, $2.6 billion could be saved from hip fractures if people over age 50 took 1200-1500 mg/day of calcium. [363]

The following increase the risk of osteoporosis:

- Smoking and Caffeine – 2 to 3 cups of coffee/day [364-369]
- Sedentary Lifestyle, Aging
- High Sodium, High Protein diet, and High Blood Acid
- Soft drinks (high phosphates).
- Steroid treatment of arthritis, asthma, inflammatory bowel disease;[370] and excessive thyroid hormones.
- Anti-depression medications: fluoxetine, fluvoxamine, paroxetine, sertraline, nortriptyline, protriptyline, de-

    sipramine, amitriptyline, desipramine, clomipramine, doxepin, imipramine, and trimipramine. [371]
  - Cadmium – a toxic metal found in tobacco smoke and also dolomite, a common calcium tablet. [372]
- Hypertension – reduced. [373]
- Alzheimer's disease risk – reduced. [374]
- Asthma flares – reduced.
- Some male infertility problems – reduced.
- Kidney stone risk – reduced. [375,376]
- Calcium carbonate is the most bioavailable form of calcium. Take at bedtime or between meals with a little orange or tomato juice. [377-379] Calcium should be taken with several other nutrients that aid calcium absorption and metabolism. Some of these nutrients, like vitamin D and vitamin C, should be taken only with food, while others, like magnesium, potassium bicarbonate, boron, silicon, threonine, and lysine, should be taken with calcium at night or between meals. [380]
- Simone recommended dose: 1500 mg per day for age 50 or older or post menopause, otherwise 1000 mg per day.

Magnesium
- Cardiovascular Disease risk and Death – reduced. [381,382]
- Hypertension – reduced. [383]
- Asthma – improved. [384]
- Low magnesium causes low levels of calcium and potassium.
- Simone recommended dose: 420 mg per day for age 50 or older, otherwise, 280 mg per day.

Iron
- Iron should not be taken unless you have an iron deficiency anemia because iron causes free radicals and excess stores of iron increase the risk of cancer in men and women. [385,386]
- Cancer risk –increased especially breast and colon. [387]
- Toxicity: Acute effects occur above 75 mg daily for adults.

- Simone recommended dose: None unless you have iron deficiency anemia, and then only in therapeutic doses for 30 days with a doctor's supervision. Avoid routine supplementation.

Amino Acids

Amino acids are the building blocks for all proteins and are necessary for brain function. We can make some in our bodies, others we cannot. The ones that cannot be made by us are called essential amino acids. All are important for our health.

Amino acid deficiencies or abnormalities can be found in:

- Athletes, Body builders, people with muscle wasting or connective tissue disorders.
- Depression, hyperactivity, attention deficit disorder.
- Substance abuse.
- Immune System disorders, Viral Infections (herpes, Epstein Barr syndrome), Allergies.
- Eating disorders.
- Surgery, Sepsis, Trauma.
- Simone recommendations include the following groups of amino acids: Essential, Branched Chain (BCAA), Neurotransmitters, Glycogenics, Urea Cycle, Connective Tissue.

Dietary Fiber

- Cancer risk – reduced. On the basis of hundreds of clinical studies, a global review of 4500 research studies, studies and statements by the US National Cancer Institute, international governmental agencies, and seven international Consensus Statements, there is little doubt that fiber lowers the risk of colorectal cancer, and other cancers.[388-391]
- Cardiovascular Disease, Diabetes, Obesity, Colon Diverticulosis risk – reduced.

Soluble fiber gets into the bloodstream and binds to and thereby decreases bile acids, cholesterol, triglycerides, sugars, poisons, and carcinogens. ***Insoluble*** and ***soluble*** fibers increase the weight and amount of stool, which dilutes and excretes carcinogens, and keeps the intestinal flora healthy.

You need about 25 to 35 grams of fiber daily for this protection: 6-11 servings of grains (cereal, rice, past, bread), 2-4 servings of fruits, 3-5 servings of vegetables, and legumes once or twice a week. However, Americans consume only about 10 grams of fiber per day. Therefore a dietary fiber supplement must be used to attain the protective effect.

- Toxicity: None. Dietary fiber is safe.
- Simone recommended dose: 25-35 grams per day.

Essential Fatty Acids

- Breast cancer risk and Cardiovascular risk – reduced.[392,393]
- Toxicity: None known.
- Simone recommendations: Linolenic Acid – 2 to 8 grams per day; Linoleic Acid – 3 to 9 grams per day.

NATURAL PROTECTORS IN FOODS

Researchers, prompted by epidemiological evidence have studied foods that can protect your health – Table 5.3.

Table 5.3 Natural Food Protectors

Protector	Food	Protective Action
Carotene Lycopene Lutein	Carrots, sweet potatoes, Yams, Pumpkins, broccoli, Kale, cantaloupe, tomato	Neutralizes singlet oxygen and free radicals Cancer risk – reduced
Indoles	Cabbage Family: cabbage, broccoli, cauliflower, mustard greens, etc.	Destroys estrogen that causes cancer.
Lignans	Flaxseed, walnuts, fatty fish	Inhibits estrogens, & certain protaglandins that promote cancer
Polyacetylene	Parsley	Inhibits certain protaglandins Destroys some carcinogens
Quinones	Rosemary	Inhibits carcinogens
Sterols	Cucumbers	Decreases cholesterol
Sulfur	Garlic	Inhibits carcinogens Lowers cholesterol
Terpenes	Citrus Fruit	Destroys carcinogens Lowers cholesterol
Triterpenoids	Licorice	Inhibits estrogens & some prostaglandins, Slows down rapidly dividing cells.

Lycopene content varies with different food sources (content in micrograms/100gram wet food): Tomato raw – 3100, tomato juice – 8600; tomato sauce – 6300; watermelon – 4100; guava pink – 5200; and pink grapefruit – 350. [394]

REDUCE YOUR RISK OF CANCER

Cancer takes decades to develop. Cancers begin and grow early in life at a time when people do not receive enough antioxidants because they are simply not eating enough of the recommended 9 servings of fruits and vegetables that might provide some of these antioxidants in modest amounts. We now have enough positive scientific data to conclude that antioxidants reduce the risk for cancer because they protect against the initiation and promotion of a cancer. **So we must begin taking antioxidants consistently early in life for long periods of time because they are protective, but they should not be used as a sole weapon to kill cancer.**

Almost 40 percent of people take vitamins, but the vitamins they take are not necessarily the ones they need.[395,396] A proper formulation should consist of four factors: the **correct nutrient**, the **correct dose**, the **correct chemical form** of that nutrient, and the **correct ratio of one to another**. Often, a person will hear or read about a specific nutrient and run to the store to buy that nutrient without knowing the correct dose, chemical form, and ratio of it to another.

President Reagan's Administration said, "This new strategy [vitamin use] holds promise for reducing the incidence of cancer more successfully than an attempt to remove from the environment all substances which may initiate the cancer process." (*Medical Tribune*, June 30, 1982). And in 1995, US National Cancer Institute researchers stated: The field of chemoprevention…is now considered to be an extremely promising approach to the prevention of invasive cancer." [397]

YOUR IDEAL SUPPLEMENT PROGRAM

I recommend taking the following combinations of antioxidants, vitamins, minerals, amino acids, fibers, and other nutrients as supplementation shown below. These nutrients can be taken daily unless otherwise specified by your physician. Pregnant or lactating women should not follow this program unless approved by their physician.

Simone Antioxidant – Nutrient Supplementation

Carotene	30 mg	**Selenium**	200 mcg
Lutein	20 mcg	**Copper**	3 mg
Lycopene	20 mcg	**Zinc**	30 mg
Vitamin A	5500 IU	Iodine	150 mcg
Vitamin D	400 IU	Potassium	30 mg
Vitamin E	400 IU	Chromium	125 mcg
Vitamin C	350 mg	Manganese	2.5 mg
Folic Acid	400 mcg	Molybdenum	50 mg
Vitamin B1	10 mg	Inositol	10 mg
Vitamin B2	10 mg	PABA	10 mg
Niacinamide	40 mg	**Bioflavonoids**	10 mg
Vitamin B6	10 mg	Choline	10 mg
Vitamin B12	18 mcg	**L-Cysteine**	20 mg
Biotin	150 mcg	**L-Arginine**	5 mg
Pantothenic acid	20 mg		

*Antioxidants are bolded

Simone Calcium Formula

Calcium carbonate	1000 mg
Magnesium	280 mg
Potassium bicarbonate	200 mg
Boron	4 mg
L-Lysine	4 mg
Silicon	4 mg
Threonine	4 mg

Simone Fiber Formula

Soluble Fiber	800 mg
Pectin, Gums (Guar, oat)	
Mucilages (kelp, psyllium)	
Insoluble Fiber	200 mg

Simone Essential Fatty Acids

Linolenic Acid	2 to 8 grams
Linoleic Acid	3 to 9 grams

I am advocating simple common sense. Modify your risk factors and thereby reduce your risk of cancer, cardiovascular, and other chronic diseases. This includes following our Ten Point Plan and taking the correct nutrients, the correct doses, the correct chemical forms, and the correct ratio of one to another according to your individual lifestyle needs.

6

Nutritional and Lifestyle Modification Augments Oncology Care

Cancer will be the number one cause of death in the United States. The successes in the treatment of cancer plateaued in the 1970s, and no real advances have been made since then. However, chemotherapy and radiation therapy continue to have a role in cancer treatment but produce morbidity. Nutritional modification, including the use of certain nutrients, and proper lifestyle can dramatically decrease the morbidity and side effects of chemotherapy and radiation therapy, and normal tissue can be better preserved. There have even been some reports that nutritional and lifestyle modification actually increases survival. Innumerable studies show that nutrients used with chemotherapy and radiation therapy can enhance tumor killing and preserve normal tissue.

NUTRIENTS AUGMENT CHEMOTHERAPY AND RADIATION THERAPY

Chemotherapeutic agents and radiation therapy reduce serum levels of certain nutrients, especially antioxidants. Supplemental nutrients given concomitantly to patients undergoing chemotherapy and/or radiation therapy can increase tumor response, reduce side effects, and even prolong survival. Since the 1970s, hundreds and hundreds of medical and scientific papers have been published about this topic. **For each section below, only representative references will be cited, however.**

CHEMOTHERAPY AND RADIATION THERAPY DECREASE SERUM NUTRIENT LEVELS OF ANTIOXIDANTS due to lipid peroxidation and thereby exhibit a higher level of oxidative stress.[1-7] Iron could be the possible intermediate cause of this oxidative stress,[8,9] and therefore supplemental iron should be given only if the cancer patient has an iron deficiency anemia.

DO VITAMINS OR MINERALS INTERFERE WITH CHEMOTHERAPY AND/OR RADIATION THERAPY? Patients frequently ask this because they have read or been advised not to take supplements during treatment since many physicians *believe* that antioxidants will interfere with the efficacy of the treatment modality that kills cells via free radical mechanism.[10,11] However, hundreds of cellular and animal studies, including scores of clinical studies, demonstrate that nutrients do not interfere with the killing effects of chemotherapy or radiation therapy, but rather actually protect normal tissues and decrease side effects from these modalities.

***IN VITRO* CELLULAR STUDIES** [12-20](close to 100 studies) **AND ANIMAL STUDIES**[21-32] (over 100) using nutrients that include vitamins C, A, K, E, D, B6, B12, beta-carotene, selenium, or cysteine as single agents or in combination given concomitantly with chemotherapy, or tamoxifen, or interferon alpha-2b, or radiation, or combinations of these modalities show the same effect: Increased tumor killing and increased protection of the normal tissues.

HUMAN STUDIES [33-94]

Antioxidants decrease the cardiac toxicity of adriamycin as determined by researchers at the National Cancer Institute. N-acetyl cysteine protected the heart and at the same time did not interfere with the tumor-killing capability of adriamycin.[33] Another antioxidant that is now a prescription medicine called dexrazoxane (ICRF-187) also was found to significantly protect the heart from damage caused by adriamycin without affecting the antitumor effect.[34-36] Dexrazoxane binds iron to inhibit iron from forming free radicals that damage the heart. Then other nutrients were tested. Scores of cellular and animal studies, and human[37-42] studies demonstrate that vitamins A, E, C, and K, as well as beta-carotene and selenium, as single agents or in combination, all protect against the toxicity of adriamycin and, at the same time, actually enhance its cancer-killing effects.

Antioxidants and nutrients increase response rates and decrease side effects of chemotherapy and radiation therapy in multiple human studies.[43-91] Over 1,960 patients were studied using single or multiple nutrients in combination with chemotherapy and/or radiation treatment demonstrating that nutrients produce a higher response rate, lower side effects, and even increased survival. Other investigators used two or more nutrients, usually antioxidants in combination or with vitamin A or the B vitamins. In each study, patients receiving nutrients with chemotherapy and/or radiation had higher response rates, and decreased side effects.

Amifostine (WR-2721), an antioxidant analog of cysteamine, was discovered by the Armed Forces and became the first broad-spectrum agent to be approved by international regulatory agencies. Studies demonstrate that amifostine (WR-2721) protects against the harmful side effects of chemotherapy and radiation, enhances the antitumor effects of these modalities, and does not interfere with the antitumor killing activity.[92-94]

Antioxidants increase lifespan. Conventional treatment alone yields a certain lifespan for each cancer. But an increase in lifespan and fewer recurrences have been demonstrated for patients who received vitamin A or antioxidants (including carotene and anthaxanthin) in combination with chemotherapy or radiation therapy. This finding is observed for patients with cancers of the breast, lung, stomach, mouth, nasopharynx, and myelodysplastic syndromes.

Folic Acid Does Not Interfere with Methotrexate

The effects of one chemotherapeutic agent, methotrexate, can be reversed with folinic acid, which is an analog of the vitamin folic acid. Folic acid itself does not reverse methotrexate's effects.[95,96] In order to reverse the effects of methotrexate, folinic acid has to be given in high doses. Folinic acid cannot be obtained over the counter, it must be prescribed.

SUMMARY. Hundreds and hundreds of studies all show that supplemental antioxidants and nutrients do not interfere with the anticancer effects of chemotherapy or radiation therapy. In fact, on the contrary, some antioxidants and nutrients used in conjunction with chemotherapy and/or radiation therapy can increase the destruction of cancer, decrease side effects, and in some cases actually increase lifespan and disease free survival.

LIFESTYLE MODIFICATION AUGMENTS ONCOLOGY CARE

BREAST CANCER – QUALITY OF LIFE IS IMPROVED WITH LIFESTYLE MODIFICATION AND NUTRIENTS. Using Quality of Life Scales, 50 patients with early staged breast cancer evaluated treatment side effects of radiation and/or chemotherapy while taking therapeutic doses of nutrients.[97,98] The patient decided if the nutrients used during treatment had improved, worsened, or made no change in her life during the treatment period. The qualities of life tested were physical symptoms, performance, general well being, cognitive abilities, sexual dysfunction, and life satisfaction.

All 50 patients had lumpectomy, axillary node dissection, and radiation therapy (4500 cGy to whole breast + 1500 cGy to tumor bed); but for 25 patients with positive nodes, 6 cycles of chemotherapy were used – cytoxan, 5-FU, and then methotrexate was added after radiation was completed. Each patient followed the Ten Point Plan as described in Chapters 2 and 27 and took nutrients as outlined on pages 71 and 72 in Chapter 5.

Patients in both groups generally indicated improvement in their quality of life, a few indicated no change, and none indicated worsening. Those who followed the Ten Point Plan and took certain nutrients in the correct doses, correct chemical form, and correct ratio of one to another, had a better quality of life while receiving chemotherapy or radiation therapy.

JAPANESE EXPERIENCE – HEALTHY LIFESTYLE INCREASES LIFESPAN. Elderly Japanese women rarely get breast cancer, but when they do, they live longer than American women stage for stage[99-106] because (1) they are less obese, (2) they eat a low-fat, high-fiber diet with vitamins and minerals, (3) they don't smoke, or drink, (4) they exercise and mentally relax. Younger Japanese women have now adopted a more Western culture and diet[102] and have a higher rate of breast cancer.

Obese breast cancer patients have a greater chance of early recurrence and a shorter life span compared to non-obese patients.[107-111] And breast cancer patients who have a high-fat intake and a high serum cholesterol also have a shorter life span than patients with normal or low-fat intake and low serum cholesterol.[112] Fat can initiate and also promote a cancer, especially a dietary cancer like breast cancer. If cholesterol intake is dramatically limited, cancer cell growth is severely inhibited.[113]

U.S. NATIONAL CANCER INSTITUTE EFFORT. Armed with this information, the US National Cancer Institute, National Institutes of Health in Bethesda, Maryland conducted a research protocol in the mid 1980s to see if a low-fat diet would increase the life span of breast cancer patients. However, in January 1988, after only a brief time and an expenditure of about $90 million, it was decided to end the proposed ten year study because: (1) Physicians did not "believe" that there was a relationship between breast cancer and fat or other nutritional factors and, subsequently, did not refer patients to the study; and (2) Once a woman was enrolled in the protocol, she subsequently "failed out" because she did not want to give up pizza, ice cream, and other high-fat foods.

HOFFER-PAULING STUDY. Professors Hoffer and Pauling asked whether therapeutic nutrition could help 129 cancer patients.[114] All ate a low-fat diet supplemented with therapeutic doses of vitamins C, E, A, niacin, and a multiple vitamin/mineral supplement, in addition to following the advice and treatment of traditional oncology care. Those who did not follow nutritional modification (31 patients) lived an average of

6 months less. The other 98 patients fell into three categories: 32 patients with breast, ovarian, cervix, and uterus cancer had an average life span of over 10 years; 47 patients who had leukemia, lung, liver, and pancreas cancer had an average life span of over 6 years; and 19 patients with end-stage terminal cancer lived an average of 10 months.

Other Clinical Studies

Other clinical studies show similar findings: Patients who undergo conventional oncology therapy generally live longer and/or have a lower recurrence rate if they modify their lifestyle, which includes diet changes, nutrient supplementation, and other lifestyle changes.[115-119]

The effect of vegetable consumption was examined over a period of 6 years in 675 patients with lung cancer. Those who lived longer ate more vegetables.[115] In another study, 200 patients who made significant dietary changes, experienced regression of their cancers without conventional treatment: 87 percent changed their diet dramatically to mainly vegetables, fruits, and whole grains; 65 percent consumed nutrient supplements; and 55 percent used a detoxification method.[116]

The effect of eating a macrobiotic diet on survival was studied in 1490 patients with pancreas cancer and 18 patients with prostate cancer.[117] Twenty-three matched patients with pancreas cancer changed to a macrobiotic diet and 12 (52%) were alive after one year; 1467 continued their high-fat, low-fiber diet and of these, 146 (10%) were alive after one year. Similarly, nine patients with prostate cancer who ate a macrobiotic diet were matched to nine patients with prostate cancer who ate their "normal" high-fat diet. Those eating the macrobiotic diet lived longer (median survival 228 months) than those who did not (median survival 45 months).

Tumor recurrence rate was decreased by 50 percent in patients with transitional cell bladder cancer who took higher than Recommended Dietary Intake (RDI) doses of certain vitamins compared to matched controls taking RDI doses.[119]

LIFESPAN IS INCREASED

• **Nutrients + Chemotherapy and/or Radiation therapy increase lifespan** in eight studies for patients who received vitamin A or antioxidants concomitantly with chemotherapy and radiation therapy compared to patients who did not receive the nutrients. This finding is observed for patients with cancers of the breast, lung, stomach, mouth, nasopharynx, and myelodysplastic syndromes.

• **Lifestyle Modification (including nutrients) + Chemotherapy and/or Radiation Therapy increase lifespan** as demonstrated in twenty studies with more than 2700 patients. The patients in these studies had the following cancers: breast, ovarian, cervix, uterus, head and neck, lung, pancreas, prostate, and bladder.

CONCLUSION

Many of the nutrients used in the above studies are antioxidants. Antioxidants neutralize free radicals. Most cancer modalities exert their cancer killing effects by generating free radicals. Therefore it would seem inconsistent that these nutrients can help the cancer patient. However, hundreds and hundreds of *in vitro* and *in vivo* studies, including scores of clinical studies have repeatedly shown that certain vitamins and minerals can enhance the killing of cancer therapeutic modalities while at the same time protect normal tissues and decrease side effects from these modalities.

How is this possible? Because cancer cells accumulate excessive amounts of antioxidants[120] due to a loss of the homeostasis control mechanism for the uptake of these nutrients. Normal cells do not have this membrane defect and do not accumulate large amounts of antioxidants. Accumulation of excessive antioxidants in cancer cells can:

- Shut down oxidative reactions necessary for making energy
- Inhibit protein kinase C activity[121] which normally increases cell division and increases cell proliferation
- Inhibit oncogene expression[122,123]

• Increase the amount of growth inhibitory growth factors[124]

With higher levels of cancer intracellular accumulation of nutrients, more of these cellular alterations occur. These changes can lead to a higher rate of cancer cell death, and a reduction in the rate of cell proliferation and induction of differentiation. These acquired changes of cancer cells due to high doses of nutrients actually override any protective action that antioxidants have against free radical damage on cancer cells.

Cancer patients should modify their lifestyles (Ten Point Plan), that includes modifying nutritional factors and taking certain vitamins and minerals in the correct doses, especially if they receive chemotherapy and/or radiation. No one should take "a multiple vitamin/mineral formula" that simply has the correct words on the label. The studies indicate that it is important to take the correct nutrients, in the correct dosages, in the correct chemical form, and in the correct ratio of one to the other.

PART THREE

The Risks

7
Free Radicals

Free radicals are made in our bodies all the time and, if not destroyed, can lead to the development of cancer and other diseases. You already are familiar with free radicals – they cause oxidation – rusty metal, rancid butter, the greenish hue on outdoor copper statues. Antioxidants, like beta-carotene, vitamins C and E, selenium, and others, can neutralize the harmful free radicals and thereby prevent disease and protect us.

By definition, free radicals are chemical substances that contain an odd number of electrons. Every atom has a nucleus and a certain number of electrons that orbit around the nucleus. This setup is very much like our solar system, with the sun in the middle and all the planets orbiting around the sun. The nucleus has a positive charge, and the electrons have a negative charge. The negative charges of electrons balance out the positive charge of the nucleus to give an overall charge of zero. Hence, the energy of a single atom is very stable at zero.

When high energy in any form (from light, radiation, smog, tobacco, alcohol, polyunsaturated fats, etc.) hits an atom, an electron is kicked out of orbit. All of the energy that forced the electron out of orbit is transferred directly to the electron, making it highly energetic and unstable. Because it is so unstable, this electron quickly seeks *another* atom to reside in. This excited high-energy electron transfers very high energy to the new atom, which then becomes extremely unstable because of the newly acquired high energy. The process is depicted below.

FREE RADICAL FORMATION CAUSING CELL DAMAGE

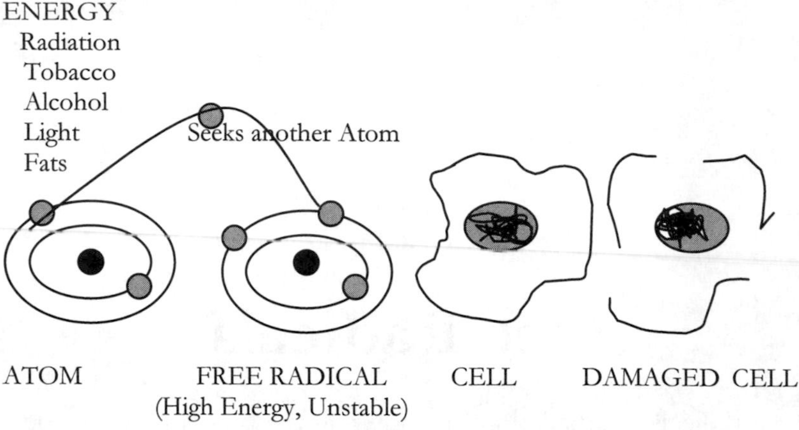

This excited high-energy atom with its extra electron is called a free radical. A free radical is unstable and must get rid of all the extra energy for the atom to become stable once again; hence the radical transfers its energy to nearby substances. All these reactions take place in a fraction of a second. When free radicals are made, the high energy is transferred to body tissues, particularly to the polyunsaturated fats found in the cell membranes, thereby causing cell damage. The more fats you eat, the more of them will be absorbed by cell membranes and the higher the risk will be for membrane disruption by free radicals. If the free radicals are not neutralized, this process can lead to cancer in the tissue affected by the radical.

FORMATION OF RADICALS

The following produce free radicals and can lead to the development of cancer:

- **Oxygen** can be activated or split with high energy into very potent damaging radicals (superoxide) or a high-energy, unstable nonradical called singlet oxygen. Singlet oxygen has extremely high energy and is very unstable, and thus is very destructive to normal body tissues and cells.
- **Polyunsaturated Fats** react with oxygen or enzymes to release their energy and thereby form a free radical. This free

radical reacts with another polyunsaturated fat to produce a hydroperoxide. The more unsaturated the fat is, the more hydroperoxides are made that produce more radicals, damage cell membranes, and can lead to the development of cancer.

• **Metals** accumulate in the body and can also initiate free radical formation by activating oxygen. Iron is one example.

• **Radiation** produces free radicals and electrons that react to yield many different kinds of free radicals. At high levels of radiation, hydroperoxides are produced in addition to all the other free radicals.

• **Sunlight (Photolysis)** produces free radicals in skin cells, which can damage the skin and lead to skin cancer, the most common of all human cancers. The three kinds of skin cancers are basal cell, squamous cell and melanoma. Chronic sun exposure in Caucasians directly damages the skin and results in wrinkling, the formation of tiny networks of blood vessels, and the appearance of discrete small raised bumps on the skin called actinic keratosis (which are precancerous). And ultraviolet light harms the immune system. Use sunscreens, sunglasses, protective clothing and don't use suntanning booths.

• **Smog** causes more tissue damage than background radiation. Ozone and other compounds of smog react with almost every type of molecule in the body to form free radicals that damage cells. Ozone in normal amounts in the air can even form radicals with polyunsaturated fatty acids.

• **Alcohol and Chloride-Containing Compounds.** Vinyl chloride, chloroprene, and carbon tetrachloride react with some liver enzymes (microsomal mixed function oxidase) to produce free radicals that damage liver cells and potentiate liver cancer.

FREE RADICALS CAUSE DISEASE

Free radicals are the main cause of many human diseases – Table 7.1.[1,2] Free radicals cause cancer by damaging the membrane and the nucleus of the cell and subsequently the DNA. When certain segments of the DNA are affected, a malignant change occurs, altering the genetic code and leading to cancer.[3-5] Antioxidants neutralize free radicals and protect against cancer.

Table 7.1 Conditions Associated with Free Radicals

Cancers: all types	**Central Nervous System Diseases**
	Senile dementia
Cardiovascular Disease	Parkinson's disease
Alcohol heart condition	Hypertensive stroke
Selenium heart condition	Encephalomyelitis
(Keshan disease)	Aluminum overload
Atherosclerosis	Ataxia-telangiectasia
Adriamycin toxicity	
Heart Attack	**Iron Overload**
Lung Disease	**Radiation Injury**
Emphysema	
Pneumoconiosis	**Kidney Diseases**
Respiratory distress syndrome	
Bleomycin toxicity	**Gastrointestinal Diseases**
Air pollutant toxicity	Free-fatty acid pancreatitis
	Nonsteroidal anti-inflam-
Alcohol-related diseases	matory drug lesions
	Liver injury from toxins
Immune System Diseases	Carbon tetrachloride injury
Glomerulonephritis	
Vasculitis	**Skin Diseases**
Autoimmune diseases	Solar radiation damage
Rheumatoid Arthritis	Contact dermatitis
Eye Diseases	**Red Blood Cell Diseases**
Cataracts	
Retinal Damage	**Aging**

Free radicals cause cardiovascular disease by damaging the cells that line the inside of all blood vessels.[6] Due to this initial injury, fats and fibrin (blood-clotting protein) and other elements of the blood ultimately form clots and block the arteries.[7] Once a person sustains a heart attack, the injury that occurs within the first twelve to twenty-four hours is secondary to free radical damage.[8,9] Therefore, antioxidants have an important role not only in the prevention of cardiovascular disease but also at the time of an ongoing heart attack. The process of aging is due to oxidation – related to free radicals.

OUR BODY'S DEFENSES AGAINST RADICALS

We know that all life requires oxygen, but sometimes oxygen can produce radicals and high-energy (singlet) oxygen. Because of this, Mother Nature has given us three major lines of defense against free radical formation to preserve our very existence and to lessen the chance of abnormal cell (cancer) development.

The first is the *protective protein coat* that lines the surface of the cell membrane and prevents oxygen from reacting directly with lipids in the membrane, a reaction that would produce many free radicals. A second defensive mechanism involves the *protective enzymes* that float around in all cell membranes and act as antioxidants. They include *superoxide dismutase*, *catalase,* and selenium-containing *glutathione peroxidase.* Vitamin E is also an antioxidant and is the third mechanism that inhibits formation of free radicals in the cell membrane.

Mother Nature did not realize just how abusive we would be to our bodies. And although these three lines of defense are important, they are simply not enough given all that we now do to generate free radicals. That's why we should take antioxidant supplements.

8
Nutritional Factors

Joyce's History

Joyce loves steak, hot dogs, pizza, and ice cream. Who doesn't? She has been eating these foods for all her 53 years. Her new mammogram shows an abnormality that was not seen on her prior three mammograms.

The National Academy of Sciences estimates that 60 percent of all women's cancers and 40 percent of all men's cancers are related to nutritional factors alone.[1-3] Overall, it has been estimated that 75 to 90 percent of all cancers are related to lifestyle: nutritional factors, smoking, alcohol consumption, occupational factors, chemicals, environmental factors, etc.

Nutritional factors are most closely associated with cancers of breast, prostate, colon/rectum, and endometrium. The number of new cancers continues to rise each year, especially diet related cancers. You can readily understand the enormous impact that proper nutrition can have in lowering the overall incidence of cancer in the United States and the world.

NUTRITIONAL EVOLUTION

The human race has existed for about two million years, and our prehuman ancestors existed for at least four million years. Today, we are confronted with diet-related health problems that were previously of minor importance or totally nonexistent. Dietary habits adopted by Western society over the past hundred years have greatly contributed to the development of coronary heart disease, hypertension, diabetes, and cancer. These illnesses have dominated the past century and are virtually unknown among the few surviving hunter-gatherer populations, like the Bantu tribesmen in Africa, whose way of life and eating habits today resemble those of people before agricultural development. Members of primitive cultures today who survive to the age of sixty or more are relatively free of these illnesses unlike their Western "civilized" counterparts.[4,5]

With the development of agriculture over 10,000 years ago, we began eating less meat and more vegetables. With less protein in our diets, our height declined by six inches. After the Industrial Revolution, the pendulum started to swing back, and we started to increase the protein content of our diets. Height increased and we are now nearly the same height as were the first biologically modern people. But our diet is still very different from theirs. We are affluently malnourished.

Animals that live in the wild have less fat than domesticated ones because they are more active and have a less steady food supply. Domesticated animals are fed high fat foods to produce tender meat. Wild game has fewer calories and more protein per unit of weight. Even modern plant foods have more fat than non-commercially grown vegetables and fruits. Table 8.1 lists the various nutrients consumed by primitive people compared with those eaten by Americans today.[6] Primitive people consumed more dietary vitamins, more protein, less harmful fats, and much more essential fatty acids.

Table 8.1 Diet Comparison of Primitive and Modern Person

Nutrient	Primitive Person	Modern American	Simone Recommendations
		Percentage of Total Calories	
Protein	34%	12%	35%
Carbohydrates	45%	46%	45%
Fats	21%	42%	20%
		Daily Consumption	
Cholesterol	591 mg	600 mg	250 mg
Fiber	45.7 g	12 g	30-45 g
Sodium	690 mg	5000 mg	1000 mg
Calcium	1580 mg	500 mg	1500 mg
Vitamin C	392 mg	80 mg	400 mg

We have created a food supply very different from that of our ancestors with the development of food technology and the chemicals used for its growth and production. This "advancement" is costly to the human race.

The vitamin and mineral content continues to decrease in our food supply because of pesticides, herbicides, processing techniques, freezing, thawing, transporting around the country, etc.

EPIDEMIOLOGICAL PATTERNS

Epidemiological studies demonstrate that a high-risk diet for cancers of the breast, colon, rectum, prostate, endometrium, as well as cardiovascular disease and other chronic illnesses is one that has high-fat, high-cholesterol, low-fiber, low intake of vitamins and minerals, more refined sugar, salt-cured, pickled, charred, smoked, or burned foods.[7-15] The more industrialized a country is, the higher is the rate of diet-related cancers.

Epidemiological studies assess cancer trends. They show a sixfold variation in breast cancer incidence in different parts of the world. High-incidence countries such as the United States are characterized by diets rich in cholesterol and animal fat. In high-incidence countries, there is a constant increase in the rate of breast cancer development with age, but in low-incidence countries the rate decreases after menopause.

- **Migration studies** show that if people emigrate from a country with a low incidence rate of a dietary cancer to a country with a high rate, they incur the higher rate fairly quickly.
  - **Japanese immigrants** to the United States, particularly the young, have the same colon cancer rate after only twenty years of consuming the American diet and have the same incidence of breast cancer after only two generations. Older Japanese would be less apt to adopt American dietary customs and therefore have less risk for these cancers. Only 20% of the daily calories in Japan is derived from fat compared to 40% in America. But now, as the diet in Japan has become more Westernized, especially among the young, the rates of breast, colon, and prostate cancer have risen.[16]

○ **Southern Italian women immigrants** to Australia adopt a higher fat diet and incur a higher breast cancer rate as well.[17]

• **Bantu** people of Africa eat a low fat, high fiber diet and have an extremely low incidence of cancer compared to people in industrialized nations.

• **Seventh-Day Adventists and Mormons** in the United States have a very low incidence of cancer and heart disease because they consume a high fiber, low fat diet.[18-20]

• **American-born Jews of European descent** are at high risk for developing colon and rectal cancer. A twenty-year prospective study conducted in Israel showed that a high-fiber, low-fat, high vitamin C diet substantially reduced the number of colon and rectal cancer cases in that group.[21]

• **Finns** have a high fat intake, mainly from dairy. They have a high incidence of heart attacks but a low incidence of colon cancer because they consume a large amount of fiber from rye that suppresses fecapentaene, a cancer-causing chemical. Fecapentaenes are found in stools of people on fiber-depleted diets. These people have a higher incidence of colon cancer. This chemical, produced by bacteria in the large bowel and then released by them when they die, is not present in fiber-eating populations who are free from colon cancer.[22,23] When fiber is added to the diet, the bacteria stay healthy, they don't die and they don't release fecapentaenes.

• **Chinese**, compared to Americans, consume 20% more calories, three times the amount of fiber (33 to 77 grams), one-third the amount of fat, less protein from animal sources, have a lower cholesterol, eat twice the amount of starch, half as much calcium (all from vegetables) as Americans yet do not have osteoporosis, and are less obese. Because of a lower fat diet, Chinese women start menstruating three to six years later than American women and have less breast cancer. [Nutrition, Environment, Health Project, Chinese Academy of Preventive Medicine, Cornell-Oxford]

Chinese people are a genetically similar population, but there are differences in dietary habits, environmental exposures, and disease rates in China from region to region. For instance, the cancer rate varies by a factor of several hundred from one region to another. The genetic contribution to cancer in China is minimal. Chinese who do eat more protein and fats have more heart disease, cancer, and diabetes. Any differences in cancer rates and other chronic illnesses, like heart disease, are attributed to dietary and other environmental exposures.

• **Diet Recall Studies** ask people what they ate every day for the last number of months or years. Can you to remember what you ate two nights ago for dinner? Most people tend to underestimate their consumption of fat and/or other unhealthy foods particularly when they know that a high-fat diet is not healthy. Despite this, most diet recall studies suggest that a high fat intake increases the risk for breast cancer.[24-31] However, the Nurses Health Study,[32] widely publicized, suggested otherwise. Many scientist-physicians agree that the study is flawed for several reasons: (1) The patients consumed a high-fat diet of 32% compared to a low-fat diet of 20% that protects against breast cancer – in fact, other investigators[33] showed that the percentage of fat was even higher than 32% - and the authors of the Nurses Health Study freely admit that a 20% or less fat diet does decrease the risk of breast cancer;[34] (2) The study involved middle-aged women and totally ignored diet earlier in life, a time critical to breast cancer development; (3) This was an eight-year study, most cancers take decades to develop.

High-fat diets are correlated with a higher risk of breast cancer and other cancers like colon, prostate, endometrium, etc. I recommend a 20% or less fat diet.

• **Breast fluid** also influences the development of breast cancer. Breast fluid secretion occurs in most women, but in varying amounts. For example, Oriental women have much less breast fluid secretion than white women. Breast fluid bathes the ductal cells of the breast gland where most cancers originate. A high blood cholesterol level increases the breast fluid level of a carcinogen called cholesterol epoxide.[35] Nicotine and its close relative cotinine appear in breast fluid within five minutes after smoking or inhalation of other people's smoke. Carcinogens get into breast fluid, bathe breast tissue for long periods of time, and increase the risk of cancer.

PHYTOESTROGENS

The belief that soy, a bean containing phytoestrogens, protects against breast cancer originates in the fact that older Japanese women have a lower incidence of breast cancer than older American women. However, this is not solely due to Japanese women's higher intake of soy. They have a lower incidence of breast cancer because of their better overall lifestyle that includes not only soy, but also a lower fat diet with little or no red meat or dairy foods, less obesity, little or no smoking and alcohol, exercise, stress modification and other healthy habits.[36]

Soy has two phytoestrogens – genistein and daidzem. They were initially thought to be weak estrogens because they bound weakly to the alpha Estrogen Receptor. Now, however, it is known that they have strong estrogen capability because they bind strongly to the beta Estrogen Receptor.[37] Animal studies have demonstrated that soy can stimulate the growth of estrogen receptor positive breast cancer cells implanted into nude mice[38] and increase DNA synthesis which represents a marker for increased cancer risk.[39]

A growing body of evidence suggests that phytoestrogens are not safe.[40] Extracts of vitex, dong quai, American ginseng, and cohosh – all phytoestrogens – bind estrogen receptors in exactly the same way as estrogens made by the body.

In animal experiments, ovaries were removed from rats so that they could not produce significant amounts of estrogen themselves. Phytoestrogens were then given to them for 30 days. A decreased blood level of luteinizing hormone (LH) was found indicating high circulating levels of estrogens were present. Since the rats had no ovaries and could not produce their own estrogen, the drop in LH could only have resulted from the phytoestrogens given to the rats. Additionally, the uterus of each rat got larger indicating that the organ responded to the phytoestrogens as it would to any estrogens.

Phytoestrogens have the same effect as estrogens produced by the body. Don't consume phytoestrogens!

FATS

In 1942 Dr Tannenbaum first showed that dietary fat significantly favored the development and growth of both spontaneous and induced breast cancer in animals.[41] Dietary animal fat is found in all four-legged animals (red meat), luncheon meats, and all dairy products, including milk, cheese, and eggs.

- **Animal fat promotes and initiates cancer**[42-62] because:
  - Fats increase sterol chemicals and bile acids that bacteria convert to carcinogens and carcinogenic estrogen.[63,64]
  - Overweight women have fatty breasts that accumulate carcinogenic estrogens and are attacked by free radicals.
  - Fats increase prolactin, a carcinogenic hormone.[65] High prolactin levels are also found in women who have their first pregnancies late in life that may account for their higher risk of developing breast cancer.
  - Fats inhibit the immune system.
- **Fats decrease lifespan and increase death rate in breast cancer patients.**[66-71]
  - Japanese women in Japan with breast cancer live longer than women in America with similar breast cancer [72-74] because of a lower fat diet.[75-78] Neither the clinical extent of disease nor histology was the basis for the differences seen in survival. Disease-free survival was also greater for Japanese women than American women.[79]
  - In Hawaii, Japanese women, given the same medical care as Caucasian women, lived longer because of their diet and lifestyle – not the treatment.[80]
  - Being overweight and having a high cholesterol decreases both disease-free survival and lifespan[81-83] because prolactin is increased,[84] gonadotropins are decreased,[85] more androstenedione is converted to estrone,[86] and sex hormone binding globulin, free androgen, and free estrogen are altered.[87]

FIBER

Dietary fiber is safe. Hundreds of studies involving tens of thousands of subjects demonstrate that 25 to 35 grams of dietary fiber daily will reduce the risk of cancer.[88] The most compelling and the most comprehensive review and evaluation of the link between diet and the development of cancer concludes that 3 to 4 million cases of cancer per year could be prevented by appropriate diet and lifestyle changes. A panel of over 150 scientists who reviewed and evaluated 4,500 research studies published their findings in a 670 page report, Food, Nutrition and the Prevention of Cancer: A Global Perspective.

Decreased cancer risk is most convincingly linked to fiber from vegetables, followed by fibers from non-soluble polysaccharides, starches, and fiber foods with carotenoids. Most Consensus Statements indicate that 25-35 grams of fiber each day is needed to protect against colon cancer. Unless a person has the time or the inclination to become a grazing animal, it would be difficult to attain the protective level of fiber each day without taking a supplement because Americans typically consume an average of only 8 to 15 grams of fiber per day. Food Guide Pyramid suggests daily: 6 to 11 servings of grains (cereal, rice, pasta, bread), 2 to 4 servings of fruits and 3 to 5 servings of vegetables daily, and legumes at least once or twice a week. Not very many of us can consume this amount without a supplement.

Breast cancer patients should increase dietary fiber because fiber increases the fecal excretion of estrogen and decreases the plasma concentration of estrogen.[89] In fact, it might be wise to extend this modified diet to other diet-sensitive cancers – colon and rectal, prostate, endometrium – in an attempt to increase lifespan and disease-free survival.

PROTEIN AND CARBOHYDRATES

High protein consumption is linked to a higher risk of breast cancer,[79,90] colon and rectal cancer,[91,92] and other cancers. A high sugar intake increases the risk for breast cancer.[93,94] Excessive carbohydrate ingestion contributes to obesity, which, in turn, increases the risk for breast cancer.

NATURALLY OCCURRING CARCINOGENS AND MUTAGENS

Some foods have naturally occurring carcinogens or mutagens. Plants have certain molecules to protect them against microorganisms and insects, and some of these are carcinogenic or mutagenic in humans.

For instance, certain foods contain nicotine. Eggplant has the highest amount of nicotine per gram of vegetable (0.1 mcg) followed by potato (0.007 mcg), then tomato (0.004 mcg).[95-98] Although there is no cotinine (breakdown product of nicotine) in these foods, it may show up in the bloodstream of people eating these foods.

Some other foods and the carcinogens they contain are: black pepper (piperine and safrole), bruised celery (psoralen), herbal teas (pyrrolizidine, phorbol esters), mushrooms (hydrazines), and all foods containing mold (aflatoxin) or certain bacteria (nitrosamines).[99] Many of these are occasional contaminants, whereas others are normal components of relatively common foods.

Mutagens are chemicals that cause DNA changes. Mutagens are found in charred foods, coffee (quinones), and horseradish (allyl isothiocyanate). Mutagens pose a minimal risk for cancer development.

DIETARY TRENDS FOR FAT AND CHOLESTEROL

It has been estimated that if Americans reduce their fat content from 40% to just 30% (still higher than the protective 20%), about 42,000 of the 2.3 million annual deaths in the United States could be deferred.[100]

The third National Health and Nutrition Examination Survey (NHANES III), conducted by the National Center for Health Statistics of the Center for Disease Control and Prevention (CDC), showed that there is a continuing decline in serum cholesterol levels among adults in the United States but still well above levels that would decrease the risk for cancer and cardiovascular disease.[101]

Studies indicate that patients fail to follow sound dietary advice.[102-106] This indicates that unless there is a strong motivating factor, and it is hard to imagine that a person's life is not such a motivating factor, people simply will not change habits even though they are told it will benefit them medically.

People who are aware of the health benefits of a low-fat, high-fiber diet supplemented with certain nutrients chose, instead, to eat high-fat snacks, and gained an average of two to four pounds a year. This "pleasure revenge," as The New York Times labels it, is seen most often among the affluent and well-educated people who previously led the health and fitness frenzy. People now are giving themselves permission to be unhealthy – not worrying about weight or smoking cessation. Consider the facts.

- Sales of high calorie foods rose: butter, beef, soda, sugar, cheese, super premium ice cream, cookies, fast-foods.
- Sales of low-calorie foods declined: margarine, diet-soda, sugar substitute, yogurt, fruit, and popcorn.
- Many diabetics eat what they want because "their medicines will take care of them."
- Fast-food chains stopped offering lean foods because people don't buy them.
- Massage is more popular than exercise.

People know what is good for their health, but many people indulge themselves and do what they want, when they want. This unhealthy trend is happening at a time when the cost for health-care is rising. Who do you think is going to pay for all this indulgence? And why should people who are striving to be healthy pay for others who indulge themselves?

Joyce's mammogram abnormality proved to be a cancer. Unlike many who don't follow sound dietary advice, Joyce did decrease fat intake and increased fiber. She is also modifying the rest of her lifestyle. These efforts will increase her lifespan.

9

Obesity

Rhoda's History

Rhoda was overweight all her life. Her parents allowed her to eat whatever and whenever even at an early age. By age 41, she developed arthritis. Heart disease soon after. And breast cancer by age 52.

Obesity affects about 45 percent of all Americans. Being obese carries with it a social stigma as well as a general health risk. One study calculated that there are 832 million pounds of excess fat on American men and 1,468 million pounds of excess fat on American women, for a total of 2.3 billion pounds.[1] More obesity occurs in middle-aged people and in people with low socioeconomic status. The percentage of African-American women who are obese is greater than the percentage of white women. Adopted children become obese if adoptive family members are obese.

The fat cell *size* is increased in all types of obesity. An increased *number* of fat cells is found in children and adults who were obese before the age of two. If children are obese before the age of two, they will likely be obese in adulthood because they already have an increased number of fat cells. Only 1 percent of obesity is caused by a disease or medical problem; 99 percent of all obesity is directly related to overeating.

Because obese individuals tend to develop a variety of diseases, some of which are life-threatening, obese adults have a higher than normal death rate for their age group. The risk of death correlates almost directly with how much a person is overweight. Even if you are only a little overweight, you still have an increased risk of death compared to a person who is not overweight.

OBESITY INCREASES RISK FOR BREAST CANCER

• Overwhelming evidence from around the world involving millions of women demonstrate that obesity increases the risk of breast cancer independently of other risk factors.[2-10]

• Weight gain from puberty to adulthood, especially between 20 and 30, increases the risk of breast cancer.[11]

• A birthweight of greater than 9 pounds increases the risk for breast cancer.[12]

• Obese postmenopausal women, especially those with a waist size larger than their hip size, have a higher rate of breast cancer.[13-19] Obese women have more estrogens circulating in their bodies because they have more fat cells, the main site of estrogen production.[20-23] Fat cells convert adrostenedione to estrone, a more carcinogenic estrogen.[24] Obese women with a large waist who lose more than 10 pounds can lower their increased risk of breast cancer by 45 percent.[25] Most obese women have lesser symptoms of menopause than thinner women because of their increased production of estrone.

• After age 35, more fat in breast regardless of weight. Breast fat then serves as a local source of estrone production. In fact, estrogen and estrone levels in breast fluid are ten to forty times the levels normally found in serum of menstruating, nonlactating women.[26,27]

• Estrogen and estrone levels can be lowered by 30 percent in three to six months when you reduce dietary fat from 35 percent to 20 percent, or by 15 percent when you reduce dietary fat modestly and add 35 grams of fiber per day.[28-31] Therefore women should reduce their weight and add fiber.

OBESITY INCREASES BREAST CANCER DEATH RATE

• Breast cancer patients who are overweight by 40 percent have a 50 percent greater risk of death.[32]

• Obesity is associated with more advanced breast cancers at the time of diagnosis, higher recurrence rates, and shorter survival times[33-39] even after allowing for other factors that do shorten survival like tumor size, lymph node involvement, etc. Originally this was explained as a result of delayed diagnosis in obese women (more difficult to find tumor, which is still, in part, true) rather than more aggressive cancer promotion from higher amounts of estrogen.

OBESITY INCREASES RISK FOR OTHER CANCERS

- Colon and Rectal Cancer
- Cervix, Endometrium, Ovary
- Gall Bladder and Biliary Passages
- Leukemia

OBESITY INCREASES RISK FOR OTHER DISEASES

- Impaired Immunity – more infections and higher death rate from infections; lower resistance to tuberculosis, malaria, and pneumonia, and decreased antibody production.
- Diabetes - a two or three times higher risk.
- Impaired breathing
- Cardiovascular disease – heart attack, stroke, hypertension, high cholesterol, high triglycerides
- Gall bladder disease
- Higher risk of death

OBESITY DECREASES LONGEVITY [40]

ATTAINING YOUR IDEAL WEIGHT

How much should a person weigh? There is no one answer, but here is a good rule of thumb. Men who are 5 feet tall should weigh 110 pounds. For every inch over 5 feet, add another 5 pounds. Thus, if a man is 5 feet 11 inches tall, his ideal weight is about 165 pounds. Women who are 5 feet tall should weigh about 100 pounds. For every inch over 5 feet, add 5 pounds. Therefore, if a woman is 5 feet 6 inches tall, her ideal weight is about 130 pounds.

Attaining your ideal weight is not always easy. Lose weight gradually. Losing one or two pounds a week is safe, and that loss will probably be maintained. Do not lose more weight than called for by the formula. Successful weight loss and maintenance of that loss will be achieved only if you totally modify your eating habits. Many people are put on high-protein liquid diets consisting of 800 calories a day and lose a great deal of weight within the first few weeks. But over time, these pounds come right back on because the person did not learn new eating habits. Eating less than 800 calories per day is dangerous and not recommended.

A person whose body weight fluctuates often or greatly has a much higher risk of developing coronary heart disease and dying than does a person who has a relatively stable body weight. Those aged thirty to forty-four were shown to suffer the most detrimental effects of weight fluctuation. These harmful effects of weight fluctuation were independent of degree of obesity or existing cardiovascular risk factors.

To lose weight, you must eat less and increase your physical activity.

Every pound of fat you have contains about 3,500 calories. Therefore, to lose one pound, you have to burn off 3,500 calories more than you eat. You will lose a pound a week if you burn off 500 calories per day more than you consume. So, if you eat a diet containing 1,200 calories per day and burn off 1,700 calories per day, you will lose one pound a week.

Before you start a physical exercise program, let a physician examine you. An exercise program should start out gradually, with new goals set every week. Walking is very good exercise. Table 9.1 shows the approximate number of calories burned by a 150-pound person performing various activities.

If you lose weight suddenly or without a good reason, see a physician. Unexplained weight loss can be a sign of cancer or another serious medical problem. Even though it is difficult to lose weight, you must try. Obesity has no benefits, and its risks are very great.

Table 9.1 Activities and the Calories They Burn

Activities	Calories Used/Hour	Activities	Calories Used/Hour
Job		*Recreation*	
Answering Telephone	50	Bowling	250
Bathing	100	Calisthenics	500
Bed making	300	Card Playing	25
Brushing teeth or hair	100	Cycling slowly (5.5 mph)	300
Chopping Wood	400	Cycling strenuously (13 mph)	660
Dishwashing	75	Dancing, slow step	350
Dressing, undressing	50	Dancing, fast step	600
Driving Automobile	120	Fishing	150
Dusting Furniture	150	Football	600
Eating	50	Golfing	250
Filing (office)	200	Handball	660
Gardening	250	Hiking	400
Housework	180	Horseback riding	250
Ironing	100	Jogging	600
Mopping Floors	200	Kissing vigorously	6-12
Mowing Lawn	250	Lovemaking	125-300
Preparing Food	100	Painting	150
Reading	25	Piano playing	75
Sawing	500	Running, fast pace	900
Sewing	50	Singing	50
Shoveling	500	Skating leisurely	400
Sitting	100	Skating rapidly	600
Sleeping	80	Skiing (10 mph)	600
Standing	140	Soccer	650
Typing	50	Swimming leisurely (1/4 mph)	400
Walking up and down stairs	800	Swimming rapidly	800
		Tennis, singles	450
Recreation		Tennis, doubles	350
Badminton	400	Volleyball	350
Baseball	350	Walking leisurely (2.5 mph)	200
Basketball	550	Walking quickly (3.75 mph)	300
Boating, rowing	400	Watching television	25
Boating, motor	150		

Source: Department of Agriculture, 1980, from data prepared by Dr. Robert Johnson at the University of Illinois.

Rhoda decided to lose weight to improve her well-being and her lifespan.

10
Food Additives, Contaminants, and Pesticides

Ashley's History

Ashley is a young mother of three small children. She thoroughly washes all fruits and vegetables but is concerned that the imported ones have extra contamination and pesticides. Is her risk higher for developing breast cancer?

The "Delaney clause" of the Federal Food, Drug, and Cosmetic Act, written because of food additives, prohibits the addition of any known carcinogens to food. Currently there are about 3,000 intentional food additives. There are over 12,000 occasionally detected unintentional additives from packaging, food processing, and other phases of the food industry.

FOOD ADDITIVES AND CONTAMINANTS

Chemical food additives and food contaminants have been extensively studied because they come into contact with our bodies. Chemicals are used to prevent contamination and spoilage of food that has to be produced in great quantities, stored, and transported. Chemicals are also used for flavoring and appearance. Chemical contaminants may develop as a result of food processing procedures such as irradiation, cooking, pickling, or smoking. The trouble with the use of chemicals in food is that we are exposed to them constantly, repeatedly, and at low doses. Therefore, laboratory investigations rather than large population studies must be done to determine whether the chemicals are potentially hazardous.

Intentional food additives are chemicals that are purposely added to food. Cyclamate, for example, has not been shown to cause cancer in humans, but it does produce testicular atrophy (shrinking) in rats. Saccharin produces bladder cancer in rats when comprising 5 percent or more in the diet,[1] but so far, there is no clear connection to human cancer.[2] Xylitol, a sweetener, causes bladder cancer in mice and adrenal cancer in rats. [3] Nitrites are used as preservatives in meats. They also add color to bacon and hot dogs. Nitrites can react with other compounds to form potent carcinogens called nitrosamines.[4] When bacon is cooked, nitrosamines form. There is a low level of nitrites in our saliva and in some vegetables, but there is no information on whether these nitrites can be activated to form nitrosamines. Vitamin C, also found in vegetables, can inhibit the formation of nitrosamines and is usually added to meat cures. Nitrites might be carcinogenic.[5]

Unintentional food additives are those chemicals used to prepare or store the food product; small amounts of these chemicals subsequently, unintentionally, become part of the food. Paraffin wax that lines many food containers, pesticides, and DES are unintentional food additives. Pesticides get into our bodies and are stored in fat cells, since they are fat soluble. These pesticide-laden fat cells can then act as reservoirs to slowly, but constantly, release the pesticide into the bloodstream. DES (diethylstilbestrol) is used to fatten cattle and has been found in trace amounts in dairy products and beef. DES causes cancer of the vagina in young women and cancer of the testicles in men whose mothers had taken DES. Keep in mind that a large amount of DES is needed to cause cancer, and only a small amount is in our food. But small amounts accumulate and do affect us.

Aflatoxin is a food contaminant that causes human liver cancer. Aflatoxin is a product of a fungus, *Aspergillus flavus*, that grows mainly on peanut plants. Other fungal products have been implicated in human cancers. *Gyromita esculenta*, a common mushroom used in cooking, contains a compound called N-methyl-N-formylhydrazine, a potent animal carcinogen.[6]

Certain food processing techniques, such as smoking and charcoal broiling, produce carcinogens.[7] Smoked food increases the risk of gastric cancer. The carcinogens that result from charcoal broiling appear to come from the fat that drips from the meat and is burned, forming the carcinogen, which then rises with the smoke back up into the meat.[8]

As yet, there are no definite proven cases of human cancers directly related to food additives, but many authorities agree that additives and contaminants do account for a small percentage of human cancers. Those chemicals implicated in animal cancers were removed from the market. However, nitrites are bothersome sources of carcinogens and should be avoided. The reduced incidence of gastric cancer in the United States is directly related to less food additives with the advent of refrigeration. Also naturally occurring food components like aflatoxins do cause human cancer and should be eliminated.

PESTICIDES

Pesticides are now in widespread use throughout the world. They control or kill pests or affect plant or animal life. There are about 1,200 pesticide chemical compounds, combined in 30,000 different formulations. Pesticides have made an important contribution to both food production and disease control. Some estimate that at least one-third of the crops in Third World countries are lost to pests.[8]

Pesticides have aided in the control of malaria, schistosomiasis, and filariasis in tropical countries, but there are still hundreds of millions of cases of these diseases each year. There is no way of knowing and no way of calculating how many lives will be saved or improved by the use of pesticides to control diseases and increase our food production. Likewise, there is no way to calculate how many lives will be lost from pesticide use. Some dangerous pesticides that are banned or restricted in North America and Europe have been unloaded on Third World countries.

Pesticides enter your body by inhalation, absorption through the skin, or ingestion. And unlike industrial chemicals, which are used in a very controlled manner, pesticides are sprayed, powdered, or dropped as pellets or granules in and around places where the general public may walk or play. In fact, pesticide residues are commonly found in human tissue in almost everyone in the United States, averaging six parts per million (ppm) in fatty tissue.[9] Pesticide residues have been found in breast milk and cow milk and have been found to cross the placental barrier to the human fetus.[10]

PESTICIDES INCREASE BREAST CANCER RISK

Because pesticides are soluble in oil or fatty tissue like that of the human breast and its milk, pesticides may be a contributing factor to breast cancer.[11] Women are at greater risk than men when exposed to the same amount of pesticides because the Allowable Daily Intake for pesticides as determined by the federal government is calculated on the basis of a 70-kilogram man, not a 50-kilogram woman with larger breast tissue.

Politicians passed the General Agreement on Tariffs and Trade (GATT) in December 1994. The GATT rules allow for substantially higher levels of pesticide residues on U.S. import produce. Specifically, 5000 percent higher levels of DDT than current U.S. standards are permitted on imported peaches, bananas, grapes, strawberries, broccoli, and carrots.

The health of American women is apparently subordinate to political pressure.

Certain pesticides, such as DDT (an insecticide), are animal carcinogens. They get into fatty tissue and are slowly released from the fat. Between 1985 and 1991, blood specimens from over 14,000 women in New York City were analyzed for content of these pesticides in the University Women's Health Study.[12-14] Women who developed breast cancer had higher levels of these two pesticides than women who did not.[15] In another study, the pesticide HCH (betahexachlorocyclohexane) was found in the breast fat of forty-four breast cancer patients and thirty-three patients with benign breast disorders.[16]

Three pesticides that have been shown to cause many types of cancer in animals were found to be 100 times as concentrated in Israeli milk compared to levels demonstrated in United States milk. It was estimated that their concentration was about 800 times greater in breast tissue than in the blood. The pesticides, alpha-BHC, gamma-BHC (lindane), and DDT were banned and a sharp drop in pesticide levels in milk was shown. Breast cancer rates have now dropped according to epidemiological and laboratory findings.[17]

Some pesticides have estrogen-like activity in the human: endosulfan, dieldrin, toxaphene and chlordane. When they are together in various combinations, they have a 150- to 1600-fold greater estrogenic affect than each alone.[18]

The implications of this are enormous. Women are commonly exposed to more than one pesticide and this synergistic action of estrogen activity increases the risk for breast cancer. The link of pesticides to breast cancer is not direct, but these findings are enough to dictate the reduction in pesticide use from a public health standpoint.

PESTICIDES INCREASE RISK FOR OTHER CANCERS

Table 10.1 lists pesticides and their roles as human carcinogens.[19-22] Pesticides are associated with, but not necessarily the direct cause of, the following human cancers:[9,23-34]

- Breast
- Brain
- Esophagus
- Leukemia
- Liver
- Lung
- Lymphoma
- Melanoma
- Multiple Myeloma
- Nasal
- Ovarian
- Prostate
- Sarcoma
- Skin
- Stomach

PESTICIDES INCREASES RISK FOR OTHER MEDICAL CONDITIONS like: Parkinson's disease,[35,36] hypertension, cardiovascular disease, abnormal blood cholesterol, allergies, liver disease, skin diseases, fertility problems as manifested by changes in the egg and sperm, and changes in the RNA and DNA.

Table 10.1 Pesticides as Human Carcinogens [19-22]

Pesticide	Definite	Probable	Possible
Aldrin and dieldrin			•
Amitrole		•	
Arsenicals	•		
Atrazine		•	
Benzal chloride			•
Benzotrichloride		•	
Benzoyl chloride			•
Benzyl chloride			•
Carbon tetrachloride	•		
Chlordane			•
Chlorophenols		•	
p-Dichlorobenzene		•	
DDT		•	
Ethylene dibromide		•	
Ethylene oxide		•	
Formaldehyde		•	
Heptachlor			•
Lindane			•
4-chloro-2-methyl acetic			•
Methyl parathion			•
Pentachlorophenol			•
Phenoxy acids			•
Dioxin		•	
2,4,5-Trichlorophenol			•
2,4,6- Trichlorophenol			•
2,4,5-Trichlorophenoxy acetic			•
Vinyl chloride		•	

Endometriosis, affecting over 5 million women in the United States, is a disease whereby tissue from the uterus travels to the abdomen, ovaries, bowels, and bladder, and causes bleeding, infertility, extreme pain, and other problems. Although specific causes of this disorder are not definite, dioxin has recently been implicated. Researchers have found that dioxin can cause endometriosis in female rhesus monkeys.

Dioxin, also known as Agent Orange, and one of its associated contaminants, TCDD, was used during the Vietnam war. Hundreds of thousands of people were exposed to these agents, and Vietnam veterans and others raised serious allegations that Agent Orange and TCDD caused malignant tumors,[23-34] sterility, spontaneous abortions, birth defects, disfiguring skin diseases, and other illnesses. Most of these studies involved a short period of time between exposure and disease. It now appears that the longer the time from exposure to TCDD, the higher the risk for the development of cancer and the higher the incidence of cancer.[37-39]

MINIMIZING PESTICIDE USE

Nature provides us with biological controls, that is, natural predators that can control insects. For example, ladybugs can fight off aphid predators. Beetles controlled weeds in the western United States in the 1950s, and parasites controlled the citrus fly in Barbados in the 1960s. Wasps have been controlled by parasites in greenhouses more effectively than with chemicals. The bacterium, *Bacillus thuringiensis,* is a good alternative to several toxic insecticides. Silicon and soap can be used in gardens as a nontoxic insecticide rather than the other commonly used pesticides for the garden. Minimize the number of pests by providing food and habitat for the pest's natural enemies.

Certain farming practices may be employed as well. Crop residues may be removed by plowing or flooding. Pest deterrents, crop rotation, proper drainage methods, and physical controls like traps or blocking of insects and/or other pests can be used.

WHAT CAN BE DONE

The number of tons of pesticides has increased thirty-three times since 1940, and their toxicity has grown tenfold. However, crop losses to microorganisms, insects, and weeds have gone up 35 percent. There are a number of reasons for this. As new pesticides are developed, insects develop resistance to them. But even more importantly, the government supports prices of various crops, which encourages farmers to produce only a single crop instead of rotating crops to inhibit the pests. By using crop rotation and biological pest control, pesticide use could be cut in half. Food prices would rise by one percent – about $1 billion a year – but the benefits would be enormous. The United States would save billion of dollars per year as a result of decreased cancers and other medical diseases, decreased damage to fish and water supplies, decreased costs of regulating pesticides, and decreased health-care costs for the 20,000 people poisoned each year from pesticides.

While chemical pesticides certainly benefit populations by increasing food production and decreasing certain diseases, it is important to use them only when they must be used and to use the pesticides that cause the least toxicity to human beings and the least damage to the environment around us.

You should learn as much as you can about any pesticides you do use. Acquiring such information is not easy but neither is maintaining good health. Acquire information and use alternatives to the current pesticides. Exposure to pesticides can be controlled. This is yet another risk factor for disease over which you have control.

Ashley is correct to avoid imported fruits and vegetables because foreign countries can use harmful/carcinogenic pesticides that have been banned in the US.

11
Smoking

Nicole L. Simone

Leslie's History
As a young child Leslie inhaled her parents' smoke and then began to smoke 1-2 packs of cigarettes each day starting at age 17. She tried quitting several times but still is smoking at age 39. Is she at risk for breast cancer and other medical diseases?

Smoking is a major health hazard. In 1995 the Brown and Williamson documents revealed that the tobacco industry knew of the harm brought on by its products.[1] About 10% of the world's deaths are related to tobacco use.[2]

The World Health Organization indicates that the annual number of premature deaths caused by tobacco will rise to 10 million by the year 2025. Over half a billion people today, including 200 million currently under the age of 20, will die from tobacco-induced disease, and half of these will be in middle age.[3] Worldwide, 1.1 billion people smoke and 330 million of them live in China. [4,5]

The WHO Conference said that the tobacco companies have targeted expansion in Third World countries, and women and girls, and young boys in the US. Smoking among children has increased dramatically. Since 1968, the number of girls between the ages of 12 and 14 who smoke has increased eightfold. Six million children between the ages of 13 and 19 are regular smokers, and over 140,000 children under 13 are regular smokers. Smoking among blacks exceeds that among whites.

More deaths and physical suffering are related to cigarette smoking than to any other single cause: over 228,700 deaths (and rising) each year from cancer, over 325,000 deaths from cardiovascular disease, and more than 50,000 deaths from chronic lung diseases. Compare these figures with the number of Americans who died in the following wars – Table 11.1. Over a ten-year period (1964-1974), research by the cigarette industry confirmed the fatal dangers of smoking cigarettes.[6]

Table 11.1 US Deaths: Wars vs. Smoking

World War I	116,708
World War II	407,316
Korean War	54,246
Vietnam War	58,151
Smoking Annually	603,700
Involuntary smoking annually	55,000

The cost of smoking-related diseases is staggering. Over $100 billion dollars a year are spent on tobacco related diseases and disability. Over $900 million are spent on prescription smoking cessation products, and close to $800 million are spent on over-the-counter smoking cessation products.[7] A great deal of this cost is paid by nonsmokers as well as smokers through ever-increasing health insurance premiums, disability payments, and other programs. Nonsmokers should not have to pay one penny for self-induced smokers' diseases.

The longer a person smokes, the greater the risk of dying. A person who smokes two packs a day has a death rate two times higher than a nonsmoker. If a smoker stops smoking, the mortality rate decreases progressively as the number of nonsmoking years increases. Those who have stopped for fifteen years have mortality rates similar to those who never smoked, with the exception of smokers who stopped after the age of 65. Cigar and pipe smokers also have an increased risk of death.

SMOKING INCREASES BREAST CANCER RISK

- Women who smoke have a higher risk for developing breast cancer,[8-18] while only a few studies show no association.[19-21]

SMOKING INCREASES LUNG CANCER RISK

- **Cigarette smoking.** The risk is increased by the amount of smoking, duration of smoking, age at which smoking starts, and content of tar and nicotine. Deaths are rising from lung cancer making it the leading cause of women's cancer deaths.
- **Marijuana smoking** also increases risk (National Academy of Sciences, "Marijuana and Health"). Marijuana smoke has 50% more carcinogenic hydrocarbons than cigarette smoke.
- **Breast Radiation Therapy + Smoking ⇒ Lung Cancer**. After about 10 years, women with breast cancer who smoked at the time they received breast radiation therapy have a 75% higher risk for developing lung cancer on the same side as the breast that was treated.[22] The overall risk for developing lung cancer in a woman who smokes and gets radiation therapy is about thirty times that of a woman with breast cancer who doesn't smoke, and over seventy-five times for the same side lung as the treated breast. If this high-risk woman is not willing to stop smoking, then maybe she should have a mastectomy instead of radiation.

TOBACCO-RELATED CANCERS AND PRE-CANCERS

- Cervix [23]
- Cervix dysplasia, a pre-cancer [24]
- Colon polyp (adenomatous, precancer) – 2.7 higher risk [25-29]
- Esophagus
- Larynx
- Kidney
- Mouth
- Nasopharnyx
- Pancreas
- Urinary Bladder

Alcohol and asbestos intensify the harmful effects of tobacco smoking. Chewing tobacco or snuff dipping in non-smokers causes a fourfold increase of oral cancers and a sixfold increase in those who smoked tobacco and drink alcohol heavily.[30] Furthermore, countries such as India, Ceylon, China, and the Soviet Union have the highest rates of death from oral cancer because the people there combine snuff and/or chewing tobacco with other ingredients such as betel nut. A chemical in the betel nut (N'nitrosonornicotine) initiates tumors in animals.

CARCINOGENS IN TOBACCO SMOKE

There are over 2,000 chemical compounds generated by tobacco smoke. The gas phase contains carbon monoxide, carbon dioxide, ammonia, nitrosamines, nitrogen oxides, hydrogen cyanide, sulfurs, nitriles, ketones, alcohols, and acrolein. The tars contain extremely carcinogenic hydrocarbons, which include nitrosamines, benzo(a)pyrenes, anthracenes, acridines, quinolines, benzenes, naphthols, naphthalenes, cresols, and insecticides (DDT), as well as some radioactive compounds like potassium-40 and radium-226. Tobacco smoke, through its many carcinogens, produces harmful free radicals.

OTHER SMOKING-RELATED ILLNESSES

- Cardiovascular illnesses[31-35]
- Osteoporosis[36]
- Emphysema and other lung diseases
- Female infertility, higher risk of miscarriage or spontaneous abortion, more genetic mutations[37-40]

SMOKING IMPAIRS THE IMMUNE SYSTEM

• **SMOKING IMPAIRS IMMUNE SYSTEM ANATOMY** by destroying hair-like structures that line the respiratory tract. These hairs normally beat upward to remove mucous and microorganisms. Without them, bacteria and viruses can grow.

Smoking also causes an increase in macrophages, cells that defend the lung against invading organisms. Macrophages secrete enzymes against the invaders, which also causes emphysema by breaking down of the walls of the respiratory tree.

• **SMOKING IMPAIRS IMMUNE CELLS** - The function of T cells, natural killer cells, macrophages, and antibody levels.[41-43]

INVOLUNTARY INHALATION OF SMOKE causes the death of approximately 53,000 people each year. A nonsmoker who is exposed to tobacco smoke has many adverse reactions and is unjustly and unnecessarily subjected to risk factors detrimental to his or her health.[44] The smoke that comes from the lighted end of a cigarette contains more hazardous chemicals than does the smoke that is inhaled by the smoker. It is virtually impossible to avoid tobacco smoke because it is so prevalent in homes, work places, and public areas.

On March 19, 1984, R.J. Reynolds Tobacco Company asserted in the *Wall Street Journal* entitled Smoking in Public: Let's Separate Fact From Fiction, that: "But, in fact, there is little evidence and certainly nothing which proves scientifically that cigarette smoke causes disease in nonsmokers." Then came the Surgeon General's report in 1986 proclaiming for the first time that involuntary inhalation of cigarette smoke by nonsmokers causes disease, most notably lung cancer.[45,46] The National Academy of Sciences reported similar findings.[47]

A movement to stop all smoking in public areas began with the ban of smoking on all domestic flights in the United States since early 1990. Forty-two states have legislated smoking restrictions in public transportation, hospitals, elevators, indoor areas, cultural or recreational facilities, schools, and libraries.

• **BREAST CANCER RISK IS INCREASED.** Involuntary inhaled smoke increases breast cancer risk.[48-56]

• **LUNG CANCER RISK IS INCREASED.**[57,58] Nonsmokers married to smokers have a 1.34 times greater risk for lung cancer than do those married to nonsmokers. This is one hundred times higher than the person exposed to asbestos for twenty years.

About 17 percent of lung cancers in nonsmokers are a result of exposure to tobacco smoke during childhood and adolescence.[49] Innocent children are at tremendous risk for lung cancer because they inhale their parent's smoke.

Smoking during pregnancy increases by 50 percent the fetus's risk of developing cancer later in childhood.[59] Infants exposed to smoke through breast milk have a higher risk of sudden infant death syndrome [SIDS].[60]

• **CERVICAL CANCER RISK IS INCREASED BY THREE-FOLD** for those who inhale smoke involuntarily for three or more hours daily.[61]

• **BLADDER CANCER RISK IS INCREASED** for nonsmokers who inhale other people's smoke.[62]

STOP SMOKING. More than 95 percent of former smokers quit on their own, usually at the recommendation of their physician. Seek help to quit smoking.

- Smoking cessation for 10 years lowers the risk of heart disease, and for 15 years lowers the risk of cancer to the same rates as a nonsmoker of that age.
- Smokers who have existing heart disease can reduce their risk of future heart attacks and death if they quit smoking, even if they are 65 or older.[63,64]
- Weight gain may occur for only a small percentage of those who stop smoking.[65] To guard against possible weight gain, follow the Ten-Point Plan in Chapter 27.

CURRENT PUBLIC POLICIES

Federally sponsored programs support tobacco prices, benefiting allotment holders (a unique monopoly situation) and tobacco growers. In addition, other federally sponsored programs benefit the tobacco industry. On the other hand, federal funds are spent to discourage smoking, to research the health effects of smoking, and to provide a great portion of the cost of medical care for people who are suffering from and dying of smoking-related diseases. Patients with *self-induced* smoking-related diseases and their families receive Social Security benefits.

The American Medical Association's official policy since 1986 has stated that it: (1) Opposes any efforts by the government or its agencies to actively encourage, persuade, or compel any country to import tobacco products; and (2) Favors legislation that would prevent the government from actively supporting, promoting, or assisting such activities. However, the AMA's Political Action Committee has been giving money to United States representatives who actively oppose the AMA's official policy and who are responsible for getting tobacco into foreign markets.[66]

TIME FOR NEW PUBLIC POLICIES

Tobacco smoke is a threat to all of our lives. It is time now to prohibit smoking in all public areas and work places.

Nonsmokers incur higher risk from involuntarily inhaling others' smoke but also have to pay higher health insurance premiums for diseases related to smoking (cancer, cardiovascular diseases, lung diseases, etc.). Moreover, nonsmokers subsidize the tobacco industry through their tax dollars. We should pressure our senators and congressmen to force the American government to stop subsidizing the tobacco industry.

The United States has adopted uncompromisingly restrictive measures concerning food additives, but only a verbal statement of caution is required on every package of cigarettes. The Delaney Clause legislation prohibits the sale of any product to the American people that has been shown to be carcinogenic to humans and animals, and thus applies to situations in which the human hazard may be minimal. Tobacco is a major risk factor for cancer, cardiovascular diseases, lung diseases, and others.

CONCLUSION

If you smoke, stop. If you have not started, don't! Seek professional help if you must, but stop smoking!

Leslie stopped smoking after we reviewed the scientific data. She knows she can lower her risk for diseases by following our Ten Point Plan. She's won her battle.

12

Alcohol and Caffeine

Holly's History

Holly drinks a glass of wine every night for dinner – sometimes two on the weekend. She likes how it tastes and how it relaxes her. However, her recent mammogram has a new abnormality.

About 100 million Americans drink alcohol, and over 28 million – 1 of every 8 Americans – are children of alcoholics. Alcohol-related costs are about $120 billion every year. Many more billions of dollars are added to this figure when you consider that alcohol is involved in 50 percent of all traffic fatalities, 30 percent of small-aircraft accidents, and 66 percent of all violent crimes. The totals are higher still when you consider the losses due to diseases aggravated by alcohol use, and losses due to alcohol-induced poor decision-making in government, industry, education, law, the military, and medicine. About 68 percent of adult Americans abuse alcohol. Alcohol-related hospitalizations among the elderly are common. All of society pays for this. Employers lose productivity, taxpayers pay the bill for programs and services, and consumers pay higher insurance premiums.

Alcohol is a risk factor for cancers of the breast, prostate, mouth, pharynx, larynx, esophagus, pancreas, liver, and head and neck. Alcohol acts synergistically with tobacco smoking in the development of other gastrointestinal cancers and urinary bladder cancer. Alcohol causes cirrhosis of the liver, the seventh leading cause of death in the US. Fifty percent of alcoholics die from cardiovascular diseases and 20 percent from accidents, suicides, and homicides.

ALCOHOL CAUSES NUTRITIONAL DEFICIENCIES

Alcoholics will consume about 20 percent of their total calories as alcohol and therefore vitamin deficiencies are common in alcoholics. Thiamine (vitamin B1) deficiency causes a severe brain disease called Wernicke-Korsakoff syndrome that can be rapidly reversed by the administration of thiamine. Folic acid and vitamin B12 deficiencies cause anemias. Pyridoxine (B6) deficiency causes peripheral nerve problems. Alcoholics have a deficiency of vitamin C because of their liver disease. Mineral deficiencies include calcium, zinc, magnesium, and iron. Some alcoholics develop the Plummer-Vinson syndrome, that is characterized by a cluster of symptoms including difficulty swallowing; a red, smooth tongue; and iron deficiency anemia. People with this syndrome have a high rate of cancer of the mouth.

ALCOHOL SUPPRESSES IMMUNITY

- Decreases the number and function of neutrophils, lymphocytes, monocytes, and natural killer cells.
- Decreases the rate of antibody production.
- Decreases the complement protein defense system.
- Increases risk for cancer, tuberculosis, viral infections.

ALCOHOL INCREASES BREAST CANCER RISK BY 200%-300%.[1-12] Women, especially younger women, who consume two to four alcoholic drinks per week, *not per day*, have a two to three times higher risk for developing breast cancer independently of other breast cancer risk factors. Twelve ounces of beer equals four ounces of wine, which equals one and a half ounces of whiskey in alcohol content. Drinking this amount will increase your risk because alcohol is immunosuppressive, carcinogenic, and, can triple your estrogen levels (also carcinogenic) for at least 5 hours after drinking.[12]

ALCOHOL INCREASES SPREAD OF BREAST CANCER. Alcohol may actually speed up an existing cancer, especially breast cancer.[13] Animals were injected with a breast cancer that always spreads to the lungs. At the time of injection, the animals were allowed to get drunk. Those with a blood alcohol content of 0.15 percent, which represents about four to five drinks an hour, later developed more than twice the number of new lung metastases compared to the animals that did not drink alcohol. Those with a blood level of 0.25 percent had eight times more tumors in their lungs.

These same levels of alcohol are seen in humans who drink excessively in one hour. Women with breast cancer who drink this amount are probably at an increased risk for developing metastatic disease.

ALCOHOL INCREASES RISK FOR OTHER CANCERS, AND OTHER DISEASES

- Mouth, pharynx, and esophagus cancers – alcohol is a topical carcinogen. People who use mouthwash that contains alcohol have a high rate of oral cancer. Alcohol and tobacco account for 75 percent of all oral cancers in the United States.
- Alcoholic liver cirrhosis increases the risk for liver cancer, varicose veins in the esophagus, ascites (fluid in the abdomen); muscle wasting; kidney failure, pancreas and heart abnormalities, and stroke.[14,15]
- Premature testicle and ovary shrinkage.
- Peptic ulcers.
- Adult brain shrinkage that may normalize after abstinence.[16]
- "Fetal alcohol syndrome" – defects in the brain, in intellectual development, physical growth, and in the facial features of infants born of alcoholic mothers.

CAFFEINE

Caffeine is the most popular drug in North America and in many other parts of the world. It is found in coffee, tea, cola beverages, and chocolate. Caffeine is linked to:

- Breast Cancer [17,18]
- Urinary Bladder cancer[19] – more than three cups per day.
- Miscarriage and Infant Prematurity – one cup per day[20-22]
- Low Infant Birth Rate.
- DNA damage – increases cancer, fetal malformations[23,24]

- Heart Disease risk – more than 5 cups per day [25]
- Osteoporosis [26]

Caffeine Concentrations in Milligrams			
COFFEE (12 oz)		**SOFT DRINKS (12 oz)**	
Brewed (drip method)	275	Cherry Cola	36-46
Brewed (percolator)	190	Diet Cherry Cola	36-45
Instant	155	Cola (all), Dr Pepper	30-46
Brewed, Decaffeinated	7	Diet Colas & Dr Pepper	38-45
Instant, Decaffeinated	5	Lemon-lime, Orange	0
TEA (12 oz)		Root Beer and diet	0
Brewed (imported)	145	Ginger Ale & diet, Tonic	0
Brewed (domestic)	95		
Iced Tea	70	**OVER-THE-COUNTER MEDS**	
CHOCOLATE		Vivarin	200
Baker's chocolate (1.5 oz)	39	No-Doz	100
Dark or semisweet (1.5 oz)	30	Excedrin	65
Hot cocoa (12 oz)	10	Vanquish	33
Milk chocolate (1.5 oz)	9	Midol	32
Chocolate Milk (12 oz)	7		

CONCLUSION

Alcohol and caffeine are two important risk factors for cancer. The decision to consume them is *yours*. You can again decide about the status of your health!

Holly's mammogram abnormality was found to be a cancer. She stopped drinking and modified her lifestyle according to the Ten Point Plan. She knows her life will be extended.

13

Hormonal and Sexual-Social Factors

Lisa's History

Lisa is 51. She start menstruating at age 11, had an abortion at age 17, and then began using oral contraceptives for 12 years starting at age 18. She never had children and just started using hormone replacement therapy 2 years ago. What's her risk?

Hormonal factors and sexual-social behavior are directly related to the development of cancer. The risk for certain cancers is increased because more hormones are used and there is a relaxation of sexual mores that increases promiscuity.

SEX HORMONES AND IMMUNE SYSTEM REGULATE EACH OTHER

• Women have higher levels of antibodies, greater response of antibodies, and a higher incidence of autoimmune diseases.

CRITICAL TIMES OF HORMONE INFLUENCE

• **Birth to 4 years, Puberty, and End of Puberty to First Full-Term Pregnancy** are times when hormones influence a female the most because: (1) Cells rapidly divide, (2) Breast tissue has more stem cells that are more susceptible to carcinogens, and (3) Mutations can be passed along.

• **After First Full-Term Pregnancy** there are: (1) Less cell division, (2) Fewer stem cells, (3) More mature cells, (4) Mature cells can repair DNA more efficiently, (5) Mature cells do not bind carcinogens as easily as stem cells.

CHILD BEARING YEARS ARE PROTECTED [1]

Between ages 11 and 19, the rates for developing certain types of cancer (epithelial types) are about 50 percent lower for females compared to males. Before age 11 or after age 19, *female sex hormones do not have a protective effect.* It may be that female sex hormones prevent the establishment of distant metastases in certain cancers. Mother Nature seems to be very protective of this child-bearing age group.

NATURAL HORMONAL INFLUENCE FOR CANCER

■ **MENSTRUAL HISTORY.** The longer the body is bathed with estrogens, the higher is the risk of developing breast cancer.

- Early start of menstruation – risk increases by 4% for every year a woman menstruates before age 17; [2] American women start at about age 11 now, but 200 years ago, it was age 17.[3] A high-fat, low-fiber diet causes the brain to release a hormone called prolactin that initiates menstruation.[4]
- Late menopause – risk increases by 4% for every year a woman menstruates after age 48.
- No pregnancies or never menstruated – threefold higher risk
- Pregnant after age 35 - threefold higher risk
- Breast cancer risk is lowered by breast feeding and having multiple pregnancies (about 5) regardless at what age – the body is not bathed with estrogen during these times.[5-7]

■ **FIRST PREGNANCY TERMINATED INCREASES BREAST CANCER RISK.** A woman who has an abortion in the first trimester of her first pregnancy, whether it was spontaneous or induced, is two and one-half times more likely to develop breast cancer.[8-19]

When conception occurs, hormonal changes induce milk duct networks to grow quickly to ultimately produce milk. During this period of tremendous growth, breast cells undergo great change and are immature ("undifferentiated") making them more susceptible to carcinogens. But when a first full-term pregnancy is completed, hormonal changes occur that permanently alter the breast network to greatly reduce the risk of outside carcinogen influence. When a termination occurs in the first trimester, there are no protective effects, and many of the rapidly dividing cells of the breast are left in transitional states.[20,21] It is in these transitional states of high proliferation and undifferentiation that these cells can undergo transformation to cancer cells.

■ **PREBIRTH EXPOSURE TO ESTROGEN INCREASES BREAST CANCER RISK** [22-26] because a daughter's mammary glands *in utero* are very sensitive to estrogen that is ten times higher *in utero* than in the adult state.[27] Symptoms related to high estrogen levels in pregnant mothers include: severe nausea, obesity, or sometimes high birthweight.

■ **BREAST-FEEDING (LACTATION) REDUCES BREAST CANCER RISK** [28-35] because it interrupts ovulation and thereby reduces the overall time that estrogen bathes the body.[36,37] Breast cancer risk is reduced by 11 percent for those who breast feed for 4 to 12 months, by 25 percent if they breast feed for 24 months or more. The younger a woman is when she breast feeds, the lower the breast cancer risk.

Women who consistently use only one breast to breast-feed have a higher risk of developing breast cancer in the unsuckled breast in postmenopausal years.[38] The Tanka people who live in boats in China breast-feed with only the right breast, probably for convenience, with the opening of the clothing on the right side. Their left breasts are smaller and softer. However, non-Tanka Chinese women who live on land and have the same style of clothing with the opening on the right, use both breasts to breast-feed. Postmenopausal Tanka women have a much higher rate of left-breast cancers than non-Tanka women. This study demonstrates that it is important to breast-feed using both breasts to confer protection to each breast.

■ **PREGNANCY DOES NOT INCREASE RISK FOR BREAST CANCER OR SPREAD EXISTING ONE** [39-44] There are not many situations in medicine that arouse the anxiety of the physician and patient as much as the discovery of cancer in the pregnant woman. Cancer during pregnancy is not uncommon. About 1 of every 1,000 pregnancies involves cancer, and about 1 of every 118 women who are found to have cancer will be pregnant at the time. The cancers most often seen in pregnant women in order of prevalence are: breast, cervix, ovarian, lymphoma, and colorectal.

Cancer and pregnancy are the only two biological conditions in which cells foreign to the mother, that is, the cancer cells and those that make up the fetus – foreign because half of the genetic make-up of the fetus is from the father – are tolerated by what appears to be a relatively normal immune system. These conditions are permitted because some aspects of the immune system are not working to peak capacity. Hormones like estrogen, progesterone, alpha fetal protein, and human chorionic gonadotropin all have an immunosuppressive effect on the mother's immune system, without which the fetus would not grow. Other changes that occur during pregnancy are depression of the cellular killers, enhancement of certain blocking antibodies, and alteration of other factors of the immune system. The hormonal mechanisms that ensure the survival of the fetus and consequently suppress the immune system are the same mechanisms that also favor a cancer.

However, pregnancy, per se, is not a risk factor for the development of cancer nor is it likely that it will cause existing cancer to spread.

Only one study from Sweden suggests a slight and transient risk for the development of breast cancer in a woman who has just given birth.[45] Poor results seen in the treatment of cancer in pregnant women have largely been due to late diagnosis or inadequate treatment.[46] Signs of cancer can often be mistakenly attributed to changes due to pregnancy or lactation and sometimes the diagnosis is delayed. If you discover you have a cancer during pregnancy, treatment should be instituted by delivering the fetus if it is viable.

Should you become pregnant after having been diagnosed with breast cancer? Pregnancy is not associated with excessive risk of cancer recurrence; hence, there is little evidence for advising against subsequent pregnancy for women who want to become pregnant and are free of any recurrences at the time. However, given the fact that most cancer recurrences appear within the first two years, it is prudent to advise a woman not to become pregnant until she has been free of cancer for at least two years. If a woman becomes pregnant before two years, the decision for a therapeutic abortion should be based on the patient's treatment program and other factors.

Most of the time, an abortion is recommended based on feelings or religious beliefs. However, clear scientific evidence runs counter to what has been taught, handed down, or otherwise believed. The data for this section involve well over 500 references and have been reviewed several times.

■ **BENIGN BREAST DISEASE** has been thoroughly reviewed in Chapter 2. A low-fat, high fiber diet with certain supplemental vitamins and minerals, together with the avoidance of caffeine, and nicotine inhalation can decrease the severity of breast tenderness and swelling after six months and breast swelling and nodularity are reduced in 60 percent of the patients.[47]

Since 1979, I have treated women with benign breast disorders, specifically lumpy breast disease. All the patients followed my Ten-Point Plan as presented in Chapter 2. Almost 90 percent of the patients had decreased breast pain premenstrually, and about half of the patients experienced a decrease in the size of their cysts. In most cases the size of the breast diminished somewhat; however, in about 10 percent of the women, the size of the breast increased slightly.

■ **PROLACTIN INCREASES BREAST CANCER RISK**[48] Prolactin is a hormone secreted by the pituitary gland during pregnancy and breast-feeding. But an early first pregnancy decreases for about 12 years the normal secretion of prolactin that subsequently decreases the risk of breast cancer.[49] However, a two-fold increase of prolactin in the non-pregnant state increases the risk for breast cancer.

ADMINISTERED HORMONES INCREASE RISK

■ **DES INCREASES RISK FOR CANCERS OF THE BREAST, VAGINA, CERVIX, AND TESTICLE.**[50-55] DES (diethylstilbestrol) was used to avert miscarriages in the 1940s and 1950s.

- Increases risk for vaginal and cervical cancer and dysplasia in women who were exposed to DES as fetuses.
- Increases risk for breast cancer for women who took it.
- Sons of DES-exposed mothers have reproductive and urinary tract abnormalities. One of these is undescended testicles, which may lead to cancer of the testes if uncorrected before the age of 6.
- Breast enlargement in children who ate meat that had DES.[56]

For women who were exposed to DES:

1. Tell your daughter or son.
2. Try to obtain the details of your DES dosage and duration.
3. Have Pap smear, breast exam by a physician, mammogram.
4. Practice breast self-exam and report anything.
5. Report any unusual bleeding or discharge from the vagina.
6. Avoid oral contraceptives, hormone replacement, etc.

For daughters of DES-exposed mothers:

1. Report unusual bleeding or discharge from the vagina.
2. Annual Pap smear at age 14 or when you begin menses.

For sons of DES-exposed mothers:

1. Have physician check reproductive and urinary systems to make certain there are no abnormalities.

■ Oral Contraceptives Increase Risk for Cancers of the Breast, Cervix, and Liver

The Collaborative Group on Hormonal Factors in Breast Cancer has analyzed the worldwide epidemiological evidence involving 54 studies with over 150,000 women and concludes that oral contraceptives increase the risk for breast cancer.[57] Other reviews show the same finding.[58-66] Women who use oral contraceptives before age 25 for four years or more, have a two-fold higher risk for developing breast cancer.[66-68] The risk for women younger than 36 is increased by 74 percent with long-term use – 8 or more years – and 43 percent with moderate term use – 4 to 8 years.[69] Oral contraceptive use accounted for 20 percent of all breast cancers among the women studied.

The incidence of cervical cancer increases from the second through eighth years of using oral contraceptives. In addition, oral contraceptive users have a higher incidence of carcinoma *in situ* and premalignant conditions like dysplasia.[70] Oral contraceptives have also been linked to primary liver cancer.[71]

The U.S. Food and Drug Administration inserts a warning in all oral contraceptive packages: Oral contraceptive use is associated with breast cancer, cardiovascular disease (heart attack, stroke), pulmonary embolus, and other illnesses.

■ PROGESTERONE INCREASES RISK

Injection of medroxyprogesterone as a contraceptive has been shown to increase the risk of developing breast cancer, cervical cancer, uterine cancer, and ovarian cancer in women.[72,73]

■ HORMONE REPLACEMENT THERAPY INCREASES RISK FOR CANCERS OF THE BREAST, ENDOMETRIUM, OVARY

Women who use hormone replacement therapy for 5 years or more have a two-fold higher risk for developing breast cancer,[74-81] an increased risk of endometrial (uterus lining),[82,83] and also ovarian cancer.[84] Estrogens administered in large amounts increased the rate of breast cancer in male transsexuals[85,86] as well as in male heart and ulcer patients.

Hormone replacement therapy is ***believed*** to:

- Protect the heart – **It does not, in fact, it increases risk** as per the American Heart Assoication.[87-89]
- Protect against stroke – **It does not.**[87]
- Decrease menopausal symptoms – **It does not.**[90,91]
- Preserve cognitive function – **It does not.**[92-94]
- Decrease risk for Alzheimer's – **It does not.**[95]
- Decrease risk for osteoporosis – **It does not**, age>60.[96]

■ ESTROGEN REPLACEMENT IS NOT RECOMMENDED FOR PATIENTS WITH PRIOR BREAST CANCER [97]

■ THYROID SUPPLEMENTS DO NOT INCREASE THE RISK OF BREAST CANCER. [98]

■ **ANDROGENS INCREASE RISK FOR CANCER AND HEART DISEASE.** Athletes use androgens to increase muscle bulk and performance. Androgens cause cardiovascular illnesses, prostate cancer, liver cancer, and osteosarcoma, as well as benign liver disease.

SEXUAL-SOCIAL FACTORS

■ **CERVICAL CANCER** is higher in women who: (1) Start having sexual intercourse before age 16 with multiple male partners, particularly those who are uncircumcised, or whose husbands were married to women with cervix cancer, or who are infected with the Papilloma virus; (2) Use oral contraceptives; (3) Smoke or inhale tobacco smoke for three hours/day – increases risk by a factor of three.

■ **AIDS INCREASES RISK FOR CANCERS OF THE ANUS, TONGUE, AND KAPOSI'S SARCOMA**

CONCLUSION

All the studies reviewed suggest a consistent theme: If a woman tampers with Mother Nature's hormonal milieu by taking hormone pills, by disrupting reproduction, or by not reproducing at all, she has a higher risk of developing certain cancers, especially breast cancer.

Lisa knows her risk for developing cancer is very high based on her hormonal and sexual-social factors alone. She is now making every effort to modify her lifestyle to decrease her risks.

14
Air and Water

Claire's History

Claire is 41 with four children. They use special filters on their vents. She feeds them well and keeps her house clean, and all chemicals locked up. They drink distilled water.

Mounting evidence suggests that our environment contains many carcinogens. The air we breathe, the water we drink, the radiation to which we are exposed, and the power lines that supply us with energy pose threats to our health. As with many carcinogens, the time between exposure to environmental carcinogens and actual development of cancer may be quite long. Therefore, the cause of a cancer initiated by trace amounts of either airborne or waterborne carcinogens years before may be attributed to an unrelated or unknown factor at the time of diagnosis. This is why we must constantly clean our environment of carcinogens.

OUTDOOR AIR POLLUTION costs $50 billion a year.

- Cancer rate is increased in cities due to: (1) more cigarette smoking; (2) more involuntary inhalation of tobacco smoke (3) occupational exposures.[1-3]
- Workers exposed to air pollutants have an increased risk for lung cancer – gas production workers (coal carbonization); steel workers at coke ovens; and roofers exposed to hot pitch
- City air pollution has more than 100 particulate carcinogens that come from the burning of any material containing carbon and hydrogen, including petroleum, gasoline, and diesel

fuel.[4] Many studies indicated that tiny particulate air pollution in cities is linked to higher mortality rates.[5-7]

- Gas phase of the air also has carcinogens: benzene, carbon tetrachloride, chloroform, and vinyl chloride, among others. [8] These carcinogens are derived from car emissions, industrial activity, burning of solid waste, forest fires, and evaporation of solvents.[9]
- Asbestos is a potent carcinogen for lung cancer and is found in roofing and flooring, car brakes and clutches, dry walls, home heating and plumbing. Family members of persons who work with asbestos or asbestos products are exposed to very high levels of asbestos also. Cigarette smoking acts synergistically with asbestos to greatly enhance the risk of lung cancer. It is *extremely* rare for lung cancer to develop in an asbestos worker in the absence of exposure to tobacco smoke.
- Diesel exhaust increases risk of lung cancer for workers exposed to diesel engine emissions.[10]

ACID RAIN is made when sulfur dioxide and nitrogen oxide are released into the atmosphere and converted into sulfuric acid and nitric acid from fossil fuel combustion and power plant emissions.

- Affects soil: releases toxic metals – aluminum, mercury, lead, nickel, cadmium, and manganese that get into the water supply adversely affecting aquatic life in 10% of Eastern lakes and streams. Reduces selenium content in soil.
- Decreases the number of red spruce at high elevations, and contributes to the corrosion of buildings and materials.
- To control acid rain – use fossil fuel with low sulfur content.

DEPLETION OF NATURAL UPPER ATMOSPHERIC OZONE INCREASES RISK FOR SKIN CANCER

The naturally occurring ozone layer in the upper atmosphere is crucial to the protection of living organisms because it absorbs harmful ultraviolet radiation. About 3 percent of the sun's electromagnetic output is emitted as ultraviolet radiation, but only a fraction of this reaches the surface of the Earth.

• Ultraviolet exposure is associated with melanoma, basal cell, and squamous cell cancer of the skin. People with fair skin, blond hair, and blue eyes who also sunburn easily are at highest risk for the development of these skin cancers. The US Environmental Protection Agency calculates that a 1 percent decrease in the ozone concentration will increase the incidence of most skin cancers by 3-5 percent.

• Ultraviolet exposure causes skin damage and skin aging

• Phytoplankton, zooplankton, and the larval stages of fish, are very sensitive to small increases in ultraviolet exposure. The resultant decrease in the food chain and in the oxygen output from the oceans' plants will have serious and dramatic repercussions on all human life.

Addressing the Problem

Chlorofluorocarbons, commonly known as CFCs, are chemical compounds that cause holes in the protective ozone layer. CFCs are in aerosols, foam blowers for items such as hamburger cartons and drinking cups, refrigerants and cooling systems, and solvents for computer circuits. In most instances, nonchlorinated substitutes are available or can be developed. Some CFCs remain in the air for over a century. For every 2.5 percent increase per year of chlorofluorocarbon, an additional million skin cancers and 20,000 deaths will occur over the lifetime of the existing United States population.

If pentane is used instead of chlorofluorocarbons as the blowing agent to produce foam products, *ozone is produced* both in the stratosphere and at the ground level. These products are less costly than paper products. A paper cup costs more to make: raw materials (wood, bark, petroleum fractions), finished weight, wholesale price, utilities needed to produce it (steam, power, cooling water), waste products produced, and air emissions (chlorine, chlorine dioxide, reduced sulfides).[11] The polystyrene cup is easier to recycle and ultimately to dispose. Here again, we have the proper technology to solve this problem.

OZONE AT GROUND LEVEL CAUSES DISEASES

• Ozone at ground level is harmful to us whereas the naturally occurring protective ozone layer in the upper atmosphere shields us from harmful ultraviolet rays. Ozone at ground level is the most widespread air pollutant in any industrialized country and is formed when car exhaust and other industrial emissions react with sunlight.

• Smog is derived predominantly from ozone as well as from carbon monoxides, nitrogen oxides, sulfur oxides, particulates, and volatile organic compounds. These compounds are derived from bakeries during fermentation; dry cleaning chemicals; paints; wood-burning stoves and starter fluid used to ignite charcoal; industries and motor vehicles using fossil fuels.

• Cities with the highest ozone: Los Angeles, New York, Philadelphia, Trenton, Baltimore, Hartford, Chicago, and Houston. Some national parks like Acadia, Shenandoah, and Sequoia national parks have higher ozone levels than some cities because of their proximity to the major cities with smog and/or the air currents around them.

• Ozone at ground level has been linked to cancer, lung and heart disease, impaired immunity, and other illnesses.

• Ozone impairs oxygen absorption.

• Ozone causes lung damage similar to that seen from smoking

• When ozone levels are high, asthmatics, cardiac patients, and older people who have respiratory illnesses do poorly.

ULTRAVIOLET SUNLIGHT has two forms: ultraviolet A (UVA) and ultraviolet B (UVB). The UVB is the more harmful causing sunburn and skin cancer. It has wavelengths between 290 and 320 nanometers. UVA causes skin cancer, skin damage, and premature aging of the skin. UVA has wavelengths between 320 and 400 nanometers, which is where the visible light spectrum begins.

Sunglasses should be used to protect your eyes from the harmful ultraviolet rays of the sun. Regardless of cost, most sunglasses filter all UVB, but not necessarily all UVA.[12]

INDOOR AIR pollution causes illnesses and the "sick building syndrome"symptoms.[13] Ventilation can eliminate this.

• **Radon** is implicated in up to 20,000 deaths from lung cancer in the United States.[14] A person living in a house with an indoor radon level of 4 pica Curies/liter has the same risk of developing lung cancer as a person who smokes half a pack of cigarettes per day.[15] Coal miners who are exposed to radon and also smoke have a higher risk of lung cancer.[16]

• **Involuntary inhalation of tobacco smoke** doubles the lung cancer rate.[17] Seventeen percent of all lung cancers are found in people who never smoked but who inhaled smoke between ages of 3 and 15. There should be no smoking in public places.

• **Stoves** without chimneys and kerosene stoves produce many pollutants, several of which are carcinogenic.

• **Heat exchangers, cooling towers**, and **leaky showerheads** provide favorable culture media for many microorganisms. These bacteria and other organisms disperse in droplets and remain airborne via mechanical or thermal air movements. *Legionella premophilia* (Legionnaires' disease) and many other organisms have been detected airborne in closed indoor situations.

• **Other indoor pollutants** come from materials that are used in the construction of modern buildings, such as formaldehyde (associated with human cancer), isocyanates, solvents, and volatile synthetic organic compounds.

WATER POLLUTION

• **Synthetic organic chemicals** amount to over 700 in our drinking water.[18] Forty of these are carcinogens, and three (benzene, chloromethyl ether, and vinyl chloride) are associated with human cancer.[19] Drinking polluted water is said by the EPA to be one of the top four health hazards in America. The EPA allows municipalities to average their water toxicities over a year. For example, much more chlorine is added to water during summer months to hold down microorganisms. In some cities, the tap water level of chlorine carcinogens exceeds the standard by 20 percent during these months. The same spike of toxicity holds true for nitrates and pesticides, both used seasonally for lawn beautification and farming.

Chlorination produces trihalomethanes – chloroform and bromohalomethane – that double the risk for gastrointestinal and urinary bladder cancers.[19-24] The EPA's safety limit of chlorine and its harmful associated carcinogens is based on the consumption of two liters of water a day, and this does not take into account increased consumption in summer, or the fact that these compounds can be absorbed during bathing.

• **Inorganic chemicals** like arsenic, chromium (certain chemical form), nickel, and lead are toxic. Lead impairs children's IQ and attention span. One in six people in the United States drinks water with higher than acceptable levels of lead.

The amount of calcium and magnesium in water determines water "hardness." It appears that soft water, water containing lesser amounts of calcium and particularly magnesium, is correlated with a higher incidence of all cardiovascular diseases, osteoporosis, hypertension, and breast and colon cancer.

• **Radioactive materials** in water varies with geography, geology, industrial wastes, pharmaceutical use, and nuclear power generation.[25]

• **Living organisms** – bacteria, viruses, and protozoa –can resist water purification, and these are responsible for 33 percent of all gastrointestinal infections in the United States.

• **Solid particulates** include clays, asbestos particles, and organic particulates.

WHO IS TO BLAME FOR THE SHAMBLES OF THE WATER SUPPLY? Probably everyone. Most states do not comply with existing standards, or comply by way of loopholes. For example, a loophole permits water suppliers to flush lead-filled water out of plumbing before testing tap water. The EPA has been lax because it only recently has imposed restrictions for radon in the drinking water.

Eighty percent of the top 1,000 superfund sites, that is, those designated as containing toxic waste and chemical contaminants, are leaching these toxic substances into the ground water. In many geographic sites in the United States, well water has been contaminated. About 10 percent of all underground tanks, which store gasoline or other hazardous chemicals, leak. Too many pesticides and fertilizers are used by farmers and homeowners. Industries dump chemicals and other harmful pollutants into our water supply, and homeowners dump chemicals into household drains.

Addressing the Problem. One of the major obstacles to clean up America's underground toxic wastes is the unrealistic requirement that has been set by government authorities throughout the nation. The problem is that the objectives are simply too difficult to be accomplished by existing technologies. If the requirement had been to reduce the contaminants from 2,000 parts per billion to, say, 10 parts, it would be possible to reduce the health hazard by 99.5 percent and leave limited funds available for twenty or thirty more of the same type of clean-up projects. It is better to clean up all the toxic sites by a significant factor like 99.5 percent than only a few sites by a factor of 99.99 percent and thereby propagate endless litigation.

A number of cities refuse to build costly processing plants and instead choose to pay less expensive fines. The EPA observes that small utilities tend to violate regulations the most, falsify documents, and even wash away evidence because of a thirty-day window given them by the state.

WATER DERIVED FROM DISTILLATION OR REVERSE OSMOSIS IS MORE PURE THAN TAP OR SPRING OR "BOTTLED"

CONCLUSION

There are documented airborne and waterborne carcinogens. It is essential for us to detect and clean our environment of as many carcinogens as possible.

Claire's doing all the right things that now includes the use of sunscreens and sunglasses.

15

Electromagnetic Radiation

Anne's History

Anne is 46 and received radiation to her face to treat acne. She also remembers putting her feet in an X-ray machine to see her feet in her new shoes. She has had 5 mammograms and sleeps with an electric blanket and clock radio near her head.

The electromagnetic radiation spectrum includes gamma rays, X-rays, ultraviolet light, visible light, infrared, microwaves, FM radio waves, AM radio waves, and long radio waves. Electromagnetic radiation with wavelengths longer than the color red (ranging from infrared to radio waves) or shorter than the color violet (ranging from ultraviolet to X-rays and gamma rays) is not visible to the eye. Radiation exposure is another risk factor for developing breast cancer.

DIAGNOSTIC AND THERAPEUTIC RADIATION

Ionizing radiation causes cancer. Mammograms, CT scans, therapeutic radiation, and other radiation exposures increase the risk for developing breast cancer. Increased risk for breast cancer was first seen among women in Japan who were irradiated during the atomic bombings. More women who had exposure during ages 10 to 25 developed breast cancer from the radiation fall-out than women who were younger or women who were older.[1] Women with tuberculosis who had multiple serial chest X-rays to follow the course of the disease also had substantially increased rates of breast cancer.[2]

MAMMOGRAM screening has been promoted as safe. However, the radiation dose from current mammographic two-view examination techniques (1-8 mGy) is extremely damaging to the glandular tissue[3] even though it is less today than before.[4]

The National Academy of Sciences and the National Cancer Institute estimate that for every 100,000 women at age 40 who are screened using mammography, there will be 10 more cancers than are normally seen in that age group due solely to mammograms. The estimate of 10 excess cases is based on the delivery of 1 cGy per mammogram per woman – the amount of radiation delivered by a technically good mammogram unit. However, as more radiation is delivered with older units or poorly calibrated units, this number will be higher based on the higher dose delivered to each patient.

CT SCANS. Almost 85 percent of the radiation to which we are exposed in developed countries is from natural sources, but 15 percent is from human-made sources. Of these, about 97 percent is from diagnostic radiology – mainly CT scans. The dose for a single chest CT scan is the equivalent of 20 mammograms – about 2 to 3 cGy.

Children commonly receive an overdose of radiation when they have CT scans.[5,6] In fact, they receive doses that are at least five times greater than necessary. Radiologists can reduce the dose without compromising image quality but they do not. The number of indications we use CT scans for children has increased dramatically. Japanese children exposed to a single dose of 5 cGy during World War II have a four times greater risk for breast cancer. **So if a child today has two or three CT scans** of the same area – each giving 2 to 3 cGy per CT scan – over the long term, **the risk of cancer is increased significantly**.

THERAPEUTIC RADIATION FOR CANCER TREATMENT. Patients who had radiation therapy for various diseases have a higher incidence of breast cancer if the radiation therapy was delivered to or near the breast, for example, chest radiation therapy to treat Hodgkin's disease.[7] The women who did develop breast cancer secondary to the radiation for Hodgkin's disease were all under the age of 40 and on average had the radiation about ten years prior to the diagnosis of breast cancer.

Four patients, 3 women and 1 man, of 910 survivors of childhood cancer developed breast cancer after having had 300 cGy of chest radiation for the treatment of Wilms' tumor between the ages of 8 and 13.[8] The number of breast cancer cases in this group exceeds the expected number; hence, these breast cancers are attributed directly to the radiation therapy.

Breast cancer. More women with early stage breast cancers are being treated with breast-conserving surgery followed by radiation therapy. **On balance, it seems that there is a slight increase risk for developing breast cancer in the breast opposite the one that received radiation treatment for breast cancer – Table 15.1.** These patients should be under close surveillance.

Table 15.1 Risk of cancer in untreated breast from scatter radiation

Total Patients	Risk
97,346 [9,10]	Slight Increase
84,620 [11-24]	No Increase

However, breast cancer radiation therapy does increase the risk for developing leukemia (particularly in association with certain chemotherapies), lung cancer (especially in smokers), and sarcomas.[24]

THERAPEUTIC RADIATION FOR NONCANCEROUS LESIONS INCREASES BREAST CANCER RISK. In the past, radiation had been given for benign lesions. This is generally no longer done.

- **Thymus Gland** radiation was given to young babies because it was thought that their enlarged thymus gland was not normal. However, today we do know it is normal. Over 1,200 women were given radiation treatment in infancy for an enlarged thymus gland and they and their 2,400 nonirradiated sisters were studied. After a follow-up of about 36 years, there were 22 breast cancers in the radiated group and only 12 in their nonirradiated sister group. For every 100 cGy of radiation given, 3.5 more breast cancer cases per 10,000 people was observed.[25]

• **Scalp** radiation given to children between ages 5 and 9 had an increased risk for breast cancer.[26]

• **Benign breast infections** that were treated with massive doses of radiation between the 1920s and 1950s in Sweden, increased the risk for breast cancer.[27]

Summary. Women have a higher risk for developing breast cancer if they have been exposed to radiation at a particularly young age – early childhood and teenage years. Low-dose radiation (CT scans, repeated chest X-ray and mammograms) produces more cancer risk than does high-dose radiation like therapeutic doses for treatment of breast cancer. High-dose radiation can slightly increase the risk for developing breast cancer in the breast opposite the one that was treated, and increase the risk for developing leukemia (particularly in association with certain chemotherapies), lung cancer (especially in smokers), as well as sarcomas.

ELECTROMAGNETISM INCREASES RISK

Nonionizing electromagnetic radiation is generated largely through electrical and magnetic fields around us that include infrared rays, microwaves, radiowaves, and alternating electrical currents. All of these, except for infrared rays, penetrate the body readily. Such radiation is found in household wiring, appliances, high-tension wires, radio transmitters, television screens, video display terminals, electric blankets, and even the Earth, which has its own electromagnetic field. In fact, this electromagnetic field is responsible for making a compass needle point in the direction of north. However, the Earth's electromagnetic fields do a flip flop, the North and South Pole fields trading places at intervals of hundreds of thousands of years. Electromagnetism produces vague symptoms of fatigue, nausea, headache, loss of libido, and increases cancer risk.[28]

An electromagnetic field is created along wires when electricity flows and is measured in gauss. The electromagnetic field is made of two components: the electric field made from the strength of the charge that starts the flow, and the magnetic field that results from the motion of the alternating currents.

The energy needed to make electricity flow is called voltage. More voltage is needed to make electricity go farther. Voltage is either stepped-up or stepped-down along transmission lines by transformers at substations or on utility poles near homes. The strength of the field is important for human health.

All electrically driven products have electromagnetic fields that, among other things, suppress melatonin, a hormone produced by the pineal gland in the brain. Melatonin regulates the immune system. Low levels of melatonin have been linked to breast and prostate cancer.[29] Postmenopausal women who use electric blankets have a higher risk of breast cancer.[30] The closer you are to a given appliance or other source, the higher is the strength of the electromagnetic field.

Table 15.2 Electromagnetic Fields of Various Sources

Source	Electromagnetic Field Strength (milligauss)*
Coffee makers	0.7-1.5
Crock pots	0.8-1.5
Refrigerators	0.1-3.0
Clothes dryers	0.7-3.0
Irons	1.0-4.0
Toasters	0.6-8.0
Garbage disposals	8-12
Dishwashers	7-14
Televisions	0.3-20.0
Washers	2-20
Desk Lamps	5-20
Blenders	5-25
Fans	0.2-40.0
Portable Heaters	1.5-40.0
Fluorescent Fixtures	20-40
Ovens	1-50
Ranges	3-50
Microwave ovens	40-90
Hair Dryers	1-100
Shavers	1-100
Mixers	6-150
Vacuum Cleaners	20-200
Can Openers	30-300
Electric wires on telephone pole	10-600
High tension electric wires	50-10,000

*At a distance of 30 centimeters

High Voltage Wires Increase Risk

- Children living near the wires have a two times higher risk of developing cancer.[31-33]
- Men exposed to electrical and magnetic fields at work have an increased risk of leukemia (especially acute myeloid leukemia), brain tumors, and breast cancer.[34-39]

Low Voltage Wires Increase Risk

- Childhood leukemia and brain cancer is increased when homes have a large amount of house wiring or are close to telephone pole power lines.[40]
- Adult have more cancers when exposed to high magnetic fields secondary to large amount of house wiring.
- Low-frequency electromagnetic fields produce weak electric fields in our bodies, affecting hormone levels, the binding levels of ions to cell membranes, certain genetic processes inside the cell such as RNA and protein synthesis, and calcium ions. Calcium ions in the cell play a major role in cell division.

Computer Monitors Increase Risk

The "extremely-low-frequency" magnetic fields produced by these monitors have been linked to cancers, breast disorders, spontaneous abortion (16 studies),[41] and other health problems. The US Environmental Protection Agency recommended that the radiation fields produced by these monitors be categorized as *probable* human carcinogens. Color monitors produce more radiation. The amount of radiation is always higher at the sides, back and top of the monitor. The more powerful the monitor, the more radiation is emitted. Workers should sit at least two feet away from the front of the monitor and stay at least four feet away from the back or sides of a co-worker's monitor. The same precautions for laser printers. Some computer makers already sell low-radiation monitors but do not advertise them as such, perhaps fearing that these would create concern and anxiety about other terminals that the company produces.

Magnetic Resonance Imaging Scans. Patients undergoing MRI scanning are exposed to three types of electromagnetic radiation: static magnetic fields, pulsed radiofrequency (RF) electromagnetic fields, and gradient (time-varying) fields. Atoms of all tissues resonate at specific frequencies within an electromagnetic field and produce signals that convert to images.

The fastest MRI scanners rely on the time-varying fields to obtain large amounts of information in milliseconds that produce a clearer image. However, time-varying fields produce electric currents in the body. These currents can cause cardiac arrhythmias or nerve stimulation. Further research is needed to determine the harm to the human body.

CELLULAR PHONES INCREASE THE RISK FOR CANCER SLIGHTLY because they produce radiofrequency radiation and therefore effect cells and tissues.[42-47]

OTHER HEALTH CONSEQUENCES.

Electromagnetic fields increase cortisol that suppresses the immune system. The fields can alter cancer cell membranes and make them resistant to the immune system.[48] Microwaves affect our circadian rhythms, which in turn affect our sleep patterns, growth, and repair mechanisms, and even IQ tests in animals.

ADDRESSING THE PROBLEM. New transmission lines should be routed to avoid developed areas and increase the distance from the lines to the houses. The problem is that little can be done to reduce the electromagnetic fields from the low-voltage lines within our cities.

Help yourself! Use computer monitors that have reduced electromagnetic radiation. Use electric blankets only to preheat the bed. Move electric alarm clocks as far away from your bed as is practical. Buy home appliances that have minimal fields. We obviously need to be wary about where we live, avoid high-tension wires, and take other common sense precautions.

Anne is making changes. She moved her clock radio, doesn't use the electric blanket, and began following the Ten Point Plan, including protective antioxidants. She will only get a mammogram if it is indicated.

16
Sedentary Lifestyle

Barbara's History

Barbara is a 56 year old woman who is in middle management corporate America working a gazillion hours a week. She has two children in nearby colleges who she tries to visit on weekends. She "doesn't have time to exercise." Sound familiar?

We have all accepted that a sedentary lifestyle or lack of exercise is a risk factor for the development of cardiovascular illnesses. A sedentary lifestyle can also suppress the immune system and increase the risk for cancer and other diseases. Doctors preach about exercise and people generally are aware of it, sometimes even putting on their sneakers to do something about it. Sales of exercise equipment have risen over the past few years, but more often than not, these treadmills, stationary bicycles, and other very expensive devices remain unused in most people's basements. More than 90 percent of all Americans older than age 18 do not exercise. People who exercise are subsidizing the health-care costs for those who do not.

EXERCISE ENHANCES THE IMMUNE SYSTEM [1-12]

- Exercise increases the number and activity of T and B cells, natural killer cells, macrophages, and lymphokine activated killer cells and their regulating cytokines.
- Exercise slightly raises body temperature leading to an increase in the production of pyrogen, an interleukin that enhances lymphocyte functions. High temperatures kill viruses and cancer cells.[13-14]
- Exercise inhibits cancer growth.[15,16]

EXERCISE DECREASES BREAST CANCER RISK [17-29]

- Prospective and cohort studies make identical conclusions.
- Leisure time activity decreases risk by 37%.
- Exercise 7 hours a week, and lower the risk by 20-30%
- Longer menstrual cycles, characteristic of physically active women, confer protection against breast cancer because there are more days during the low-risk interval. Earlier studies showed that women with breast cancer have significantly shorter menstrual cycles than women without cancer. Females who begin training in ballet, swimming, or running before puberty are more likely to begin menstruating at a late age and have long and intermittent menstrual cycles.

EXERCISE LOWERS RISK FOR OTHER WOMEN'S CANCERS [21]

- Women who engaged in college sports had a lower incidence of cancers of the breast, ovary, cervix, vagina, and uterus.

EXERCISE DECREASES NEGATIVE SIDE EFFECTS OF BREAST CANCER TREATMENT [30]

- Women who exercise during breast cancer treatment have fewer side effects from the treatment(s).

EXERCISE DECREASES COLON CANCER RISK

- Men who have sedentary jobs have a 1.6 higher risk of developing colon cancer, especially in the descending colon, than their colleagues who have more active jobs.[31]
- People who work at a sedentary job for more than 40 percent of their work years developed colon cancer two times more frequently compared to those who never have.[32]
- The risk of getting colon cancer was 1.3 times higher for those in sedentary jobs than for those in active jobs (1.1 million men in Sweden, 19 year study).[33]

Increased physical activity causes more motility of the gastrointestinal tract and more frequent evacuation of the colon. The longer the stool remains in the colon, the longer a carcinogen (fecapentaene) in the stool has to exert its effect on the colon. Consequently, the higher is the risk for cancer.

WALKING DECREASES CARDIOVASCULAR RISK [34,35]

- Brisk walking and vigorous exercise each produce a similar and substantial decrease in cardiovascular disease among women. Even moderate walking speed decreases the risk.

LIFESTYLE ACTIVITY vs STRUCTURED EXERCISE

- Lifestyle activity (household chores, stair climbing, and walking for 30 minutes a day) is as effective as structured exercise for weight loss, decreasing blood pressure and the risk of cardiovascular disease (500 women and men).[36,37]

EXERCISE DECREASES CARDIOVASCULAR RISK[38-41]

- Exercise performed at frequent intervals over a long period of time decreases cardiovascular risk and sudden heart attack by strenuous exertion. However, bouts of heavy exertion pose a significant threat for sedentary people who have coronary artery disease or risk factors for it (331,000 people).
- Even small improvements in physical fitness produce a significantly lower risk of death (2014 men, 22 year follow-up).
- Exercise reduces borderline or mild hypertension.

FUTURE PROJECTIONS. What will happen to future generations as our jobs become more service related? Children are less physically active and physically fit than their counterparts of twenty or even ten years ago. Forty percent of children aged 5-8 exhibit signs of obesity, elevated blood pressure, and high cholesterol levels, according to the American Alliance for Health, Physical Education, Recreation and Dance. Our schools must help get our children into shape. However, only four states require all students to take a specific amount of physical education in all grades, kindergarten through twelfth: Illinois, New Jersey, New York, and Rhode Island. Only Illinois requires that all students take physical education classes every day. With a decrease in exercise, an increase in obesity, an increase in junk food, and the other risk factors that we have already discussed and will discuss, the incidence of cancer and other diseases will continue to spiral with each succeeding generation unless we dramatically alter our lifestyles.

BEGINNING AN EXERCISE PROGRAM

The one most important factor likely to initiate and increase a person's physical activity is the physician's recommendation.[42] Physical activity promotes health, affords a longer life, and decreases the risk for cancer, cardiovascular disease, hypertension, diabetes, osteoporosis, obesity, mental health, musculoskeletal disorders, and immunological abnormalities.[43,44]

Everyone, young or old, should exercise and increase their lifestyle activities. People are more likely to engage in low-intensity activities since they are more comfortable, convenient, and affordable, as well as safer. However, you must begin your exercise program slowly working up to the desired level. You should not start a heavy physical exertion program particularly if you have been sedentary because you can have a heart attack.

Because of the risk of sudden death associated with beginning to exercise, anyone 35 or older, or less than 35 with cardiac risk factors, should be medically screened with a full history and physical exam, and an electrocardiogram (ECG). A stress test is indicated if you have symptoms of heart disease.

An exercise program should be individualized because abilities and motivations differ. Your heart rate should be monitored. Of course, you should be warned to stop exercising immediately if you experience chest pain, severe shortness of breath, palpitations, or other cardiac symptoms. You should contact your physician at once if any of these occur. And finally, it is well known that people who continuously engage in a heavy exercise program, like marathon runners, are more susceptible to getting upper respiratory infections. Heavy exercise can suppress the immune system and hence should be avoided.

New athletes often consult with their physicians about exercise and nutrition. Athletes realize that proper nutrition plays a major role in their performance. Over 7 million high-school athletes are in an age group that has the highest risk of nutritional deficiencies. An adequate diet, with the proper vitamin and mineral supplementation is a must for all athletes. Athletes who attain their ideal weight may require additional calories for the extra energy they need. They can monitor this by weighing themselves regularly. Athletes must not increase muscle mass by taking any hormones – these cause many diseases including cancer. Exercising the muscles will increase muscle mass.

TAKE CONTROL

The benefits of exercise are enormous. Exercise lowers the risk for cancer, cardiovascular disease, hypertension, stroke, diabetes, obesity, depression and other diseases.[45-47] The immune system is enhanced.

My recommendations are simple: For 20-30 uninterrupted minutes 4 to 5 times a week, you should walk briskly, do everyday household chores, and/or climb stairs. These activities require no fancy warm-up suits, no fancy leotards, and no membership fees. In inclement weather, you simply go to a shopping mall to walk. Virtually everyone can walk. All age groups benefit from brisk walking. Climbing stairs for 15-20 minutes is also beneficial. During repetitive stair climbing, each individual step increases life by about four seconds.[48]

For decades, cardiac rehabilitation exercise programs have been commonplace. The same should be true for patients with cancer. In most instances, walking can be tolerated by all.[49]

There is no excuse for not walking or stair climbing. Check with your physician first and gradually build an exercise program. Again, exercise is another risk factor over which you have absolute control.

Barbara decided to walk briskly 20-30 minutes four times a week. After hearing the data, she knows she will live longer by making this small investment in time and effort.

17
Stress and Sexuality

Linda's History

Faced with being a 42 year-old single parent, working mom, Linda came to me full of anxiety, stress, and loss of libido. She told me she was worried that she may develop a breast cancer. She was going through a contentious divorce and her three teenage children were acting out. She said she had similar severe and prolonged stress at age 15 when her brother died in a car accident.

STRESS

As early as the second century, Galen, the physician who systematized medical learning, said that psychological factors contributed greatly to the development of cancer. He believed that melancholic women were more likely to develop cancer than those who were not. Other physicians of the eighteenth and nineteenth centuries observed the same relationship between emotional trauma and the development of cancer.[1]

NERVOUS SYSTEM AND IMMUNE SYSTEM COMMUNICATE with each other by way of nerve chemicals and special proteins made by immune cells. Special neuroendocrine cells have been found in important immune structures, and specialized T cells have been found at the ends of large peripheral nerves.[2] The nervous system can influence the immune response and the immune response, in turn, can alter nerve cell activities. Cells from the immune system can send messages to the brain, relaying information about invading microorganisms or other problems that might not otherwise be detected by the classical nervous sensory system.

The nervous system sends fibers to the thymus gland, the immune organ in which T lymphocytes are matured. The nerve fibers form a very specific pattern in this organ.[3] The spleen, lymph nodes, and bone marrow also contain very specific patterns of nerve fibers. The nerves follow the blood vessels into the organ and branch out into areas that contain T cell lymphocytes and not in areas that contain B cells.

The immune system influences the nervous system with proteins and hormones. One of the hormones produced by the immune system, called thymosin alpha 1, acts on the hypothalamus and pituitary gland in the brain to increase production of cortisol. Cortisol depresses the immune system by decreasing the number of lymphocytes, decreasing the mass of the spleen, and decreasing the size of the peripheral lymph nodes, among other things.[4] Early in life, thymosins protect T lymphocytes from the immunosuppressive effects of cortisol and allow them to mature normally.

STRESS IMPAIRS HUMAN IMMUNE SYSTEM[5-25]

- **Stress + Inability to Cope = Impaired Immune System**
- Stress and depression inhibit the function of lymphocytes, helper T cells, natural killer cells, and antibody production. These studies were done on medical and dental students who are routinely under great stress.
- Hypnosis and meditation can suppress the immune response.
- We can condition ourselves to suppress our own immune system by a variety of triggers.

STRESS INCREASES CANCER RISK[26,27] FOR:

- Children who had a significant stressful change a year before, including personal injury and/or change in the health of a family member.[28]
- People who experience the loss of a loved one.[29]

- People who are widowed, divorced, or separated; individuals who express a sense of loss and hopelessness; and those who have an inability to cope with the stress of separation.[30-32]
- People who are unable to express negative emotions and who also have reduced aggressive behavior.[33-35]
- People with an inability to cope,[36-38] People with depression.
- People who have stress and a precancer.[39]
- Swedish people who had serious aggravation at work had a 5.5 times greater risk for colorectal cancer than those without such pressure. People who work in high pressure situations, over which they have little control, face the highest risks.[41]

Detection of a cancer occurs many years after the first cell changed into a cancer. When people are asked about a past stressful event after being told that they do have cancer, their perception of that stressful event may be very different from what actually happened.

STRESS IMPAIRS MEMORY[42] After several days of stress, some aspects of memory is impaired in healthy people.

STRESS IMPAIRS WOUND HEALING[43]

STRESS INCREASES NEURAL TUBE DEFECTS[44]
Severe emotional stress during pregnancy especially that related to death of a child, increases the risk for neural crest defects.

STRESS CONTRIBUTES TO DIABETES as a cause of it because it raises blood sugar and increases obesity.[45,46]

STRESS INCREASES ASTHMA ATTACKS [47]

A PERSONALITY PRONE TO BREAST CANCER

Is there a cancer-prone personality? The evidence suggests that a person who is unable to cope with stress may have a higher risk for the development of cancer. Those who can cope better have less of a risk. Therefore, learn to cope, learn relaxation techniques (see inset) and techniques like meditation and biofeedback, and use any other techniques that you think will make you better able to cope and deal with stress.

One of the earliest observations that there may indeed be a personality prone to breast cancer was a study of women with breast cancer who were found more likely to control feelings of anger than an age-matched group of women with benign disease.[48] A review of over twenty separate studies shows that emotional control is implicated as a real risk factor in either causing cancer or causing its progression.[49-51]

Breast cancer patients in particular show a behavioral type; many breast cancer patients are characterized by suppression of emotional reactions, especially anger, and by conformity and compliance. Patients with breast cancer are also characterized as having poorly organized neuroses or psychoses, excessive self-esteem, hysterical disposition, and unresolved recent grief.[52] Emotional suppression is probably a real risk factor for developing breast cancer and not simply a reaction to having breast cancer. It is quite clear that emotional suppression in particular is linked to symptoms of depression and anxiety among breast cancer patients.[53]

Relaxation Technique

Get into a very comfortable lounging position. Concentrate on "feeling" every part of your body with your mind. You can begin by thinking about your right foot, then your right ankle, right leg, right thigh, then left foot, etc. Then move to your hands up to your shoulders and neck, and so on. Now, start to tense specific muscle groups as hard as you can, hold them tense for twenty or thirty seconds, then relax them. Again, start with your feet muscles (tense, relax), the leg muscles (tense, relax), and so on. You may repeat the entire sequence once or twice. While you are doing this, tell yourself that you are tightening your muscles each time you do so, and, provided that your effort is exhausting, you will look forward to relaxing each muscle group. While this is happening, you can think of a pleasant place that invokes fond memories. This sequence should produce relief and relaxation, and decrease your anxiety levels. Stress is another risk factor over which you have a great deal of control. Seize control of stress!

BREAST CANCER CAUSES STRESS

One-third of women with breast cancer have pronounced anxiety, a fifth become depressed, and a third experience sexual dysfunction.[54] Women with breast cancer have to deal with many losses – health, breast, femininity, and confidence. They often focus on death anxiety; living with uncertainty; fear of recurrence; understanding complex treatments; body and self-image; sexuality; relationship with doctor, partner, family and friends; changes in lifestyle; and setting goals for the future.

STRESS REDUCTION PROLONGS SURVIVAL AND DECREASES RECURRENCES [55-63] and also:

- Anger toward disease increases survival.[62]
- Breast cancer patients who have at least one confidant live longer than those who do not. Patients who confided in a nurse or physician lived even longer.[64]
- Belief system is linked to survival. The deaths of 28,000 adult Chinese-Americans and 400,000 "white" Americans were studied. Chinese-Americans, but not whites, die significantly earlier than normal (one to five years) if they have a disease, and their birth year is considered ill-fated by Chinese astrology and medicine.[65] The more strongly a person is attached to Chinese traditions, the more years of life are lost.

SEXUALITY

Being sexually active can enhance your immune system.[66] More than 100 undergraduates between the ages of 16 and 23 were asked how frequently they had sexual occurrences. An antibody (IgA) of the immune system was measured in their saliva and found to be the highest for those who had sexual occurrences one or two times per week. The antibody IgA was lower for those who had more sexual occurrences – three or more times a week. In another study, promiscuity actually impaired the immune system.[67]

Masturbation is a sexual occurrence that is practiced by 92% of men and 58% of women in the US, and 82% of men and 75% of women in Britain.[68,69] The percentages are probably even higher than reported. Self-masturbation is described as having sex with the person you love the most or having sex with the only person whose sexual history you can trust completely. It is safe. Masturbation has a very colorful history. It is written that the ancient Egyptians' Sun God, Atum, masturbated to create the first couple. Ancient Judaic teaching, however, was that it was a crime worth the death penalty. Onan, committed the Biblical sin by spilling his seed on the ground. St Thomas Aquinas said it was a sin worse than adultery or rape. The Kellogg Cereal Company developed a special breakfast cereal designed by Mr. Kellogg to prevent masturbation.

CONCLUSION

Constant depression, anxiety, and uncontrollable stress are risk factors for developing a cancer. Stress depresses the immune system If you develop a cancer and believe that you will do badly, studies show that you *will* do badly. If you develop a breast cancer and think that you will do well and you deny that you have the illness, studies show that you *will* do well.

You will learn in the chapter on Quality of Life and Ethics that physicians are obligated by law to tell the patient the life expectancy for his or her particular illness. A significant number of patients who, after hearing that they have a finite period of time to live – three or six or nine months – go home, circle a day on the calendar, and proceed to die on that day. Since psychological factors have a tremendous influence on overall survival, perhaps a physician should not pronounce an exact sentence for an individual based on statistics of thousands of similar patients who were simply treated "conventionally." Based on many studies, a modified lifestyle that includes psychological support, as in our Ten-Point Plan, will give a patient a better quality of life and increased survival.

Linda and I reviewed the issues. We set goals for stress reduction and behavior pattern guidelines for her children. With time, the household settled down, Linda had less stress, and her immune system became enhanced.

18

Lack of Spirituality

Charles B. Simone, II

Jessica's History

Jessica is 37 years old, was raised in a religious household, but stopped attending religious services and praying years ago. She developed breast cancer and turned to prayer.

SPIRITUAL TRENDS

When asked about religion, most Americans say they are religious, they do believe in heaven and hell, and they believe that prayer has healing power.[1-3]

April 1998 CBS News poll:

- 80% believe personal prayer can help medical treatment
- 22% say they have been cured by prayer
- 63% believe doctors should join their patients in prayer
- 34% believe prayer should be part of medical practice
- 60% say they pray at least once a day
- 64% say they pray for their own health and 82% say they pray for the health of others.

March 1997 CNN/USA TODAY/GALLUP POLL:

- 61% believe that religion can answer all or most of today's problems, but 20% believe that religion is old-fashioned
- 30% attend church or synagogue once a week, 13% almost every week, 17% about once a month, 30% seldom

February 1996 USA Weekend Faith and Health Poll:

- 79% believe faith can help people recover from illness

- 56% say their faith has helped them recover from illness
- 49% of 18 to 34 year olds say their faith helps them heal and that number rises to 62 percent in the 45-54 age group
- 63% want doctors to talk to patients about spiritual faith
- 10% say a doctor has talked to them about spirituality

June 1996 TIME/CNN poll:

- 82% believed in the healing power of prayer
- 73% said praying for someone else can help their illness
- 77% said God sometimes intervenes to cure people
- 64% said doctors should join their patients in prayer

SPIRITUALITY AND DISEASES

ARTHRITIS [4]

- Many arthritic patients believe that prayer reduces pain and improves their quality of life.

BLOOD PRESSURE [5]

- People who attend religious services regularly and prayed or studied the Bible at least daily had lower blood pressure than those who did so less frequently or not at all (4,000 people).
- Nine other studies demonstrate similar findings (thousands of people).

CANCER [6-11]

- 93% of 736 women with gynecological cancer said that their spirituality helped to sustain their hopes to fight the cancer.
- Over 75% of spiritual people are better able to cope with their deadly malignant melanoma.
- When told they have cancer, many people turn to God.
- Numerous studies find that for cancer patients, religious, spiritual, and quality of life are most important.
- Spirituality helps both the physical and mental well being of the terminally ill patient.

CARDIAC CONDITIONS [12-16]

- Spiritual patients heal more quickly after open heart surgery
- Patients who had heart attacks have less complications if others pray for them.

DEPRESSION AND MENTAL HEALTH [17-34]

- Among 1,900 women twins, those who were more religious had lower rates of depression, smoking, and alcohol abuse.
- The National Institute on Aging found that older adults who attended church weekly or more often, had half the depression rates compared to those who did not.
- Multiple other studies involving thousands of patients demonstrate similar results: those who used their religious faith to cope were significantly less depressed and had better mental health.
- Schizophrenics were less likely to be hospitalized if they continued religious worship.

IMMUNE SYSTEM [35]

- Elderly church goers (1,718 studied) have an enhanced immune system as measured by elevated levels of interleukin-6.

LIFE SPAN, GENERAL HEALTH, AND DECREASED HOSPITAL STAYS [36-55]

- Attending religious services and spirituality are associated with increased lifespan and better health (thousands of patients studied over decades).
- Hospitals stays are shorter for those who are spiritual.
- Coping skills are increased for those who are spiritual.
- Spirituality acts as a bridge between hopelessness and meaningfulness in life for terminally ill patients with AIDS.
- Attending religious services regularly increases life span by 7 to 14 years for African Americans – 24,000 adults.
- Those who never attend services have a 50 percent higher risk of mortality and are about four times as likely to die from respiratory disease, diabetes, or infectious diseases.

- Reviews and meta-analysis confirm that spirituality and religious involvement is a protective factor against disease.
- Death after heart surgery is 14 times less likely if the elderly patient is socially active and finds strength in her/his religious faith.

QUALITY OF LIFE [56-64]

- Multiple studies demonstrate that people who attend religious services weekly or read the Bible or pray daily have a better quality of life with or without an illness. These people include teenagers, divorcees, acutely ill persons, and others involved in stressful life events.

SMOKING [65]

- People who attend religious services weekly or read the Bible or pray daily are 990% less likely to smoke.

SUBSTANCE ABUSE [66]

- People who attend religious services weekly or read the Bible or pray daily are less likely to abuse alcohol or drugs.

Jessica turned again to prayer and religious services in her time of need. During stressful times, some people make deals with their God, …"if you let me live, I'll do this, this and this…" Jessica found her religious strength and thereby enhanced her immune system and decreased her risks for disease.

19
Genetics and Breast Implants

Sharon's History

Sharon is 39 years old, has breast implants that were placed at age 28. Her mother had breast cancer at age 62, and her aunt had breast cancer at age 58. Does Sharon have a genetic risk for breast cancer and do her implants pose a significant risk for breast cancer as well?

Inherited genetic factors make a minor contribution to the causation of cancer.[1] Only about 5 percent of all breast cancer patients have an inherited basis for this disease.[2] There is no genetic basis for all other breast cancer patients. Breast cancer in these other people is due to the risk factors that we have discussed. Chance alone may account for some clustering of breast cancer cases seen in some families because breast cancer is a very common malignancy, affecting one in eight women. However, in other families, clustering of several cases of breast cancer may be related to an inherited mutation in a specific gene.

ONCOGENES AND TUMOR SUPPRESSOR GENES

Every person has a set of oncogenes and tumor suppressor genes. Oncogenes promote tumor growth only when they are turned on. Tumor suppressor genes actually inhibit tumor formation when they are turned on. What activates these genes? Certain vitamins and minerals turn on tumor suppressor genes and, at the same time, suppress oncogene activity. Many other factors like dietary fat, tobacco, alcohol, etc. activate oncogenes.

What we do to ourselves will determine whether oncogenes will be turned on or not.

However, certain people may have a predisposition to having the oncogene turned on more quickly than the tumor suppressor gene. For example, some people who smoke do not necessarily develop cancer. Hence, some exposed individuals may genetically resist the carcinogen effect. Other people, however, may show an increased susceptibility to a given carcinogen. The majority of people are in between those who are resistant and those who have an increased susceptibility. This situation, therefore, is not based on true genetics but simply on a predisposition for activating existing genes that can promote or suppress tumors.

HEREDITARY CANCER

Six features characterize most hereditary forms of cancer:

1. Early age when the cancer is found.
2. Multiple cancers occurring in the same person at the same time with specific patterns within families or patients.
3. Physical signs and markers in hereditary cancer syndromes.
4. Characteristic pathological features.
5. Longer survival when compared to people who develop the same cancers without a hereditary basis.
6. Mendelian inheritance patterns of cancer transmission.

These features do not all apply all the time to a specific patient because there are variable expressions and penetrance (degree of expression as time goes on) of the affected genes. However, these six features will help guide the clinician in identifying a hereditary variant of many hereditary cancer syndromes.

Besides strict Mendelian genetics, traits can be passed along by non-Mendelian genetics and by genomic imprinting.[3,4] Genomic imprinting is the phenomenon whereby the expression or nonexpression of a gene is determined by the parental origin of that gene. Many factors modulate genomic imprinting, non-Mendelian traits and genotypes: dietary factors including antioxidants, free radicals, fats; estrogens; androgens; environmental pollutants, and other factors.[5] Other than strict Mendelian genetics, all the other forms of genetic influences are rare and have little influence on the majority of our diseases.

Breast Cancer Genetics

As has been stated, only about 5 percent of all breast cancer patients have an inherited basis for their cancer.

BRCA1 and BRCA2. The first BReast CAncer gene, BRCA1, was discovered in a patient who had early onset breast cancer. BRCA1 was also found in patients with ovarian cancer. This gene is linked to a region on chromosome number 17q21.[6-9] If a person has the BRCA1 gene, the risk of developing breast cancer by age 50 is 59% compared to about 2% in the normal population for this age; and the risk for a 70 year old with this gene is 82% compared to 7%. This shows that the gene is highly penetrant, which means that it is expressed more forcefully as time goes on.

The breast cancer gene can be carried either by the mother or the father; however, male carriers generally do not develop breast cancer. Both male and female carriers are at an increased risk for developing colon cancer and male carriers are also at an increased risk for developing prostate cancer.[10-12]

BRCA1 is associated with cancers of the breast, ovary, colorectal, and prostate. BRCA2 is associated with cancers of the breast (including male breast cancer), and prostate.[13]

Patients with BRCA1 or BRCA2 who do not have breast cancer or ovarian cancer live from 2.9 to 5.3 years longer if they have prophylactic mastectomies, or 0.3 to 1.7 years longer if they have prophylactic ovary removal.[14] However, a woman who develops breast cancer and is found to have BRCA1 or 2 has the same survival and number of recurrences as the person without the gene.[15]

NEU Oncogene is related to the family of epidermal growth factor receptors. A mutation causes more of the NEU receptors and proteins that cause a progression of breast cancer.

p53 Gene – the Prevention gene. On the same chromosome number 17, there is another area called the p53 region. The p53 protein is the leader in the body's antitumor army.

When the p53 gene has been *mutated* or *changed* or *altered* by free radicals or other agents, cancers and other illnesses develop.[16] The p53 gene is the most commonly altered gene in human cancer. It is one of the most important members of the tumor suppressor oncogene family. Of the 7.5 million people worldwide who are annually diagnosed with cancer, about half of them have the p53 mutation in their tumors.[17,18] A mutated or altered p53 is found in about 25% of breast cancers, 12% of brain cancers, 12% of soft tissue sarcomas, 6% of leukemias, and 6% of osteosarcomas.

The *P* stands for Protein but really denotes *P*revention because the action of p53 is to help prevent cancer by acting as a tumor suppressing gene. The p53 protein or suppressor gene puts the breaks on cell growth and division so when a cell starts to grow too rapidly or divides too many times, it will push that cell into a program of self-destruction and prevent multiplication of the cell. This is called apoptosis. Apoptosis is part of normal cellular development and is triggered by DNA damage from radiation, chemicals including chemotherapy, and free radicals. The p53 gene normally binds to other genes and thereby controls their expression.

CANCER-RELATED GENETIC SYNDROMES

The Li-Fraumeni Syndrome describes an early onset breast cancer and all the subsequent cancers early in life that develop from a mutated p53 gene.[19] This syndrome is inherited with an autosomal dominant trait (a single gene acting alone to produce an outcome) that obeys strict genetics. The early age of onset and the very high frequency of second cancers in a single individual were observed in these families and are quite consistent with features of hereditary forms of cancer.

Cowden Syndrome is a rare disorder that is characterized by multiple sores and other changes (hamartomas) of the mouth and skin. Women who have Cowden Syndrome have a higher risk for breast cancer, thyroid cancer, and thyroid goiter.

Muir Syndrome is characterized by autosomal dominant genetics and a higher rate of breast cancer in women as well as gastrointestinal cancers, and many skin tumors.

Proliferative Breast Disease (PBD)[20] is a benign (not cancerous) growth of epithelial cells in breast ducts of women who do not have cancer but whose relatives did. Proliferative breast disease may increase the risk for breast cancer but, unlike the other genetic diseases above, does not mean that this woman will develop breast cancer.

GENETIC COUNSELING

Currently, women who are in high-risk families should:

- Examine their breasts routinely beginning in their late teens.
- Have a physical exam twice a year starting at age 20.
- Perhaps have annual mammograms starting between the ages of 20 and 25 – this will not change lifespan.
- Perhaps have ovarian cancer screening with ultrasound and possibly serum CA-125 level – this will not change lifespan.
- Perhaps get tested for the BRCA and the mutated p53 genes.
- Above all, maintain intensive surveillance, and strict modification of lifestyle factors as per our Ten Point Plan.

Whether family members are genetically affected or unaffected, they experience tremendous psychological consequences. Unaffected family members often feel relief but, at the same time, tremendous guilt. After affected or nonaffected patients receive genetic information, they require intensive psychological support. In addition, once this information is known to the patient, insurance companies may use the information to deny that person life and health insurance.

After a breast cancer is apparent, other oncogenes become evident in the bloodstream as well. They include erB, erB2, erB3, H-ras and many others. But these have not been good predictors of outcome. However, one dominant theme is certain – when the short arm of chromosome number 17 is lost, the breast cancer behaves very aggressively.[21]

SUMMARY

Inherited genetic factors make a minor contribution to the causation of cancer.[1] Only about 5 percent of all breast cancer patients have an inherited basis for this disease.[2] However, your existing normal genes, like p53, can be altered by free radicals or other means. Once these genes change, once the tumor suppressor genes no longer work, or once the oncogene gets turned on, a tumor cell can grow uninhibited.

It is important to modify your lifestyle early enough in life so that these changes in oncogenes and tumor suppressor genes never occur. Furthermore, if you do have breast cancer, it is imperative to modify your lifestyle so that no further free radicals are formed and tumor promotion does not occur. Change your lifestyle factors now.

BREAST IMPLANTS

About 175,000 American women undergo breast augmentation yearly. About 90 percent of these are purely for cosmetic reasons and the rest for reconstruction. Approximately 2 million women in the United States have had breast implants. Augmentation procedures have included: simple injections of liquid silicone not encapsulated, implants of various materials, and self-tissue transplantation. Since there was concern as to whether breast implants can cause cancer or other diseases, the FDA banned implants. Women with implants have sued manufacturers over the years alleging that the implants leaked silicone and caused cancer or systemic immunological diseases.

But the facts show no harm according to the 1999 report of the Institute of Medicine.[22] **Implants** filled with silicone gel:

- **Do not cause Cancer.**[23-28] The only cancer attributed to silicone is connective tissue sarcoma in rats[29], but no human sarcoma has been demonstrated.[30]
- **Do not cause Lupus, Scleroderma, Arthritis or other Immunological diseases.**[31-41]
- **Do not cause Neurological disease.**
- **Do not cause other Chronic Illness.**

- **Do not pose a risk to infants who breast feed** from mothers who have implants.

Silicone implants do cause the following complications:

- Contractures
- Rupture
- Obscures abnormality on mammography
- Breast pain
- Infection
- Implant Migration

Women with breast implants are more likely to drink alcohol (greater than 7 drinks per week), be younger at first pregnancy, be younger at first birth, have a history of terminated pregnancies, have used oral contraceptives, and have had a greater lifetime number of sexual partners.[42] All these risk factors increase their risk for developing breast cancer.

Women who desire to have implants should have a right to do so as long as informed consent is obtained about the risks and that the informed consent is without bias.[43] Without being given this opportunity, women will leave the United States to have the implant procedure performed elsewhere.

Sharon learned that her breast implants and her inherited genetic make-up do not increase the risk for developing breast cancer, but her lifestyle can alter her protective p53 gene. She decided to change her lifestyle to minimize any risk.

PART FOUR

Breast Cancer: Detection to Conventional Treatment

20
Breast Cancer Detection

Breast self-examination, physician examination, and mammogram + ultrasound are the main tests to detect a breast cancer.

Does early detection of breast cancer and therefore subsequent earlier treatment, increase the length of life?

BREAST SELF-EXAMINATION

After properly being taught, every woman can perform breast self-examination (Figure 20.1). Patients find about 90 percent of breast cancers, either accidentally or by self-examination. Eighty percent of lumps are benign. Only 40 percent of women actually perform Breast Self Exam. A woman who examines her breast incorrectly may have a false sense of security when she finds no masses. About 20 percent of women were proficient at detecting about half of the lumps in a model of a breast with seven lumps in it. Breast Self Examination should be done by both men and women and in conjunction with an annual physician's examination.

MONTHLY EXAMINATIONS should be done a few days after the menstrual period begins because the breasts are not swollen or tender at that time. After menopause, you should pick a particular date each month to examine your breasts.

HOW TO EXAMINE: LOOK, THEN FEEL. The first step in breast self-examination is to stand in front of the mirror without clothing from your waist up and lean forward. You must look for any changes in the shape or size of your breast, for

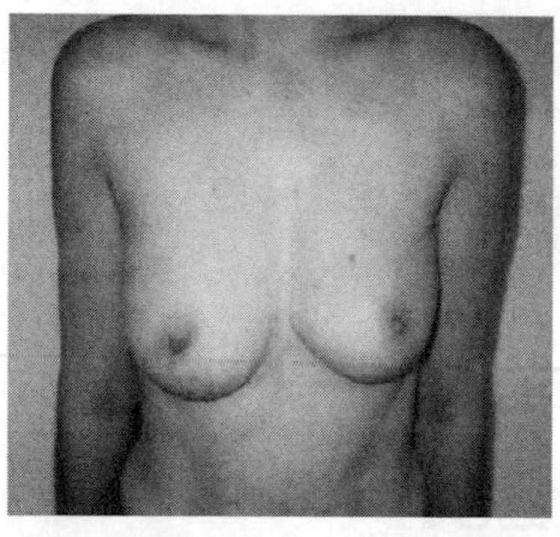

Before beginning, read the detailed instructions.

a. Stand in front of mirror and lean forward. Look for changes in size or shape of breasts, discharge, or pulling inward of nipples, for changes in skin appearance.

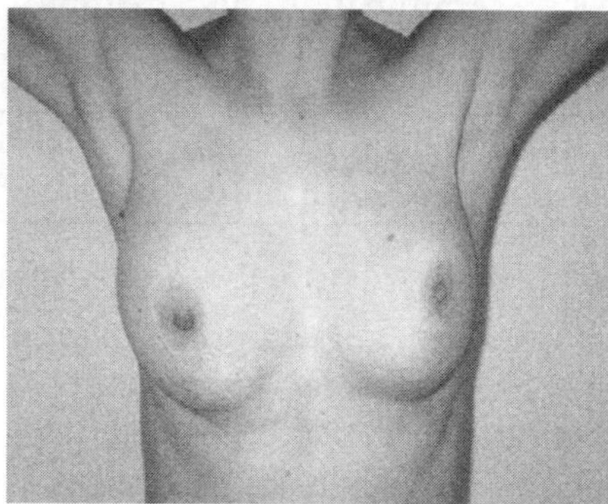

b. Place hands behind head. Repeat your observations.

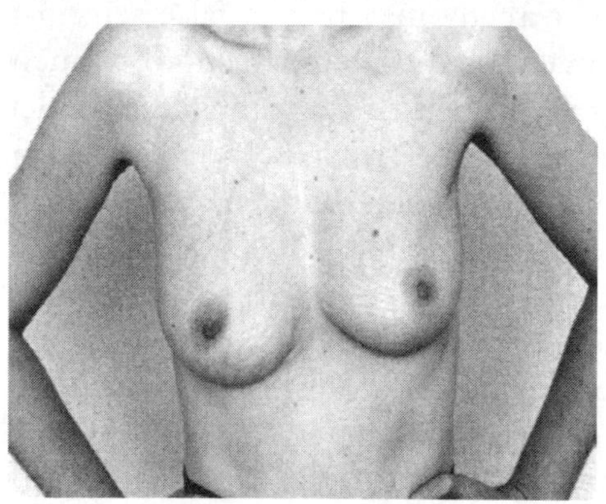

c. Push down on your hips. Repeat your observations.

Figure 20.1 Breast Self Examination

d. Lie on your back and examine each breast. Gently but firmly feel for masses.

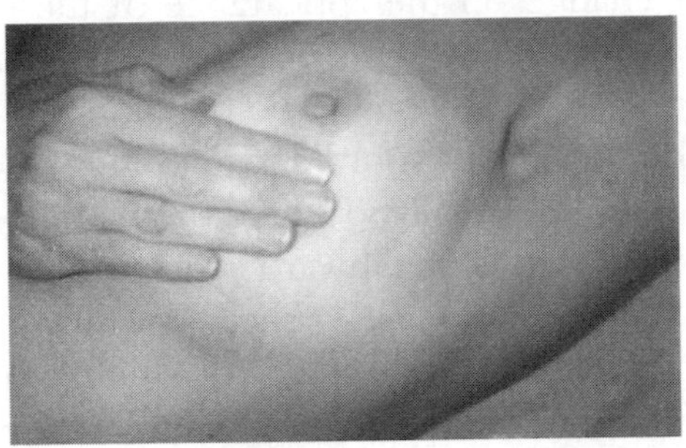

e. Examine axilla (armpit area) in the same manner, gently but firmly feeling for masses.

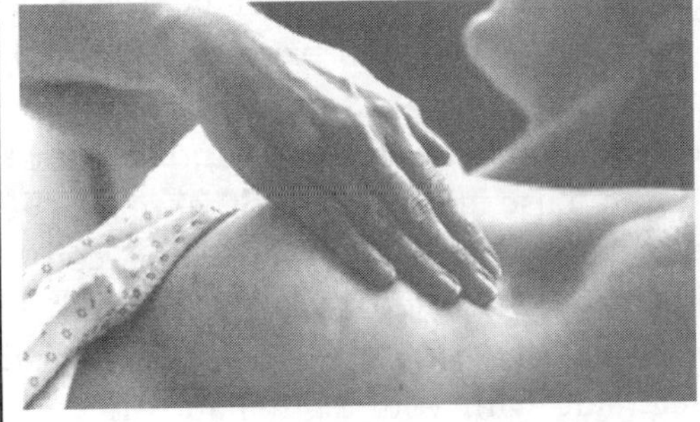

f. Squeeze nipple. Look for discharge, changes in shape, size, or skin of nipple.

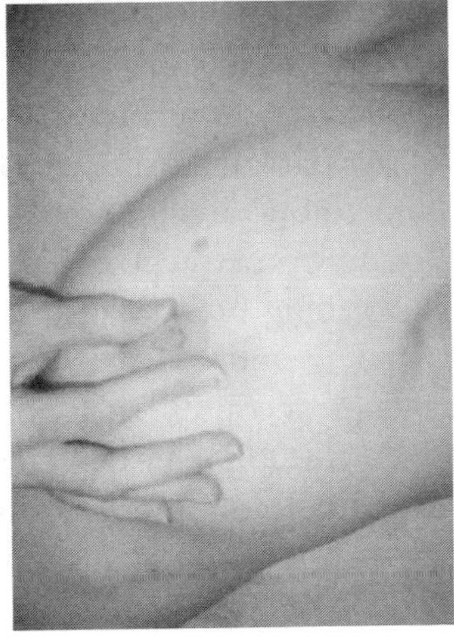

discharge from the nipples, for pulling inward of the nipples, or for changes in the appearance of the skin, like dimpling or an orange-peel appearance. Since changes in the breast may be accentuated by changing the position of your body and arms, you should next put your hands behind your head and observe your breasts; and finally, observe them after you place your hands on your hips, pushing inward on your hips with your hands.

The next few steps begin with lying on your back and placing a folded towel under your right shoulder if you have large pendulous breasts that hang off to the side of the chest. The towel acts to tilt the chest, allowing the breast to lie flat on the chest for easier examination. Now, put your right hand and arm behind your head. Use your left hand, elbow raised and fingers flat on breast. Move your fingers in a circular motion around your breast, working in from the outer edge of the breast to the nipple, in order to explore for masses. Do not pinch your breast between your thumb and fingers because this may give you the false impression of a mass. Feel gently but firmly. Thoroughly examine the area between your breast and axilla (underarm) because this is the location of some of the lymph nodes that drain the breast. Now, repeat the process on the opposite side with your right hand. If you think anything is abnormal, contact your physician.

Memorize the location of your lumps, if you have lumpy breasts. Also divide each breast into four imaginary quadrants. In this way you can easily "map" the location of the lumps. Since there is more breast tissue in the upper outer quadrant, the upper part of the breast located closest to the axilla, you will find more abnormalities in this area if they are to be found.

Young women who find asymptomatic benign breast lesions by performing breast self-examination are exposed to unnecessary anxiety and unnecessary medical investigations, including invasive procedures and potential risks of false reassurance.

Breast Self Examination does Not Increase lifespan Large randomized trials of Breast Self Examination have failed to show any impact on length of life, or on the extent of disease, or the size of the cancer when detected. These studies include randomized and cohort trials from Shanghai (267,040 women),[1] Russia (122,471 women),[2] US (450,156 women),[3] Sweden (548,000 women),[4] the World Health Organization,[5,6] England, and others.[7-9] Breast Self Examination seems to be as effective as mammography with regard to lifespan.[10]

PHYSICIAN EXAMINATION

Examination by a competent physician is important. Generally, physicians who spend the most amount of time doing the examination find the most lumps, and this was not linked to level of training or experience.[11] OB/GYN physicians found less lumps compared to internists, family practitioners, or any other physician who spent more time in doing the examination. It is difficult, however, to feel lumps that are less than 1 cm in size unless they are superficial. Since mammograms can miss 10 to 15 percent of all cancer lumps, some of which are quite large, physician's examination is important to detect cancer.

A good examination, as shown in figures 20.2 and 20.3, can take from ten to fifteen minutes. It should be done in a well-lighted room because changes in skin texture and color tend to be quite subtle but significant. The physician should first check for symmetry of the breasts, differences in size and shape, and ask the patient if any differences occurred recently. The breast surface should be inspected for dimpling or flattening, discoloration, ulceration, erosion, or dilated veins. Examination of the nipples should include determination of inversion, crusting or discharge, or deviation of one nipple compared to the other.

I first examine the patient seated on the examining table. With one hand underneath the breast, my other hand is pressing gently from the top of the breast and rolling the breast tissue back and forth to determine if there are any palpable masses in the breast between my two hands. The same type of examination can be done with hands on each side of the breast compressing together, again feeling for any masses that might be within the breast but between the two hands.

Next, the patient should put her hands on her hips and push down on her hips with force. If there is a malignant mass that is attached to the deep muscles, the mobility of the breast when the physician attempts to move it from side to side will be se-

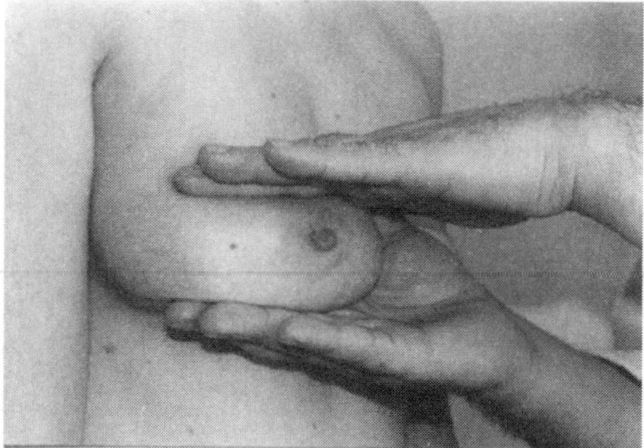

a. Physician rolls breast back and forth between hands

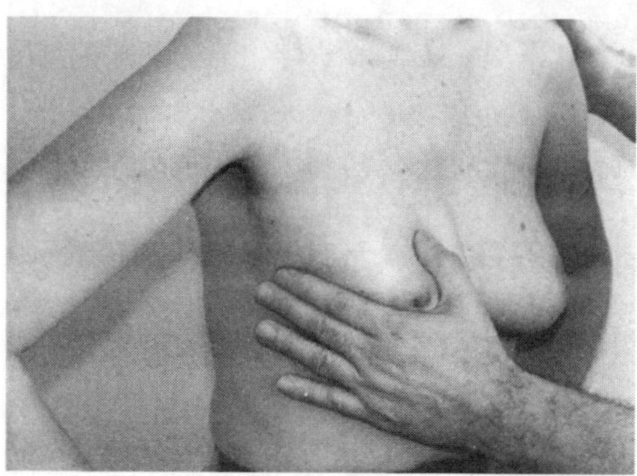

b. Breast mobility checked when patient pushes on her hips.

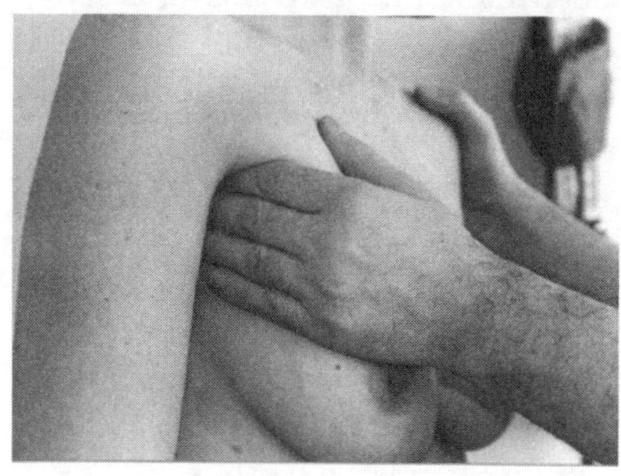

c. Axilla examined

Figure 20.2 Physician's Examination of Seated Patient

a. Physician examines breast with gentle circular motion.

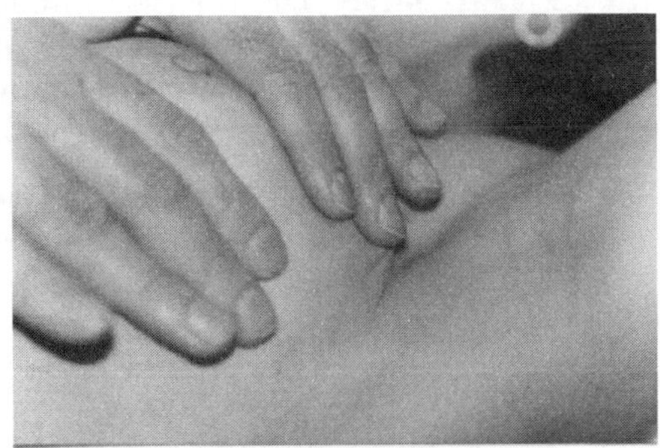

b. Physician examines areola. Fat and glands stop at margin but ducts attach under it.

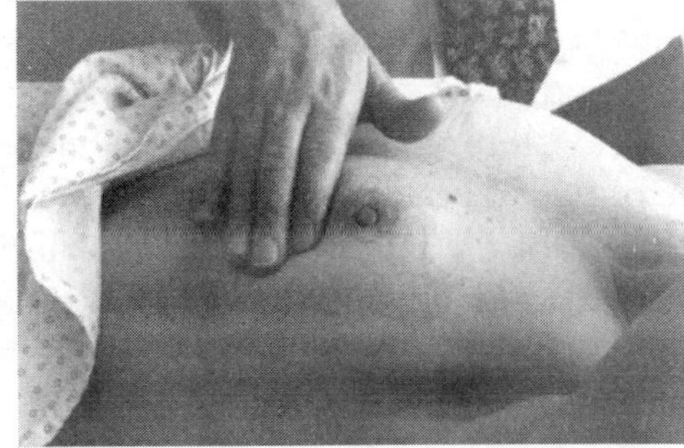

c. Physician examines ductal system by applying pressure with both hands. Possible discharge and its location on nipple are observed.

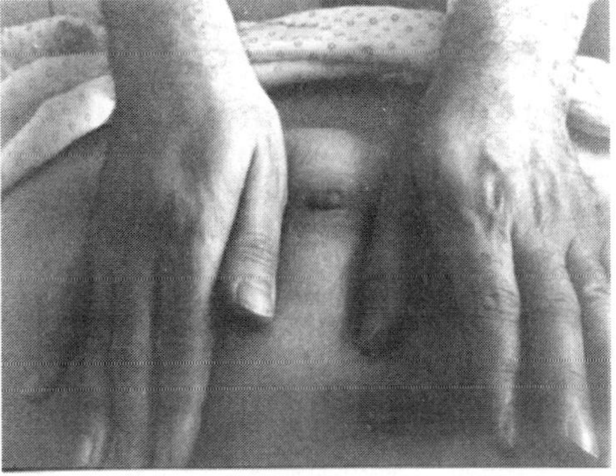

Figure 20.3 Physician's Examination of Reclining Patient

verely limited. For the next maneuver, the patient raises her arms above her head. The physician inspects the under portion of the breast, which is called the inframammary fold region. While in this position, the patient leans forward slightly so the physician can look for early nipple or skin retraction. Now, the patient puts her arms down along her sides in a relaxed position, and the physician examines the axilla. While doing this, the physician's fingertips should roll underneath the pectoralis muscle to ensure the examination of the lymph nodes underneath that muscle high up in the axilla. Examination of the supraclavicular region, the region above the collar bone and near the neck, should be done at this point.

Now, the patient should be in a reclining position. The patient's arms should be over her head and, if the breasts are large and pendulous, one hand of the physician should hold the breast on top of the chest wall while the examination is being performed. The method I find best is to plant my fingers on one area of the breast and, without lifting my fingers, examine that area for lumpiness or masses by pulling the breast in a circular motion with those fingers. Examination must be done gently; hard palpation can obliterate any sensation of small lumps beneath the examiner's fingers. After this region of the breast is thoroughly examined, the physician's hand should be lifted, put on to another place on the breast, and the motion repeated until the entire breast is examined. If a lump is felt in the breast, it should be sequestered between two fingers and evaluated for hardness, buoyancy, and mobility. The inframammary fold area, the bottom most part of the breast, is sometimes difficult to examine because it normally is thickened and hardened in women who have larger breasts. Examination of this region must be thorough so that a small mass is not missed. Although breast cancers are infrequent in this region, time must be spent here.

Care and attention should also be given when the areola (the colored, circular area around the nipple) is examined since the consistency of the breast tissue is very different here. The fat and glandular material of the breast generally stops at the margin of the areola. Finally, the physician should examine the nipples for any discharge. To see if there is discharge, both hands should be used to form a concentric ring several centimeters away from the nipple and pressure should be applied. During the application of pressure, the physician's hands should roll toward the nipple, thereby expressing any discharge from the ductal glands if, indeed, there is one.

Physical examination, not mammogram, was the main reason for the reduction of breast cancer mortality in the Health Insurance Plan Study which compared mammography to physical examination as a screening tool (used when a patient has no symptoms or obvious findings).[12-14] In some studies, the physical examination is more accurate than a mammogram in indicating a breast mass that turns out to be cancer.[15,16] Other studies show that the physician's physical examination is equal to that of mammography for the detection of cancers.[17]

MAMMOGRAPHY – a $4 Billion a Year Industry

In this section, I review mammography as a screening test of asymptomatic patients. However, if a woman has signs or symptoms suggestive of a malignant process in the breast, they are candidates for mammography regardless of their age.

The objective of a screening mammogram is to detect a breast cancer before it has a chance to spread to other organs of the body. While this is certainly a noble pursuit, does it work? And, importantly, what age groups should be screened by mammography knowing that about 76% of all breast cancers are in women aged 50 and older.[18]

AGES 40 TO 49: SCREENING MAMMOGRAMS DO NOT PROLONG LIFE

This issue is a subject of great emotion, anger, and tremendous anxiety for women in their 40s who have always thought that a mammogram is their protective shield but are now being informed there is no role for mammographic screening in this age group. So emotionally charged is this subject that every self-serving institution has jumped on one side or the other.

In October 1991 an analysis of a Canadian study of women 40-49 were presented to the NCI and concluded that screening mammograms did not extend life – this was published in November 1992. Five other randomized trials concurred. In February 1993, the NCI convened an international workshop that concluded: "The randomized trials of women ages 40 to 49 are consistent in showing no statistically significant benefit in mortality after 10 to 12 year follow-up….no reduction in mortality from breast cancer that can be attributed to screening."[19] The NCI endorsed this conclusion.

But on November 22, 1993, the National Cancer Advisory Board (NCAB), members who are scientists and non-scientists appointed by the President of the United States to "advise" the NCI Director, told the NCI to "defer action on recommending any changes in breast cancer screening guidelines at this time."[19] This was despite what the NCI's Division of Cancer Prevention and Control said, "In a meta-analysis of eight randomized studies done in different countries at varying screening intervals, one sees consistency in showing no statistical benefit in mortality after 10-12 years of follow-up.[20]

Despite NCAB's advice, the NCI Director on December 3, 1993, recommended that women between the ages of 40 and 49 ***not*** have routine screening mammography by issuing the following statement: "To date, randomized clinical trials have not shown a statistically significant reduction in mortality for women under the age of 50."[19] Then on February 23, 1994, the National Cancer Advisory Board told the NCI to stick to its primary mission of research and "not involve itself independently in the setting of health care policy."[19]

The NCI director was summoned to the Senate to explain the NCI's flip-flop position on March 9, 1994. He said, "Two principles need to guide us whenever possible: the consensus of scientific peer groups and clinical trials as the instrument for consensus."[19] But this subject is so politically charged that he also said, "What I would do as an individual is recommend annual mammograms, but I can't recommend it to the public because I don't have the facts."[21] He also said that the "current NCI position is in close alignment with positions of several public and private organizations – e.g., the National Women's Health Network, the U.S. Preventive Services Task Force, the

American College of Physicians, and the American Association of Family Practitioners."[19] This is simply ***not true*** for all except the first. In fact, the latter three organizations and others cried out for a change in the guidelines because the scientific data show absolutely no benefit for the 40 to 49 year old group.[22,23]

In an attempt to settle the confusion, the National Institutes of Health, the parent to the NCI, convened a Consensus Conference on January 21, 1997 and issued the following concluding statement: "Evidence from randomized controlled trials indicates that for women ages 40-49, during the first 7 years following mammography, breast cancer mortality is no lower in women who were assigned to screening than in controls."[24]

Then political trouble began. Senator Arlen Specter (R-PA), chairman of the subcommittee who controls the NIH's purse strings, pressed the NIH to reverse its position. That failed, but the US Senate issued a "Sense of the Senate" resolution that the NIH Consensus Statement "caused widespread confusion…and reinforced barriers and negative attitudes that keep women from being screened." The US Senators, contrary to the conclusions of the scientists, said that there was benefit to screening and "strongly urged" the NCAB to issue guidelines recommending that all women be screened.

Specter held hearings. NCAB said it needed two months. Specter wanted quicker action and wrote to the new Director of the NIH and the new Director of the NCI. Three weeks later, after multiple letters and phone calls to NCAB members, NCAB issued its recommendations: "It is prudent to have mammograms every 1 to 2 years." Remember now, who serves whom. The NCAB serves to "advise" the National Cancer Director, who is subordinate to the Director of all the Institutes – National Institutes of Health. Despite the scientific conclusions reached by the Consensus Conference of the entire NIH, political pressures won, politically appointed people like the Directors of the Institutes became sullied, and the scientific process was dismissed.

As I have previously mentioned, the mortality rate, or life span, for patients with breast cancer has remained unchanged since 1930, which means there has been no progress in the treatment of breast cancer. That information is startling to most people because they hear from the news media that the medical profession has one triumph after another, one miracle breakthrough after another.

Cancer charities and organizations report these "breakthroughs" to the media and ask for dollars directly from you or the Congress. They say that with a few more dollars, they will hand you the real cure to this illness, to this cancer; just look at all the triumphs to date. Hearing all these marvelous accomplishments from the media, a typical person wonders who the heck can be dying of breast cancer these days. What we have done is improve the quality of life, somewhat, for patients with breast cancer. So the oncology community has had to turn its attention to another area – early detection using mammography, which was portrayed as the next ray of hope. However, it takes approximately eight years of growth before a breast cancer can be found on a mammogram. During those eight years, many things happen, including the dissemination of those cancer cells to other organs by way of the bloodstream.

A good physician-scientist must dispassionately examine the scientific data as it evolves. Let us now review the scientific data which leads to the conclusion that routine screening mammography affords no survival benefit whatever to women aged 40-49. In New York in the 1960s, a randomized controlled trial began that indicated for the first time that screening for breast cancer using mammography resulted in benefit.[25] However, international committees recommended the study be repeated before any mass screening took place.[26,27] Consequently, clinical trials began in Sweden,[28] Canada,[29] Scotland,[30] England,[31] the Netherlands,[32] Utrech,[33] and Florence, Italy.[34] An analysis of longer term was conducted by the New York HIP (Health Insurance Plan of Greater New York)[35] and investigators independently analyzed these studies.[36-38] Each study had problems with design and none of them looked at specific age groups. But even so, **the overall survival or lifespan was unaffected despite earlier detection by mammography**.

In 1991, the Canadian National Breast Screen Study (published 1992), the first specifically designed for women ages 40 to 49, demonstrated that these women and others who had undergone routine mammography and physical examination had a higher death rate from breast cancer than women who had undergone only a single physical breast examination.[39-41]

Although the Canadian study had faults,[42-44] its results combined with Swedish studies,[45,46] the Edinburgh Trial,[47] the UK Trial of Early Detection of Breast Cancer,[48] and other published randomized controlled trials demonstrate that screening mammography does not benefit women 40 to 49.[49-55] The Edinburgh Trial stated: "No breast cancer mortality was observed for women whose breast cancers were diagnosed when they were younger than 50 years." Most of the cancers that were detected in the first screen in women aged 40-49 were *in situ* carcinomas and other lesions of low malignant potential. Less than half of these would develop into invasive cancer.

These are simply the facts and no emotional lobbyist, marches, US Senate, and no vested interest group can change the facts. Rather than continuing to focus on mammograms, all patients, including those aged 40 to 49 should be screened with the use of the Self Test in Chapter 3. The resulting risk assessments should be combined with a pathological breast biopsy report if available to make an overall assessment of risk. Women with a high overall risk should be followed closely.

MAMMOGRAM RATE OF FALSE ALARMS IS HIGH. About one third of women screened had abnormalities requiring additional evaluation, even though no breast cancer was present.[56] About 20 percent of all false alarms could be avoided by ***not*** performing routine physical examination before the age of 45, breast self-examination before the age of 35, and screening mammography before the age of 60.[57] Breast pain and nipple discharge are usually not symptoms of breast cancer, and this accounted for another 30 percent of the false alarms.

QUESTION: DOES DETECTION BY MAMMOGRAPHY EXTEND LIFE? ANSWER: NO.

One study concludes that screening of 10,000 women annually for 10 years would on average extend all 10,000 women's lives by 2.5 days.[58]

In another study the following questions and answers were developed by John M. Lee, M.D.[59] to simplify the morass of statistical information concerning the use of screening mammography in women aged 40-49:

- *Question:* What are a 40-year-old woman's chances of getting breast cancer in the next ten years?
- *Answer:* 13 per 1,000.
- *Question:* Of these 13, how many would survive without screening?
- *Answer:* 5. Some cancers are so slow-growing that mortality is not increased by waiting for symptoms. A cancer detected by screening does not always equal a life saved.
- *Question:* Of the 8 per 1,000 destined to die without screening, how many do studies indicate would be saved by screening with an annual physical examination plus mammography?
- *Answer*: One-quarter or 2.3 per 1,000. False negatives account for a portion of the unavoidable deaths as do aggressive cancers that develop and metastasize between screenings.
- *Question*: How many false positives (from both the physical exam and the mammography) will have to be evaluated to save 1 life in this age group?
- *Answer:* 150.
- *Question:* What is the cumulative 10-year risk of a false positive screening result?
- *Answer:* 13 percent at 3 percent per year. The woman must be aware of the possible medical and psychological harm of a false positive result.
- *Question:* After submitting to an annual physician's examination, how much does a 40-year-old woman increase her chance of dying of breast cancer by not getting an annual mammogram screening?
- *Answer:* By 1 in 1,250.
- *Question:* By skipping mammography 1 year?
- *Answer:* By one in 12,500.

- *Question*: How much extra life can the average 40-year-old woman expect if she adds mammography to an annual physical examination for the next 10 years?
- *Answer*: 7 days.

MULTIPLE REVIEWS CONCLUDE THAT SCREENING MAMMOGRAMS ARE NOT JUSTIFIED [60-62]

AGES 50 TO 59: SCREENING MAMMOGRAMS DO NOT PROLONG LIFE [63]

In women aged 50-59 years, the addition of annual mammography screening to physical examination has no impact on breast cancer mortality.

AGE 60 AND OLDER: SCREENING MAMMOGRAMS DO NOT PROLONG LIFE [45,49,64]

There are no reliable data to suggest that routine mammographic screening can reduce the death rate or mortality in this age group.

WHAT TO DO? YOU CAN PREVENT BREAST CANCER BY FOLLOWING THE TEN POINT PLAN IN CHAPTER 27. SCREENING MAMMOGRAMS ARE NOT THE ANSWER, PREVENTION IS. IF YOU DO HAVE A BREAST CANCER, YOU CAN EXTEND YOUR LIFE BY FOLLOWING THE SAME TEN POINT PLAN.

BREAST IMPLANTS OBSCURE MAMMOGRAM READING in 20 to 85 percent of the breast tissue, making cancer detection difficult. There is a 41 percent rate of false negatives, and a higher rate of axillary nodal metastatic disease in patients with augmented breasts. When silicone leaks from the implant, mammograms are of limited value, and the physician's breast examination becomes critical.[65,66]

MAMMOGRAPHY INCREASES THE RISK OF SPREADING OF CANCER CELLS[67,68] Studies show more deaths and earlier deaths among women with breast cancer who had dense breasts compared to women whose breasts were not dense.[69,70] Women with dense breasts required a five-fold increase in compressive force for the mammogram in an attempt to flatten the breast and thereby have more visualization on the X-ray picture.[71]

LOW FAT DIET REDUCES AREAS OF MAMMOGRAPHIC DENSITY [72-74]

HORMONE REPLACEMENT THERAPY INCREASES AREAS OF MAMMOGRAPHIC DENSITY. [75]

OTHER DIAGNOSTIC TOOLS

• **Ultrasound** can be used to differentiate fluid filled cysts from solid masses and also can be used to guide a needle into a mass for aspiration. Ultrasound should be used in conjunction with either physical examination and/or mammography. Ultrasound cannot identify malignant lesions less than 1 cm in diameter or microcalcifications.

• **Thermography** is based on the fact that the temperature in the region of a breast cancer is elevated. An abnormal thermogram is associated with large tumor size, high grade, positive lymph nodes and large regional vessels.[76,77] Thermography is risk free and should be used in conjunction with either physical examination and/or mammography.

• **Translumination** is a technique of shining light through the breast. Although this technique has been around since 1929, it has not been very efficient at detection of cancers. More recently, technology has improved the light source and, therefore, the detection rate. However, at this point, translumination should be considered quite experimental.

• **CT and MRI Scans** both detect tumors, but are expensive.

• **PET Imaging** (Positron Emission Tomography) detects radioactive compounds that are preferentially taken up by cancers. PET scanning may eventually eliminate the need for surgical removal of axillary lymph nodes because it will be able to detect whether lymph nodes are involved with cancer. PET scanning can also detect cancer in other sites of the body.

DOES EARLY DETECTION OF BREAST CANCER AND THEREFORE SUBSEQUENT EARLIER TREATMENT, INCREASE THE LENGTH OF LIFE? ANSWER: NO

This is the question posed at the start of the chapter. How could the answer be NO? If we detect a breast cancer early why does it not increase the length of life? The answer is simple. By the time our technology can detect a cancer, it has already spread to other parts of the body by way of the bloodstream via angiogenesis (Chapter 21).

SUMMARY

The physician's physical examination seems to be as good or better than a screening mammogram. The emotionally charged widespread use of screening mammograms has cut deeply into much needed health-care dollars for no gain. Clinical scientists should make recommendations and set policy based on scientific facts and not emotions or wishes. It is a disservice to give false hope to young women about the value of mammograms. Only the truth should be given to people.

Many women will advocate mammograms no matter what – they erroneously believe that the risk of cancer is greatest at young ages, or that mammograms are "all they've got," or that mammograms prevent breast cancer.

A female physician in her forties and co-chair of the international screening workshop, sums it up:

> "If mammography were a treatment, we would have to call it an unproven treatment for women in their 40s. I believe we owe the American woman the honesty of telling her the truth – that the benefit of this test for women in their 40s is not proven."[78]

My recommendations for asymptomatic women:

- Physician breast examination – all women starting at age 40.
- Take the Self Test and follow the Ten Point Plan Modification as outlined in Chapter 3 and 27. If overall breast cancer risk assessment is high, then mammogram should be obtained based upon clinical judgment.

21

Cancer Angiogenesis

Every day approximately 350 billion normal cells divide in your body to form new ones. Every time one of these cells goes through the reproductive cycle, there is always a possibility that it can go awry and transform into a cancer cell, especially if you have multiple lifestyle risk factors. But usually, if the immune system is working properly, these transformed cells are killed.

But if just one of these transformed, cancerous cells escapes the immune system, it starts to grow into a small colony of cancer cells. This is called an *in situ* cancer - it remains in one site. This is usually a cancer of a millimeter or so in diameter.

Avascular Cancer Mass

At this point, the cancer is usually harmless because it has no blood vessels to remove the cancer's wastes or to supply it with oxygen and nutrients. Hence, this *in situ* cancer cannot grow. Oxygen, nutrients, and wastes are diffused to and from blood vessels. So unless blood vessels are intimately in contact with the cancer cells, even the most aggressive cancer cells may remain dormant for months or years.

Vascularization of the Cancer

For the small colony of cancer cells to grow into a large detectable cancer, it must become vascularized - a process known as *angiogenesis* – the formation of (*-genesis*) new blood vessels (*angio-*). This happens when cancer cells release a chemical substance, called tumor angiogenesis factor (TAF), that induces new blood vessels to form.[1-3] Many substances induce or inhibit angiogenesis.

Inducers of Angiogenesis	Inhibitors of Angiogenesis
Estrogen	Tamoxifen, Medroxyprogesterone
Prostaglandins E1, E2	Aspirin
Interleukin 8	Interferon, Severe Infection
Vascular endothelial growth factor	Methotrexate, Bleomycin
Transforming Growth Factor-B	Mitoxantrone, Bisantrene
Angiotensis II	Retinoids, Vitamin D3 analogs
Plasminogen activator	Hyperthermia, Radiation Therapy
Substance P, Fibroblast growth factor	Minocycline, Suramin

Existing blood vessels that are near the small group of cancer cells are stimulated by TAF to produce and send to the cancer cells small new blood vessels, capillaries that penetrate the cancer. These newly formed blood vessels feed the cancer with oxygen and nutrients, and, in addition, remove wastes. Now the cancer grows rapidly and becomes pink because it is being fed, oxygenated, and its wastes are removed.

Cancers can generally be detected by our technology only when they are the size of about a centimeter (half inch) diameter sphere or more (one cubic centimeter). This small spherical mass contains about one billion cancer cells.

Angiogenesis and Metastasis

As the vascularized cancer grows, it invades and destroys local tissues as well as more distant sites in the body. For a cancer to metastasize or spread to other parts of the body, it must first invade the local tissue and then the bloodstream, and finally land in a distant organ and begin the process of growth and angiogenesis all over again at that site. Cancer cells manufacture a complex series of enzymes and other proteins necessary to accomplish all this.[4,5]

Angiogenesis is an integral part of the ability of the cancer cells to gain access to the bloodstream initially and then flourish in distant organs. In fact, many studies have shown that if angiogenesis does not occur, the cancer cannot metastasize.[6]

This leads to a very important fact. **When a cancer is large enough to be detected in the primary site, as with mammography, it has already developed angiogenesis and hence its cells have already spread to other organs.** The colonies in these distant organs are usually not large enough to be detected but are capable of growth and angiogenesis.[7]

A high number of blood vessels in the cancer as seen under the microscope, correlates well with a high likelihood of spread to other organs at the time of biopsy, especially breast cancer, prostate cancer, lung cancer, and melanoma.[8-12]

Angiogenesis and Leukemias

Until recently, scientists thought that angiogenesis only played a role in the growth and spread of solid cancers like breast, prostate, colon and rectal, uterus, and many others. Now it seems likely that leukemias also depend upon angiogenesis for growth. Patients with leukemia had high urine levels of an inducer of angiogenesis, and as the leukemia was successfully treated, these urine levels fell to normal.[13]

Age Alters Angiogenesis

Usually, young people have more aggressive cancers compared to older people because they have a greater and more rapid angiogenic response.[14] Also, older animals are unable to efficiently support the growth of the new blood vessels once the process started.

Severe Infection Inhibits Angiogenesis

Observation in humans and animals suggests that severe infection inhibits angiogenesis and thereby shrinks cancer.[15]

Steady State for Normal Blood Vessels

The vascular system in humans is designed to remain quite dormant for relatively long periods of time – weeks in women and decades in men.[16] The creation of new blood vessels occurs regularly every month as part of the menstrual cycle and also during the time of pregnancy. The placenta (tube connecting the fetus to the mother) manufactures a protein called placental proliferin that stimulates angiogenesis. This ensures that the fetus will be fed. And after a while, since *new* blood vessels are no longer needed because the existing blood vessels are adequate, the placenta manufactures another protein to inhibit angiogensis, called proliferin-related protein.[17] Men, however, do not have a need for new blood vessel formation regularly.

Emily decided to take one 325 mg aspirin every day to help prevent angiogenesis.

22

Establishing the Diagnosis and Stage

Sue's History

While caring for her husband with prostate cancer and her mentally handicapped son, Sue came to see me for routine examination. I found no breast lumps but only a dime-size area of the breast skin that did not feel just right – it felt a little leathery. Mammogram and ultrasound were negative. She wanted to stop there. I did not. With great reluctance, she and her husband came with me to a competent breast surgeon who did not want to perform a needle aspiration. At my insistence, and to the grumbling of all, it was done and was found to be nondiagnostic. All wanted to end the investigation there – all but me. I almost had to find another surgeon. Medically there was no reason to proceed. To make a long story short, the biopsy was positive and she did well with conservative management. The bottom line – if you have a good reason to pursue a work-up despite initial negative findings and attitudes, keep pushing.

If you feel a lump, generally, your doctor will recommend that you observe the lump through one menstrual cycle and if it reduces by day four or five of menses, it is usually a benign cyst. If it does not reduce in size, see your physician.

A pathologist establishes the diagnosis of breast cancer after examining breast tissue under the microscope. Then other factors must be assessed: sentinel or axillary lymph nodes, tumor size, estrogen and progesterone receptors, and several others. The next step is to determine the "stage," i.e., find out with our limited technology if the cancer is confined to the breast or has already **noticeably** spread. All this information is used to predict prognosis and determine treatment options.

PROCEDURES

■ **NEEDLE ASPIRATION** can be performed on any breast mass without local anesthesia in a physician's office; a mammogram is not necessarily done first.

A cyst can be silent or painful and, depending upon the amount of fluid within the cyst, it can either be soft and fluctuant with low pressure and a low amount of fluid, or tense and-hard and may feel like a solid mass if it is completely filled with fluid. If the palpable mass is cystic and needle aspiration removes fluid from it, the cyst will collapse. This generally precludes the diagnosis of cancer and biopsy is not required.

If the cysts are relatively new, the fluid that they contain is thin and straw-colored. If the cysts are older, the fluid may be thicker and darker in color, from brown to greyish green.[1] Unless the fluid is bloody, there is no value in sending it to the laboratory for analysis.[2,3] There is no evidence to suggest that analysis of breast cyst fluid could accurately predict the development of future breast cancer.[4] If a cyst recurs, it may simply be aspirated again if indicated. About 20 percent of simple cysts will refill and less than 9 percent will refill after two or three aspirations. Repeated aspirations do not increase the risk of future cancer or cause tumor cells from the aspirated mass to track along the needle tunnel.[5,6] One should be suspicious of an intracystic carcinoma or another type of cancer within the cyst if the aspiration contains blood, or if a palpable mass remains when all the fluid is withdrawn, or if the cyst repeatedly refills, or if a mammographic density persists.

Aspiration of a solid mass is done by inserting the needle into the mass and applying more backward pressure on the plunger of the syringe. A core biopsy is thus obtained through the needle. However, the range of false negatives (anywhere from 1 to 35 percent) and false positives (up to 18 percent) is high and must be kept in mind when a report comes back. If, however, the result is read as "nondiagnostic" and the mass is still present, then an open biopsy must be performed.

■ **INCISIONAL BIOPSY** is the removal of a portion of a mass that is either too large to be totally removed or is done when the patient is inoperable.

■ **EXCISIONAL BIOPSY** is the removal of the entire mass. If the mass is near the areola, then an areolar incision may be made and tunneled down to the mass. If, however, the mass is located more in the periphery of the breast, a curvilinear (Langer's lines) incision should be made, as part of a small segment of a concentric circle around the breast. A radial incision, which would look like part of a spoke of a wheel, should not be used because it causes a poor cosmetic outcome. It is important that a small drain be put in any excisional biopsy to avoid the accumulation of a large amount of blood and hematoma that can cause scar tissue, possible dissemination of cancer cells that are left behind, and poor cosmesis. The drain used can be as small as a small rubber band. Many physicians do not put in a drain and I have seen it take weeks for a large hematoma to resolve that, ultimately, produces poor cosmetic outcome. Margins of the removed specimen should be marked so that the pathologist may determine where tumor has been left behind in the breast, if at all. Excellent surgeons inadvertently leave cancer cells in the breast about 33 percent of the time, requiring re-excision.

■ **BIOPSY OF NONPALPABLE LESIONS** detected by mammogram should be done when there is (are):[8,9]

- The presence of a solitary mass, especially if spiculated or margins not well defined.
- The presence of a specific mass that is significantly different in size or contour compared to the others in the breast.
- Microcalcification clusters.
- Calcifications in or adjacent to a nonpalpable mass.
- A distorted area of breast tissue that is not seen in the other breast mammographically.

About 70-80 percent of all lesions removed are benign. However, when a patient hears that there is a suspected lesion on the mammogram, her immediate reaction (and her attorney's reaction) is to have the lesion removed. But, if the mammographic findings are "soft," it would be prudent to delay biopsy until another mammogram is obtained four to six months thereafter. By waiting, the woman can avoid a biopsy and scar tissue and still not jeopardize her medical situation. And, in fact, surgical scars that result from breast biopsies can give rise to breast cancers.[10]

■ **DELAY IN DIAGNOSIS BY FOUR TO SIX MONTHS DOES NOT AFFECT LIFESPAN** when mammographic findings are ambiguous or equivocal (soft) and a cancer is later proved.[11-14] However, the news media, consumer groups, cancer charities, and ultimately the attorneys, force immediate biopsy. There has been no change in lifespan for breast cancer since 1930, which means everything that we have done to date – screening programs, early detection, chemotherapy, radiation therapy, surgical techniques – has done nothing to increase the survival of any patient with breast cancer. So waiting four to six months to repeat a mammogram to ascertain whether an equivocal mammographic lesion has progressed, represents little or no time at all and, in fact, has no impact on survival. It takes about 4 to 6 months for a change to be seen on mammogram.

No mammogram should be thrown away, patients should always hand carry films to physicians, and serial mammograms should be done using similar equipment.

Breast biopsies are not emergencies. However, once a biopsy has been recommended and a woman has made the decision to go ahead with the biopsy, somehow, emotionally, it has to be done yesterday. But waiting two or three weeks has absolutely no effect on the ultimate outcome. And a biopsy for a nonpalpable lesion requires scheduling and planning. It is localized using a needle in the breast, which is guided by mammographic films. Then the patient is taken to the surgical suite so the surgeon can make an incision by following the needle to the lesion identified. If the lesion is composed of calcifications, the excised tissue is X-rayed to ensure that all calcifications are removed. A frozen section is not indicated in this procedure. The biopsy site is closed using a drain. No sutures are placed in the breast; sutures are to close the skin only. About 20 to 30 percent of nonpalpable lesions as shown on mammography turn out to be cancer.[8,12] Once the diagnosis of cancer is established, the patient and family review the options with her physician.

DETERMINE IF CANCER HAS SPREAD

A chest X-ray, bone scan, and liver function tests are necessary. Clinical examination of the axilla prior to biopsy may be negative, but one-third of these cases ultimately will be shown to have cancer in the lymph nodes. If the clinical examination and the blood tests of the liver are normal, it is unlikely that there are liver metastases (less than 1%). If any one of the above tests is positive, the tumor has metastasized from the breast to another organ, and the work-up is stopped. There is no need for surgical intervention other than the initial biopsy, and the patient can then be considered for systemic and/or local treatment. If the metastatic workup is negative, a radiation oncologist should see the patient to determine if she is eligible for radiation therapy before any further surgery is done.

PATHOLOGY – MICROSCOPIC CLASSIFICATION as per the Armed Forces Institute of Pathology and the World Health Organization. There are two groupings of breast cancer, one that invades tissue (invasive or infiltrating), and one that does not (*in situ*).

CARCINOMA *IN SITU* (NON-INVASIVE)

These cancer cells are localized to one site and this *in situ* cancer has an eight- to tenfold risk of developing a subsequent invasive cancer. It may involve the ducts or the lobules.

■ **Ductal carcinoma *in situ* (DCIS)** – is a group of cancer cells localized in the breast duct. However, when these patients have a mastectomy, 60% of their disease is ductal carcinoma *in* *situ*, and 15-25% is invasive cancer. With more mammograms being done, more ductal carcinomas *in situ* cases are found.

Clinical Presentation. More than half have a palpable breast lump and some women have Paget's disease of the nipple, or a bloody nipple discharge.

Pathological Types

- Comedo carcinoma – produces firm masses.
- Ductal carcinoma *in situ.*
- Predominant intraductal with an invasive component.
- Papillary
- Tubular
- Mucinous (colloid)
- Medullary with lymphocytic infiltrate

Prognosis. About 15-20% develop a local recurrence in five years; about 50% of these will develop invasive breast cancers.

Treatment. In the past, most patients were treated with mastectomy. But because tumor recurrence or death occurred in only about 1 percent of these patients, a more conservative approach was instituted – excisional lumpectomy, axillary node dissection, and then radiation therapy. Mastectomy is still indicated if there are two or more sites of disease in the breast or diffuse microcalcifications throughout the breast.

Ductal carcinoma *in situ* is unlikely to recur if completely excised. Margin width is the distance between the boundary of the cancer and the edge of the excised specimen. **If the margin around the tumor is at least 10 millimeters or more in each direction, the risk of a local breast recurrence is very low and there is no need for postoperative radiation therapy.**[15] More surgery should be done if the margin is less than 10 mm. If the margin is less than 1 millimeter despite additional surgeries, postoperative radiation treatment should be given.

■ **Lobular Carcinoma *In Situ*** never forms a palpable mass and is considered a premalignant process. It is found primarily in premenopausal women and may involve multiple areas of the same breast. Lobular carcinoma *in situ* is found 25% of the time if a mirror image biopsy is performed in the other breast. Calcifications are rarely seen on mammograms.

Pathological Type **–** only lobular carcinoma *in situ.*

Prognosis. About 20-25% of all patients who have an initial diagnosis of lobular carcinoma *in situ* will develop an invasive cancer in one or both breasts after 25 years. The second cancer is usually ductal carcinoma *in situ*, invasive ductal carcinoma, or both. The risk for progression to an invasive cancer from lobular carcinoma *in situ* is about 1% per year, and from ductal carcinoma *in situ*, about 2% to 3% per year.
Treatment – three options: (1) Careful and close observation. (2) Mastectomy with biopsy of the opposite breast. (3) Bilateral mastectomies should never be considered unless the patient is extremely uncomfortable about having a higher risk for developing a cancer in the future. There seems to be no role for radiation therapy in the management of this disease. Just one final note: Remember this diagnosis is an incidental finding when a breast biopsy is done for another reason entirely since nothing on a mammogram can reveal a lobular carcinoma *in situ.*

■ **Paget's Disease** is an *in situ* cancer of the nipple that may be associated with a noninvasive or invasive breast cancer.
Clinical Presentation is usually redness, crusting, discharge, or eczemoid changes of the nipple. Over 50 percent of the cases may have a palpable breast mass as well.
Pathological Types - Only Paget's disease.
Prognosis The five-year survival data: nipple involvement 85%; nipple involvement + postive lymph nodes 46%; breast mass only 68%; and breast mass + positive lymph nodes 22%.
Treatment – breast-conserving surgery with or without radiation therapy.

■ **Cystosarcoma Phyllodes** is a rare breast disease that is generally benign and does not spread to lymph nodes. However, about 25 percent of these cases are malignant.
Presentation – a large and bulky mass that is smooth, multinodular, and rounded. It can grow rapidly to a very large size. Prominent veins appear on the breast's skin surface.
Pathological Types – benign or malignant.
Prognosis. Local recurrence is 20% for benign cystosarcoma phyllodes because it was not completely removed initially. One-

half of patients with recurrences have aggressive metastasis to the chest wall and chest cavity. Local recurrence is 8% for malignant cystosarcoma phyllodes because it is treated aggressively from the outset. About 15% of patients have positive lymph nodes. Spread to lungs and bone occurs in 66% and 28% of cases, respectively. The average survival time is thirty months for all cases. The longest survival time recorded for someone with metastatic disease is 14.5 years.

Treatment – very wide excision or mastectomy cures most patients unless the surgical margins are positive – then the risk of a local recurrence or metastases is high.

INVASIVE CANCERS

■ **Invasive or Infiltrating Ductal Carcinoma** – 80% of all breast cancers. The terms invasive and infiltrating are synonymous. These cancers are quite hard and commonly metastasize to the axillary lymph nodes. Women generally present with a thickening or a swelling in the breast. Invasive lobular carcinoma accounts for only about 5 to 10 percent of all invasive carcinomas. However, both invasive lobular and ductal cancers have similar prognoses. Invasive ductal carcinoma metastasizes more frequently to bone or other organs like lung, liver, and brain but lobular invasive carcinomas metastasize mainly to the surfaces of organs.

■ **Tubular Invasive Carcinoma** – 2% of all breast cancers. Patients present with a small palpable breast mass and skin retraction or fixation in about 15% of the cases. Tubular invasive carcinoma has a better prognosis than invasive ductal carcinoma. Metastasis to the axilla is quite rare. Two treatment options: (1) mastectomy; or (2) excisional lumpectomy, axillary node sampling, and radiation therapy. Local recurrences – less than 5% of patients. Metastatic disease outside the breast region – only a few patients have been reported.

■ **Medullary Carcinoma** – 5 to 7% of all breast cancers, grows rapidly, but generally has an excellent prognosis unless it is atypical. Sixty percent of patients who have medullary carcinoma are younger than fifty.

■ **Mucinous or Colloid** Carcinoma – 3% of all breast cancers. They are slow growing and become bulky masses that the patient finds. A woman may also have nipple discharge, fixation, and skin ulceration. Prognosis is also more favorable than for an invasive ductal carcinoma.

■ **Inflammatory Carcinoma** is a diagnosis made when the physician clinically observes and examines the breast. The breast, or some portion of it, is red, warm and the skin has ridges appearing pitted because of its edema and swelling – called *peau d'orange.* There may or may not be a palpable breast mass. This condition is often mistaken for an infection and may initially be treated as such by physicians. To reiterate, this is a clinical diagnosis and a biopsy will support the diagnosis if there are cancer cells in the small lymphatic channels of the skin. The signs and symptoms of inflammatory breast carcinoma are actually due to the cancer invading these lymphatic channels in the skin or to capillary congestion.

Inflammatory breast carcinoma has the poorest survival of all the breast cancers. When various modalities are combined – chemotherapy first, then preoperative radiation therapy, then mastectomy, and then maintenance chemotherapy – a 25-40% five-year survival rate is obtained.

There are other very rare invasive breast cancers that include: papillary carcinoma, metaplastic carcinoma, apocrine carcinoma, adenoid cystic carcinoma, squamous carcinoma, secretory carcinoma, and several others.

PROGNOSTIC FACTORS (FACTORS THAT PREDICT OUTCOME) and the extent of disease (stage) determine the patient's treatment options and prognosis. We know, however, that by the time we can actually detect a breast cancer, tumor cells have already spread to other parts of the body through the bloodstream.

■ **Cancer Size** is one of the most important prognostic factors, especially in patients who have negative lymph nodes. The larger the size of the cancer, the lower is the survival. Ninety-nine percent of women live 5 years if their cancer is less than 1 cm; 85% are alive at 5 years if their cancer is 3 cm.

Best Prognosis: Less than 1 cm cancer diameter.

■ **Sentinel/Axillary Lymph Node Status.** Eighty-five percent of patients who have negative lymph nodes live at least five years compared to less than 40% who have four or more positive lymph nodes. However, about 30% of all patients with negative lymph nodes will have a recurrence and die of their disease. So other factors are important as well.

Best Prognosis: Negative lymph nodes

■ **Pathological Classification.** When the size of the tumor is combined with the unique pathological type, a decision to treat or not to treat with systemic therapy in patients with negative lymph nodes is clear-cut. For instance, approximately 25% of all patients who have tumors less than 1 cm or whose tumor is either ductal carcinoma *in situ*, pure tubular carcinoma, papillary carcinoma, or typical medullary carcinoma have recurrence rates ranging from 1-10%. There is no need to use systemic therapy in these patients as determined by the National Institutes of Health Breast Cancer Consensus Conference of 1990. Patients whose tumors are larger than 3 cm have a recurrence rate greater than 50 percent and systemic therapy is generally given. The majority of the patients (50 percent) have tumors ranging from 1-3 cm in size with recurrence rates, generally, of 30 percent. And the majority of these patients are "cured" without ever having any systemic therapy. Other prognostic factors help the clinician decide whether systemic therapy in patients with negative lymph nodes should be given or not.

Best Prognosis: Ductal carcinoma *in situ,* Tubular carcinoma, Papillary carcinoma, or Medullary carcinoma.

■ **Histological or Nuclear Grade** – determines aggressiveness. Grade 3 affords the worst prognosis.

Best Prognosis: Grade 1.

■ **Breast Lymphatic Vessel Cancer Invasion** heralds a very high recurrence rate and eventual death from the disease.

Best Prognosis: No cancer cells in breast lymphatics.

■ **Breast Blood Vessel Cancer Invasion** heralds a very high recurrence rate and eventual death from the disease.

Best Prognosis: No cancer cells in breast blood vessels.

■ **Estrogen Receptor (ER), Progesterone Receptor (PR)** Generally, but not always, patients with estrogen receptor negative tumors have a higher rate of recurrence independent of nodal status or size of tumor. A positive progesterone receptor predicts the time of recurrence for patients who have positive lymph nodes. However, estrogen status and tumor size are the most important factors to predict disease-free survival in patients with negative lymph nodes. False negative receptor status occurs if: (1) The breast specimen is not frozen within 15 minutes; (2) The breast specimen is not large enough to be tested; (3) The body has mounted a defensive reaction of normal cancer-fighting cells around the cancer thereby decreasing the number of cancer cells in the specimen; (4) The cancer is *in situ*; (5) The patient is taking exogenous hormones (pills) or producing enough estrogen in her body to bind the available receptor sites so they cannot be detected in the lab assay.

Best Prognosis: Positive estrogen and progesterone recep tors (greater than 15 femtomoles/mg)

■ **Ploidy and S-Phase Fraction** determines aggressiveness of cancer cells. Cancer cells with the normal amount of DNA are called diploid. An abnormally high DNA content is called aneuploidy, and the prognosis is usually poor. Aneuploidy is seen in about 60-70% of all early breast cancer patients. The S-phase fraction, which denotes how quickly the cells turn over, is a more important prognostic factor to determine survival than ploidy status or nuclear grading. The higher the S-phase number, the more aggressive the cancer cells are, and the more likely the patient is to have recurrent disease and die earlier. In other words, patients who have fast-growing tumors have more frequent events and earlier death. A high S-phase fraction is also linked to a high expression of certain oncogenes and the loss of the p53 tumor suppressor gene. This also may be one of the reasons the high S-phase fraction can predict early recurrence and earlier death.

Best Prognosis: Diploid status; DNA index =1.0; S-phase < 7%.

■ **HER-2 neu** is related to the family of epidermal growth factor receptors. A mutation causes more of the NEU receptors and proteins that cause a progression of breast cancer.

■ **Cathepsin D** is an enzyme that is higher in amount than normal for breast cancer patients. A high level is correlated with a high recurrence rate and death. Breast cancer patients who have negative lymph nodes in the axilla but whose tumors are aneuploid and have high levels of Cathepsin D have a recurrence rate of 60 percent in five years.

Best Prognosis: Low Cathepsin level (<50 units)

■ **Other Potential Prognostic Factors** include: pS2, Ki-67, epidermal growth factor receptor, stress proteins, NM23, plasminogen activators, markers of angiogenesis, and many others. Ki-67 is specific for all aggressive cells in a cancer.

■ **Circulating Tumor Markers** include CEA (carcinogenic embryonic antigen), LSA (lipid associated sialic acid), CA 15-3, and others. They often don't correlate very well with the clinical status of the patient. Sometimes these tests are negative or low when there is obvious cancer in the patient. And sometimes when the patient is perfectly healthy, these tests may be elevated, which forces "million dollar work-ups" searching for a cancer recurrence that may or may not be present.

STAGING OF BREAST CANCER is done after a biopsy to determine whether the cancer has spread to other parts of the body. Treatment and prognosis are determined by the stage of the patient.

■ **Carcinoma *in situ*** is an early form of breast cancer that accounts for about 5-10% of all breast cancers. These are found only in the one area of the breast tissue without spreading to adjacent structures.

■ **Stage I** – the cancer diameter is 2 cm or less and has not spread outside the breast.

■ **Stage II**

- Cancer diameter is 2 cm or less and has spread into the axillary lymph nodes; or
- Cancer diameter is between 2 and 5 cm, and the cancer has either spread to the axillary lymph nodes or not; or
- The cancer diameter is larger than 5 cm but not spread to the axillary lymph nodes.

■ **Stage III**

- Stage IIIA – the cancer is less than 5 cm and has spread into the axillary lymph nodes that have grown into each other or into other attached structures; or cancer diameter is larger than 5 cm and spread into the axillary lymph nodes.
- Stage IIIB – the cancer from the breast has spread into nearby structures like the chest wall (ribs and muscles); or, the cancer has spread to lymph nodes near the collar bone.

■ **Stage IV** – the cancer has spread to other organs of the body that may include the bones, lungs, liver, or brain, etc.

Inflammatory Breast Cancer This classification has already been discussed and is considered inoperable initially.

CONCLUSION

Now that you have all the information about your cancer including tissue type, nodal status, prognostic factors, extent or stage of disease, you can explore the best treatment options available for your case.

Sue had a Stage II invasive breast cancer with excellent prognostic factors. She modified her lifestyle according to the Ten Point Plan to improve and extend her life.

23

Localized Treatment Options for Breast Cancer

Judy's History

Judy just found out she had breast cancer. She wanted to preserve her breast, make sure the cosmetic outcome of her breast was good, and at the same time, not jeopardize her lifespan.

Once the diagnosis of invasive breast cancer has been made, treatments are considered. Localized treatment is intended to eradicate cancer in the breast itself and adjacent structures, like lymph nodes. Breast cancer spreads by way of lymph node channels and also by way of the bloodstream to almost any site in the body. This is why systemic treatment is considered as well (Chapter 24).

Radical mastectomies were the norm until 1970, then modified radical mastectomies, and finally, lumpectomies and axillary node dissection/sentinel node biopsies. Let's define terms:

- **Radical mastectomy** (almost never done) – removal of the entire breast, chest wall muscles and its coverings, and all axillary lymph nodes. The patient has a flattened chest wall.
- **Modified radical mastectomy** – removal of the entire breast, some of the axillary lymph nodes, the lining over the chest muscles, and usually a small muscle of the chest wall.
- **Total mastectomy** – removal of the entire breast plus the cover of the chest wall muscle but not the muscle itself. No lymph nodes are removed.

- **Lumpectomy** – removal of the breast mass with margin of tissue around it.
- **Axillary node dissection** – removal of the nodes from underneath the arm, the area called the axilla.
- **Sentinel Lymph node biopsy** – removal of one or a few nodes that first drain the breast identified by injecting blue dye or radioisotope. Sentinel lymph node biopsy reliably predicts axillary node status in 98% of all patients and 95% of those who are node-positive.

Since 1930 the lifespan of a breast cancer patient has not changed. And over the last 100 years, the results are not improved when more aggressive surgery is done, like radical mastectomy. Lumpectomy is as effective with regard to outcome. Axillary lymph node dissection had been done to determine prognosis, provide local control, and plan treatment – not as an attempt to cure the patient. A negative sentinel node biopsy has a 95-100% likelihood of correlating with negative axillary nodes. It is now fashionable to do a sentinel node biopsy rather than axillary node dissection/sampling even though it is technically difficult. PET scanning might help determine whether the lymph nodes are involved with cancer or not and, hence, obviate the need for any surgical nodal evaluation. However, the **breast tissue itself provides all the information needed to determine prognosis and treatment options, whether nodes are positive or negative.**

MASTECTOMY, OR RADIATION TO KEEP BREAST?

Once the diagnosis of breast cancer is made, the entire breast must be treated to decrease the risk of other non-detectable cancers from growing. That's done either by removing the breast, or using radiation to treat the intact breast if suited.

CONTRAINDICATIONS FOR BREAST CONSERVATION

Radiation treats the entire breast and preserves the cosmetic appearance of the breast – critically important. There is no role for conservative management of the breast if the patient ends up with a mound of tissue on her chest wall rather than having a cosmetically pleasing outcome. Contraindications include:

• Breast cancer greater than 5 cm; however, patients who have larger breasts and who have lesions larger than 5 cm may be adequately treated if the ultimate cosmetic outcome is acceptable to the patient.[3]

• More than one cancer in breast as shown on mammogram.

• Multiple positive surgical margins despite re-excision.

• A predicted poor cosmetic outcome – small breast with very large cancer that when removed will leave a large defect in the modest-sized breast; or patients who have collagen vascular diseases such as scleroderma or lupus.

• Clinical inspection of the axilla before axillary node dissection that reveals lymph nodes matted onto each other.

LUMPECTOMY + RADIATION THERAPY IS AS EFFECTIVE AS MASTECTOMY FOR LOCAL CONTROL AND OVERALL LIFESPAN, AND PROVIDES GOOD COSMESIS. [4-14]

ABOUT 2 CM OF HEALTHY BREAST TISSUE AROUND THE CANCER SHOULD BE REMOVED – MORE REMOVAL YIELDS POOR COSMETIC OUTCOME, [15,16] does not extend life and defeats the purpose of conservation for cosmesis.

It must be noted that separate incisions have to be made for performing the lumpectomy and for performing the axillary node dissection. This enhances the functional and cosmetic outcome, and also prevents contamination by cancer cells from one field into the other.

RADIATION DOSE: ENTIRE BREAST RECEIVES 45-50 GY AT 1.8 GY PER DAY; CANCER BED RECEIVES 10-15 GY (BOOST) using electrons from radiation machine, or from an implant using radioactive seeds placed in the breast itself. These seeds are removed after a certain period of time that has been calculated to deliver a certain dose. No radiation is given to the axillary nodes if they are negative.

RADIATION DECREASES BREAST RECURRENCE RATE TO 10% COMPARED TO 40% IF YOU JUST HAD LUMPECTOMY.

AXILLARY NODES DO NOT HAVE TO BE REMOVED because they do not influence lifespan or the need for systemic treatment. Systemic therapy is recommended for patients who have the following factors known at the time of lumpectomy: positive estrogen receptor in a postmenopausal woman, aneuploidy, high S-phase fraction, high Cathepsin D level, a large-size tumor, and multiple microvessels in one microscopic field.[17]

SYSTEMIC TREATMENT IS SOMETIMES GIVEN BEFORE SURGERY TO SHRINK A LARGE BREAST CANCER.

THE PHASE OF THE MENSTRUAL CYCLE AT THE TIME OF SURGERY DOES NOT INFLUENCE SURVIVAL.[18]

BREAST CONSERVING SURGERY IS NOT IN WIDESPREAD USE except in the northeastern states where physicians are required by law to disclose all options.[19,20] The way information is presented to a patient can influence her decision: "If it were my wife, if it were my mother. . ." Younger women are offered breast-conserving surgery more often than older women.[21] Also, because patients are not properly educated, there is a belief among them that if you remove the breast, you remove the problem forever. That is simply not true. The chance of recurrence and length of life is the same for the two procedures.

There may also be financial considerations – charges for breast-conserving surgery, i.e., lumpectomy, axillary node dissection is about 60 percent of the $7000 cost of mastectomy. When radiation therapy costs are added to costs for breast-conserving surgery, the total costs can be up to $28,000.

THE CHEST WALL SHOULD BE TREATED WITH RADIATION WITHIN WEEKS OF MASTECTOMY IF:

- Breast cancer diameter is greater than 5 cm.
- Four or more positive axillary lymph nodes.
- The breast cancer mass was very close to the chest wall.

Once there is a chest wall recurrence, treatment is of little help. Surgical excision should be done but recurrence may come again. Chemotherapy does not help. Radiation controls only about half of those treated. When radiation is combined with surgical or chemotherapy for the recurrence, the control rate does not improve. Once a chest wall recurrence grows, other symptoms ensue such as ulceration, bleeding, odor, pain, and weeping from the cancerous wound. If the breast cancer recurs in one of the lymph node regions, local treatment is not effective and growth of the cancer there may lead to involvement of nerves, pain, and swelling of the arm in addition to erosion, and ulceration.

BREAST RECONSTRUCTION AFTER MASTECTOMY is an option for those who: (1) were not suitable candidates for breast conservation; or, (2) desire a reconstruction several years after having had a mastectomy. The most common way of doing a reconstruction consists of either inserting an implant or transferring a flap of tissue containing muscle and skin from another site of the body. To improve the cosmetic outcome, a nipple and areola may be reconstructed or tattooed on the skin. Also, the opposite breast may need to be changed to make it symmetrical with the reconstructed one.

WHEN IS THE BEST TIME TO RECONSTRUCT A BREAST? If reconstruction is done immediately, patients feel "whole" and this decreases anxiety and depression. But there is a down-side to immediate reconstruction. If a breast cancer recurs at all on the chest wall, it usually does so within the first two years of initial diagnosis. A reconstructed flap or implant makes it more difficult to detect a recurrence by physical examination and by mammographic means. Given this problem, many physicians recommend waiting two years for reconstruction.

PROPHYLACTIC MASTECTOMY if done at all, must be done completely to avoid any residual breast tissue. Pectoral fascia, the nipple-areola complex, the axillary tail, and a sample of the lower axillary lymph nodes must be removed, otherwise the patient will be left with the same risk.

Patients with BRAC 1 or BRAC 2 who don't have breast cancer or ovarian cancer live from 2.9 to 5.3 years longer if they have prophylactic mastectomies, or from 0.3 to 1.7 years for prophylactic oopherectomies. All other high-risk patients do not benefit from prophylactic mastectomies. Instead of prophylactic mastectomy, a patient at high risk must follow a healthy lifestyle, be examined by a physician twice a year, and get a mammogram, depending on the indications.

SIDE EFFECTS OF SURGERY AND RADIATION

• **HEMATOMA** (blood), **SEROMA** (fluid in a sac), **INFECTION**.

• **SKIN DESQUAMATION**, dry or moist – like a sunburn reaction, during the third or fourth week of radiation therapy may occur, particularly underneath a large breast. Since the bra rubs against the skin and acts as sandpaper, the use of a bra should be minimized or eliminated during this time. Patients should use aloe vera gel, not aloe vera cream, three or four times a day during radiation therapy. Patients are often told by radiation oncologists not to put anything on the skin because they are concerned that the dose delivered might be higher if something thick is placed on the skin. A gel however, which gets into the skin very rapidly, does not have this effect and, in fact, will protect the skin. Certain antioxidants also protect the skin.

• **FATIGUE** is not due to radiation *per se*, but mainly to the fact that: (1) Patients have been told they may experience fatigue during radiation; (2) They travel to and from the radiation therapy unit daily, five days a week; (3) They have anxiety and depression associated with their newly diagnosed cancer and with seeing physically ill patients who have advanced cancers.

• **POOR COSMESIS** and higher risk of **PNEUMONITIS** is seen when adriamycin or methotrexate chemotherapy are given concurrently with radiation.

• **RIB FRACTURE OR PNEUMONITIS** may occur in 1% or 2% of people treated with radiation. The pneumonitis may manifest with low-grade fever, shortness of breath, and sometimes a cough. In less than 5% of the patients, a chest X-ray may reveal fibrosis in the region of the lung that was partially treated underneath the breast. This will not be a clinical problem.

• **ARM EDEMA** is found in 8-10% of all the women treated with axillary node dissection, chemotherapy, and radiation therapy. This is generally related to how vigorous the surgical procedure had been as well as concurrent use of chemotherapy and radiation therapy. The arm swelling can be relieved temporarily with a compression sleeve and sometimes physical therapy.

• **MONDOR'S SYNDROME – THROMBOPHLEBITIS OF AXILLARY OR BREAST VEINS** can develop in the axillary vein (vein in armpit) or a superficial vein on the intact breast surface approximately two to four weeks after a biopsy, axillary node dissection, or mastectomy. This condition is not common; hence, it is often not recognized or treated. This causes severe pain and limits the arm motion. Proper treatment includes one aspirin daily and warm moist compresses (not dry heat) applied to the inflamed venous cord three to four times daily for twenty minutes at a time. Be careful not to burn your skin.

• **SECOND MALIGNANCY RISK** to breast(s) or chest wall is higher if radiation is combined with chemotherapy.

• **PAIN SYNDROME** can manifest itself months or years after mastectomy. The pain is quite real and treatable. The physicians (surgeon, oncologist, or primary care physician) don't often recognize this syndrome. Pain is often described as radiating, shooting, burning, sharp, or constricting, and occurs about 5-10% of postmastectomy and lumpectomy patients. Pain can be effectively treated with a variety of analgesics, or if severe, a TENS (transcutaneous electrical nerve stimulation) unit.[22]

HYPERTHERMIA, temperatures above 41-42C° (approximately 106F°) for a certain length of time, has a direct killing effect on both normal and tumor cells. Heat can sometimes kill cells that would otherwise resist the effects of radiation. High temperatures can also potentiate a variety of chemotherapeutic drugs like bleomycin, cisplatin, cyclophosphamide, melphalan, mitomycin C, and nitrosoureas.

Hyperthermia is effective for small and superficial cancers that can be implanted with heating elements. Recurrent breast cancer on the chest wall is an ideal setting for the use of hyperthermia and radiation therapy. When the two are combined, tumor masses decrease dramatically. The problem, however, has been technical difficulties in assuring adequate delivery of an even amount of heat for all the tissues. Only a few centers have efficiently performed hyperthermia because of these technical stumbling blocks.

CONCLUSION

Review this chapter with your own condition in mind. Next, turn to Chapter 24 to learn if you need systemic treatment.

Judy had options. She chose lumpectomy and radiation therapy, had an excellent cosmetic outcome, and modified her lifestyle to optimize her lifespan.

24
Conventional Systemic Treatment for Breast Cancer

Elizabeth's History

Elizabeth is a menstruating mother of two and needs systemic treatment for breast cancer. She already had lumpectomy, sentinel node sampling and radiation to her left breast. The cosmetic outcome is very good. Can she improve her lifespan if she chooses chemotherapy, hormonal therapy, or a combination of both, and/or modifies her currently poor lifestyle?

The medical profession had deluded itself for over a century in thinking that breast cancer was a surgical disease and the more tissue removed, the more women would be cured. We now realize that by the time a breast cancer is detected and then removed surgically, it has already disseminated to other parts of the body. Thus we turned our attention to systemic therapies that enter the bloodstream and travel throughout the body to theoretically kill cancer cells anywhere. Systemic therapy includes hormonal therapy, chemotherapy, treatment with biological response modifiers, and anti-angiogenic agents.

HORMONAL THERAPY kills cancer cells that depend upon hormones to grow. Estrogens are growth promoters for many cells including breast cancer. Breast cancer cells may have estrogen receptors that act as doorways for estrogen to enter the breast cancer cell and thereby feed it. About 50% of all breast cancers are estrogen receptor positive, which means they depend on estrogen to grow. If estrogen is unavailable, those cancer cells will die. Estrogen positive (ER+) cancers are seen in 30% of menstruating women, 60% of postmenopausal women and 20% of women entering menopause, perimenopausal. Those with ER+ cancers have a 50%-60% response to a hormonal treatment, and up to 20% of patients with estrogen negative receptors have a response to hormonal treatment.

- **If you change the hormonal milieu of the patient, you can expect to see a response.**
- **During the first few weeks of a hormonal treatment there may be a flare of pain in the areas of the body that have cancer – this indicates that the treatment is working.**
- **Patients who initially respond to a hormonal therapy and then become resistant may have continued disease regression if the therapy is abruptly stopped.**
- **Responses to hormonal therapy last 6-12 months or longer.**

■ **ORGAN REMOVAL** of both **ovaries** (castration) by surgery (oopherectomy – immediate depletion of estrogen) or by radiation treatment (20 Gy given over 3 days – gradual depletion of estrogen over 1-2 months) produces a 50-60% response for those who are estrogen receptor positive – that means 50-60% of the women will have cancer regression. All patients have a 30-40% response, regardless of estrogen receptor status. Metastasis to bone, soft tissue, lymph nodes, and lung generally respond to hormonal manipulation like castration, but metastasis to liver or brain rarely respond. **If a woman responds to one hormonal manipulation like castration, 40-50% of the time she will respond to another hormonal modality.** Patients who respond to hormonal manipulation generally live about two years longer than those who do not. Surgical removal of the **adrenal glands** or **pituitary gland**, independent of other procedures, produces about a 30-40% response. A drug, called aminogluthethimide, stops the production of hormones by the adrenal glands, including estrogens, and yields a 35-50% response.

■ Individual Hormone Therapy

• **Estrogen** at high doses (Premarin 10 mg three times a day) produces a 30% objective response lasting over a year, and when the estrogen receptor is positive, there is over a 50% response in some cases.[1,2] Patients who initially respond to this estrogen therapy and then become resistant may have continued disease regression if the therapy is abruptly stopped (30%), and then, a subsequent hormonal manipulation generally works. A large body of clinical evidence indicates that estrogen treatment is superior to all other hormonal therapies with respect to response rate, response duration, or survival.[3]

• **Androgens**, male hormones, produce a 20% response for all postmenopausal women with advanced breast cancer. There may be a brief response to androgens in premenopausal women if they had their ovaries removed. Mechanism is unknown.

• **Progesterone Agents**, like Megestrol (Megace), at 40 mg four times a day, exerts an antiestrogen effect and can produce remissions for about seven months in 30% of all patients.

• **Tamoxifen** is an antiestrogen that blocks the doorway, the estrogen receptor, to a cancer cell so that estrogen, which feeds the cell, may not enter. The usual daily dose is 20 mg. For patients who have bony metastasis, there is a flare of bone pain and a transient elevation of calcium during the first few weeks of treatment, indicating the drug is working. Tamoxifen produces about a 40% response rate, and this is slightly higher for postmenopausal women. Premenopausal women have a lesser response unless they have positive estrogen receptors, and then they can have up to about a 75% response. But castration seems to be superior to tamoxifen in premenopausal patients who have negative estrogen receptors. Tamoxifen is superior to androgen therapy and has largely replaced other individual hormones as well as adrenalectomy and hypophesectomy in postmenopausal women.

• **Other Antiestrogens– Inhibitors of Estrogen Synthesis (Aromatase Inhibitors like Arimidex, Femara)**. Arimidex is as effective as Megace. Responses range from 25% to 35% when the cancer is estrogen receptor negative.

■ **TREATMENT OF CHOICE FOR PREMENOPAUSAL OR PERIMENOPAUSAL PATIENTS WITH METASTATIC DISEASE IS HORMONAL:** Oopherectomy, tamoxifen, or hormones that stop the ovaries from functioning (LHRH agonists).[3] Responses range from 25% to 40%; and from 60% to 75% when the cancer is estrogen receptor positive. Premenstrual women with ER+ cancer have a worse prognosis and do even worse if they continue to menstruate after chemotherapy.

■ **HORMONAL TREATMENT FOR POSTMENOPAUSAL PATIENTS** is 20 mg of tamoxifen a day. Once tamoxifen stops producing a response, other hormonal agents can be used.

Ovarian ablation or tamoxifen or chemotherapy produce similar lifespans and similar recurrence rates regardless of your age, or whether you are menstruating or not, or whether your estrogen receptor is positive or negative, or whether your lymph nodes are positive or negative.[4-11]

CHEMOTHERAPY might be considered for rapidly progressive cancers, or rapidly progressive liver metastasis, or for inflammatory breast cancer, or for lymphangitic spread in the lungs. Combination chemotherapy came into being in the mid to late 60s and initially produced remarkable results in otherwise fatal and extremely rare tumors. The subspecialty of medical oncology was born. Since the 1970s in the United States, combination chemotherapy has been used for premenopausal and postmenopausal women with positive lymph nodes.

The following are the most commonly used combinations of drugs for breast cancer treatment: **CMF** (cyclophosphamide, methotrexate, 5-fluorouracil); **CAF** (cyclophosphamide, adriamycin, 5-fluorouracil); **CMFVP** (cyclophosphamide, methotrexate, 5-fluorouracil, vincristine, prednisone), and **taxol** combinations. Methotrexate, 5-fluorouracil, and adriamycin are given intravenously on days 1 and 8 of a 28 day cycle. Cyclophosphamide is given orally on days 1 through 14. CMF, CAF, CMFVP generally produce about a 50 percent response rate in almost all sites of breast cancer metastases including liver, bone, soft tissue, and other organs. The duration of response varies from 12-18 months, and the length of survival is between 24 and 30 months. When patients relapse after receiving combination chemotherapy, second-line chemotherapeutic agents are not very effective. A hormonal manipulation can be used in patients who have a recurrence of disease after combination chemotherapy.

Chemotherapy has little or no influence in diminishing the rate of bone or other organ metastases.[12,13] And no matter what combination of drugs is used, chemotherapy does not improve the survival rate (lifespan).

■ **CHEMOTHERAPY COMPARED TO HORMONAL THERAPY**

- Ovarian ablation is superior to chemotherapy in premenopausal women with ER+ cancers.[6,14,15]
- Ovarian ablation + tamoxifen is superior to chemotherapy.[16]
- Tamoxifen is superior to chemotherapy in node positive women 50 years old or older (lifespan is same).[17]

■ **HIGH DOSE CHEMOTHERAPY IS NOT MORE EFFECTIVE THAN CONVENTIONAL DOSE CHEMOTHERAPY.**[18-22] It produces a higher rate of death and many more side effects.

■ **CHEMOTHERAPY GIVEN BEFORE SURGERY OR IMMEDIATELY AFTER SURGERY OR WITHIN A FEW WEEKS OF SURGERY PRODUCES THE SAME OUTCOME.** [23-25]

■ **CHEMOTHERAPY GIVEN AT NIGHT IS IMPRACTICAL BUT MORE EFFECTIVE** because normal cells are best protected since they are in a repair mode and cancer cells are more vulnerable at night.[26-28]

ADJUVANT SYSTEMIC THERAPY FOR BREAST CANCER PATIENTS WITH POSTIVE NODES OR OTHER HIGH RISK PROGNOSTIC FACTORS. General conclusions can now be made:

- **LIFESPAN** – same for chemotherapy or hormonal therapy.

- **DISEASE-FREE INTERVAL** – period of time in which there are no disease events – longer in women who receive adjuvant systemic therapy.
- **OVARIAN ABLATION** is more effective in premenopausal women and perimenopausal.
- **OVARIAN ABLATION PRODUCES THE SAME LIFESPAN AND RECURRENCE RATES AS CHEMOTHERAPY** suggesting that the benefits of chemotherapy can be attributed to interfering with the hormones produced by ovaries.
- **TAMOXIFEN** is more effective in postmenopausal women and should be used for two or more years.
- **TAMOXIFEN ALONE IS AS EFFECTIVE AS TAMOXIFEN PLUS CHEMOTHERAPY** for lifespan and recurrences, and has less side effects and better quality of life.[29]
- **COMBINATION CHEMOTHERAPY** is better than single-agent and is more effective in premenopausal women than it is in postmenopausal women.
    - **There is no additional benefit in using chemotherapy for more than six months.**
    - **Continued menstruation after chemotherapy heralds a poor prognosis**
- **BIOLOGICAL RESPONSE MODIFIERS** or other immune system enhancers have shown no benefit.

In 1992, the Early Breast Cancer Trialists' Collaborative Group published a report involving 133 randomized trials with 75,000 women who had early breast cancer and received systemic treatments consisting of hormonal therapy, chemotherapy, or immunotherapy.[6] Analysis of these data revealed the overall survival benefit is quite small. For every 100 Stage II breast cancer women (positive axillary nodes) treated, about 12 women more than expected became 10-year survivors.

Adjuvant systemic therapy lowered the relative risk of death by about 25% meaning that the real benefit translates to about 4% for a person who actually has a 10-20% risk of dying from breast cancer in the first five years. Obviously, as her risk of dying from the cancer increases, i.e., if she has multiple high-risk prognostic factors that contribute to a poor prognosis, the real percent of benefit rises but only slightly.

Two-thirds of all the patients had benefit from receiving hormonal systemic therapy compared to one-third of the group who had benefit from receiving combination chemotherapy.

What these articles don't discuss is the fact that we are able to detect the breast cancers earlier with better mammographic technique compared to even ten to fifteen years ago. So if we can detect cancers earlier, we are simply starting the five-year clock or the ten-year clock sooner. The end point is always the same, but it simply appears that the patient is living longer. For instance, if breast cancer is a fifteen-year disease from start to end, and we previously detected breast cancers by mammogram or clinical palpation around year eleven or twelve, patients lived only three years thereafter. Now we are detecting the cancers earlier – around years seven or eight – hence, it **appears** that the patients are living longer but this is not the case in reality. That is why these 133 trials and other randomized trials have not shown any difference in overall survival benefit.

ADJUVANT SYSTEMIC TREATMENT FOR BREAST CANCER PATIENTS WITH NEGATIVE NODES

About 70,000 women in the United States will develop breast cancer and have negative nodes; 65,000 do not need systemic treatment, and about 5,000 will have improved disease free interval if they receive systemic treatment (less disease events during their life span but no increased survival). So in May 1988, without hard clinical data, the National Cancer Institute proclaimed an urgent Clinical Alert calling for the routine use of systemic therapy for these patients.[30] It meant that about 75% of the women would be unnecessarily treated. Four studies then ensued that should have been conducted before such a Clinical Alert was issued.[31-35] The results: **The lifespan was the same for those who received treatment and for those who did not.** To achieve the benefit of less disease events for the above 5,000 patients, the other 65,000 would have to be treated and would receive no benefit. The total cost - $340 million per year (1989 dollars). The analysis does not consider toxicity and a possible 50-100 treatment-related deaths for these 5,000.

In June 1990, the National Institutes of Health convened a Consensus Conference to provide guidelines for these patients.[36] After reviewing ten randomized trials the panel concluded that adjuvant systemic therapy reduced the rate of recurrence by one-third but did not increase lifespan. However, the panel failed to issue guidelines and in fact dumped it back into the laps of the practicing physician. So how do you decide who needs systemic therapy? The answer is found in Table 24.1.

Table 24.1 Prognostic Factors That Define Low- or High-Risk for Recurrence and Shortened Life in Patients with Negative Nodes [37,38]

Low-Risk	High-Risk
Cancer diameter < 1 cm	Cancer diameter >3 cm
Cancer 1-3 cm, no high risk factors	Negative Estrogen Receptor
Ductal carcinoma *in situ*, Pure tubular, Mucinous, Papillary, Adenoid, Invasive lobular (all <2cm)	
Typical medullary, <3cm, high S-phase	
Grade I	Grade III
Low S-phase	High S-phase (>7%)
Diploid	Aneuploid
Age > 50	High Cathepsin D
Healthy Lifestyle	High-fat, Low-fiber, Obesity, No antioxidants or B vitamins, Smoker or inhales others' Alcohol: 3+/week, Sedentary Use of Hormones, Stress

Prognostic factors are assigned to either the low-risk category or the high-risk category based on their individual five-year recurrence rates – Table 24.2. For instance, the five-year recurrence rate for having ductal carcinoma *in situ* is 1%, which means only 1% of the people with this diagnosis will have a cancer recurrence in the first five years. If a patient has a tumor less than 1 cm in size, the five-year recurrence rate for that prognostic factor is only 6%, which is the same rate for having a nuclear grade I.

Table 24.2 Five Year Recurrence Rates With or Without Adjuvant Systemic Treatment for Prognostic Factors in Negative Node Patients

	Five Year Recurrence Rates	
Prognostic Factors	**No Treatment**	**Treatment**
Ductal carcinoma *in situ*	1%	0.75%
Cancer < 1.0 cm	6%	4.5%
Grade I	6%	4.5%
Low S-phase	10%	7.5%
Diploid	12%	9.0%
Cancer 1-3 cm	12%	9.0%
Grade II	25%	18.75%
Positive Estrogen Receptor	26%	19.50%
Aneuploid	27%	20.25%
Grade III	28%	21%
High S-phase	30%	22.5%
Negative Estrogen Receptor	35%	26.25%
High Cathespin D	50%	37.5%
Aneuploid + high Cathespin D	60%	45%

Remember, the review of 133 randomized clinical trials demonstrated that systemic adjuvant treatment reduced the odds of recurrence by 25%. So the reduction is greatest when the patient has prognostic factors consisting of aneuploid and high Cathespin D levels. Her five-year recurrence rate is 60%, which means that if she receives no treatment, she has a 60% chance of having a recurrence in the first five years. That 60% is reduced by one quarter to 45% if she receives adjuvant systemic treatment. It would, therefore, make sense to treat this patient but certainly not a patient with ductal carcinoma *in situ.*

ADJUVANT CHEMOTHERAPY GIVEN TO PATIENTS WITH NEGATIVE NODES DOES NOT IMPROVE QUALITY OF LIFE[39,40]

ALTERNATIVE THERAPIES DO NOT IMPROVE SURVIVAL OR DISEASE-FREE SURVIVAL FOR BREAST CANCER PATIENTS.[41]

TREATMENT OF LOCALLY ADVANCED BREAST CANCERS (greater than 5 cm) is usually done with surgery and/or radiation using 60 Gy followed by a boost to cancer mass. This provides good control of the breast region, but side effects occur in about 20% of the patients and survival is not increased. Systemic therapy should be used because of the high likelihood of metastasis.

Patients who have bleeding and fungating masses through the skin may be treated with large doses of radiation over a course of only two to four days. Radiation will stop the bleeding and start killing the cancer cells quickly so that the mass is no longer weeping, and the foul smell will subside.

SIMULTANEOUS CANCERS IN EACH BREAST. If there is no evidence of disease elsewhere in the body (normal bone scan, chest X-ray, and liver function tests) and the patient is deemed to have early stage breast cancers in each breast, each breast is then independently treated. For instance, if a woman is a candidate for bilateral lumpectomies, node samplings followed by radiation therapy, then the same procedure can be applied to both breasts at the same time. Or if she elects to have mastectomies, they can be done simultaneously as well. Another patient may require a mastectomy on one side and yet a breast-conserving procedure may be an option for the opposite side. But each breast should be considered independently with appropriate options given.

TRANSPLANTATION – HIGH DOSE CHEMOTHERAPY PLUS AUTOLOGOUS STEM CELL OR BONE MARROW TRANSPLANTATION DO NOT IMPROVE SURVIVAL BUT DO INCREASE SIDE EFFECTS AND DEATH COMPARED WITH CONVENTIONAL DOSE CHEMOTHERAPY.[42-47]

The Government Accounting Office reported that about 4000 women undergo these transplants each year at a cost between $80,000 and $150,000 – much more than the cost of standard treatment of $15,000 to $40,000. Despite the fact that these procedures do not extend life, insurers reluctantly cover them because of fear of litigation – multiple cases have settled for huge sums because patients were denied coverage (one case settled in 1993 for almost $80 million).[48]

Anxieties and emotional outcries will continue from patients who have been told by the media, organizations, and physicians that their only hope is transplantation. These procedures simply do not work.

IMMUNOLOGICAL METHODS: CHEMOTHERAPY + HER2 ANTIBODY DELAYS DISEASE PROGRESSION BY ABOUT 2 MONTHS BUT DOES NOT EXTEND LIFE. [49]

ANTI-ANGIOGENESIS – New Blood Vessel Inhibition

Normal cells do not have the capability to perform angiogenesis. They may secrete low amounts of molecules known to induce angiogenesis, but they secrete much greater amounts of anti-angiogenic molecules that inhibit the inducers. Production of high-levels of these anti-angiogenic substances is what is thought to maintain vascular quiescence in healthy tissue. New cancer cells produce angiogenesis inducers but very little of the angiogenesis inhibitors.

Many substances have anti-angiogenic activity. Some neutralize the enzymes manufactured by the cancer cell that burrow a hole in the tissue to allow room for a new blood vessel. Others interfere with the building blocks of new blood vessels.

Mammals produce natural inhibitors of angiogenesis that include: interferons, steroids, proteins from platelets (thrombospondin and platelet factor 4), enzyme (protease) inhibitors, vitamin A, and metabolites of vitamin D_3. And drugs that were developed for other purposes, have anti-angiogenic activity. Anti-angiogenic agents do not interfere with chemotherapy or radiation therapy.

Table 24.3 Anti-Angiogenic Agents

Anticancer Drugs	Cancer Treatment	Antibiotics
Antiestrogens – Tamoxifen	Radiation Therapy	Minocycline
Interferons, Retinoids	Hyperthermia	Suramin
Bleomycin, Methotrexate		Herbimycin A
Bisantrene, Mitoxantrone		D-Penicillamine
Other		
Aspirin, other inhibitors of prostaglandin synthetase		
Vitamin D_3 metabolites		
p53 Suppressor gene		
Captopril, Megace		

Table 24.4 Theoretical Comparison of Chemotherapy and Anti-Angiogenic Therapy

Variable	Chemotherapy	Anti-Angiogenic Therapy
Target	Cancer Cell	Blood Vessel Cells
Affects Primary & Mets	Yes	Yes
Specificity	Low	High
Resistance Develops	Yes	No
Duration of Therapy	Moderate	Long
? Chemoprevention	No	Yes

Anti-angiogenic agents have been around since 1970 without any real successes so far.

TREATMENT OF OLDER BREAST CANCER PATIENTS[50-53] should be assessed in the same way as other breast cancer patients, realizing, of course, they may have chronic illnesses, like heart disease, etc., that influence the choice of treatment. Some general statements can be made.

- Breast cancers in older patients tend to be less aggressive.
- Breast-conserving surgery plus radiation can be an option.
- Tamoxifen instead of lumpectomy or mastectomy can be used to treat early stage breast cancer. No survival difference. Using tamoxifen as an initial therapy may be the best option for patients who have poor health or abundant local-regional disease or metastatic disease at time of initial diagnosis.
- Tamoxifen should be used for metastatic disease regardless of estrogen receptor status.
- Tamoxifen and combination chemotherapy produce the same survival and disease-free survival so there is little indication for chemotherapy in older patients especially if they have compromised liver, kidney, or cardiac status.
- Probably the only indication for using chemotherapy in older patients is for rapidly progressive cancer or liver metastases.
- A response to a hormonal manipulation lasts about a year, at which time another may be used. A person who responds to one hormonal manipulation is likely to respond to others.

Low Dose Estrogen Should not be used By Breast Cancer Patients because, as you learned (page 128), estrogen can feed a cancer and does not relieve menopausal symptoms, or lower the risk of stroke, heart disease, or Alzheimer's.

TREATMENT OF METASTATIC DISEASE

Breast cancer may metastasize to various organs including liver, bone, brain, eye, soft tissues like the skin, and other sites. Treatment is directed to the symptoms that are produced by these metastatic lesions.

- Radiation is used to treat the brain, or a single area of bone pain, or even the eye (5-10% of all breast cancer cases).
- Hormonal treatment may be used for any site that has metastatic disease. It works less well if liver or brain is involved.
- Combination chemotherapy can be considered for patients who have liver metastases or disease that is unresponsive to hormonal treatments. Survival is unchanged in all cases.

FOLLOW-UP FOR BREAST CANCER PATIENTS [54,55]

- **Laboratory and Imaging Studies – Not recommended** by the American Society of Clinical Oncology because they don't change the outcome. These include imaging studies like bone scans, chest X-rays, etc., blood work, tumor markers (CEA, CA 15-3, CA 27.29), and liver tests. Cost of these unnecessary tests is $1 billion per year.
- **History and physical examination** every 3 to 6 months for 3 years, then 6 to 12 months for 2 years, then annually.
- **Annual mammogram and pelvic examination**.

Once patients develop metastases, they are incurable.[56-59] Complete remissions are rarely seen.[57] And, curiously, the interval of time between initial management of the early breast cancer and the diagnosis of metastases is just about the same whether the patient is undergoing follow-up or not.[60,61] Therefore, follow-up after surgery and primary treatment does not lead to earlier detection of metastases nor does it affect the overall survival.[62,63] Recurrences are detected 86% of the time by the patient or by the physician during examination.

Besides an erroneous belief system, patient desires, the media and various organizations that say early detection is best, the driving force behind intensive follow-ups may be the threat of malpractice suits. A malpractice case is composed of two issues: deviation from the standard of care and "proximate cause." Based on the hard scientific data, the standard of care must be minimal surveillance. Proximate cause simply asks the question: Does a potential delay in a diagnosis of metastases make any difference in the ultimate outcome or survival? Proximate cause also would not be applicable because a patient is incurable once a recurrence is detected.

TOXICITY OF SYSTEMIC THERAPY

Table 24.3 Systemic Therapy Toxicities

Organ	Commonly Used Breast Cancer Therapies					
	Cyclopho Phamide	Metho trexate	5-FU	Adria mycin	Taxol	Tamoxifen
Eye	Yes	Yes	Yes	Yes		Yes
Lung	Yes	Yes		Yes	Yes	
Heart	Yes*		Yes**	Yes	Yes	
Liver	Yes		Yes			Yes
Bone Marrow	Yes	Yes	Yes	Yes	Yes	
Gastrointestine	Yes	Yes	Yes	Yes	Yes	
Nausea/Vomiting	Yes	Yes	Yes	Yes	Yes	
Nerve Damage					Yes	
Brain Dysfunction	Yes		Yes			
Skin / Hair Loss	Yes	Yes	Yes	Yes	Yes	
Leukemia Risk	Yes			Yes		
Bladder Cancer Risk	Yes#					
Endometrium Ca Risk						Yes

*Only with high doses not commonly used in breast cancer care
**With high dose continuous infusion, generally not used in breast cancer
#Drink 8 to 10 large glasses of water a day to prevent bladder bleeding and decrease the risk of bladder cancer.

TAMOXIFEN increases the risk for endometrial cancer, liver dysfunction, and ocular problems[64,65] in only 1 or 2 of every 1000. The benefit far outweighs risk.[66] No routine surveillance is needed as was once thought,[67,68] even if endometrial thickening exceeds 8 mm. Symptoms like vaginal bleeding should be checked if they arise.

DECISION-MAKING: BREAST MASS TO TREATMENT

BREAST MASS FOUND

Evaluation of Breast Cancer Risk Factors

Wait one menstrual cycle – look for change

OFFICE NEEDLE ASPIRATION

No Fluid

Bloody Fluid or Mass does not Disappear

Clear or Dark Fluid or Mass Disappears

No further workup unless mammogram indicated

MAMMOGRAM

Mass

Microcalcifications

Ultrasound

Suspicious

Benign Apppearing

Cystic-Workup done

Solid Mass

Repeat Mammogram 4-6 mo.

Suspicious

Stable - repeat 1 yr

EXCISIONAL BIOPSY

Benign

Invasive Cancer

Ductal Ca *in situ*

Lobular Ca *in situ*

Metastatic Work-up

Gross Disease

Microscopic

Positive

Negative

Systemic Treatment

Radiation Consult

No treatment, just follow

Candidate for conservative surgery + radiation RT – can choose

Not a Candidate

Breast Conserving Surgery + RT

Mastectomy ± Reconstruction

Negative Nodes

Positive Nodes

Negative Nodes → Low Risk Prognostic Factors → No Systemic Treatment

Negative Nodes → High Risk Prognos Factors → Adjuvant Systemic Treatment

Positive Nodes → Adjuvant Systemic Treatment

Adjuvant Systemic Treatment → Hormonal

Adjuvant Systemic Treatment → Chemotherapy

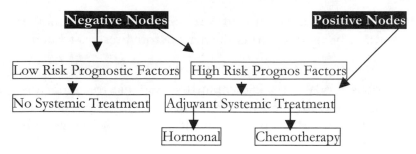

BREAST CANCER TREATMENT BY STAGE (page 201)

STAGE 0

- **Ductal carcinoma *in situ*** and **Lobular carcinoma *in situ*.** No systemic treatment is needed. Refer to pages 194 and 195.

STAGE I

- Breast local-regional treatment is mandatory with choice of:
  Lumpectomy, node sampling, radiation **OR** mastectomy
- Adjuvant systemic treatment if you have multiple high-risk prognostic factors – Table 24.2. No systemic treatment if your cancer is <1 cm or you have low-risk factors.

STAGE II

- Breast local-regional treatment is mandatory with choice of:
  Lumpectomy, node sampling, radiation **OR** mastectomy
- Adjuvant systemic treatment
  - *Positive nodes*
    Postmenopausal women – tamoxifen for 2 to 5 years. Disease-free survival is improved.
    Premenopausal patients – hormonal treatment (ovarian ablation) or chemotherapy produce identical results.
  - *Negative nodes* Postmenopausal and premenopausal women – treatment indicated as per Table 24.2.

STAGE III

- Breast local-regional treatment is mandatory with choice of:
  Mastectomy **OR** Radiation pre-operatively to shrink mass, **OR** Radiation post operatively to treat the chest wall.

- Systemic treatment is mandatory – Hormonal or chemotherapy may be used to shrink the mass before breast is treated.

INFLAMMATORY BREAST CARCINOMA.

- Various modalities are combined – systemic treatment first, then preoperative radiation, then mastectomy if possible, followed by more systemic treatment – a 25-40% five year survival rate is obtained.

STAGE IV

- Systemic treatment is primary modality. There is no need to treat the local-regional area of the breast unless there is an ulcerating mass.
- Premenopausal and postmenopausal women – ovarian ablation, tamoxifen, or chemotherapy as indicated.
- If there is rapidly progressive cancer or cancer involving the liver – chemotherapy as well as tamoxifen.
- Radiation – to palliate localized bone pain, brain metastases.

SURVIVAL – STAGE, SIZE, NODES. As the tumor size increases with positive lymph nodes, survival decreases.

Table 24.4 Percent Survival Based on Stage, Cancer Size, Node Status

			Percent Survival		
Stage	**Cancer Size (cm)**	**Nodes**	**5 Year**	**10 Year**	**20 Year**
Stage 0	0	Negative		95	
Stage I					
	<1 and special cell types table 24.1	Negative			95
	<1	Negative		90	86
	1-2	Negative		80	70
Stage II					
	<2	Positive		70	
	2-5	Negative		65	
	2-5	Positive		50	
	>5	Negative		40	
Stage III					
	<5	Pos & Fixed	13		
	>5	Positive		35	
	Cancer fixed to chest	Positive	5		

FACTORS THAT IMPROVE SURVIVAL

• **COMPETENT IMMUNE SYSTEM INCREASES LIFESPAN** for patients with Stage I or II breast cancer.[69,70] Patients with breast or ovarian cancer live longer if they have had a previous infection with tuberculosis and a positive tuberculin test.[71]

• **PROPER DIET AND LIFESTYLE (TEN POINT PLAN) INCREASES LIFESPAN** – Chapter 6, 28.

• **ANTIOXIDANTS AND OTHER NUTRIENTS ENHANCE IMMUNE SYSTEM.**

"UNPROVEN" TREATMENT COMPARED TO CONVENTIONAL TREATMENT PRODUCE THE SAME LIFESPAN AND QUALITY OF LIFE[72]

• Patients from an unconventional cancer clinic in California were matched with patients treated conventionally at a traditional academic cancer center in Philadelphia, Pennsylvania. The Philadelphia investigators hypothesized that survival time would be the same for both groups on the assumption that the unproved remedy is no more effective in patients with end-stage disease than conventional care, itself largely ineffective. Results: Lifespan and quality of life were the same for both.

People seek unproven treatment because it has little or no toxicity and conventional treatment produces toxicity without increasing lifespan. Many of the agencies and/or "benevolent" charities in the United States have developed a "hit list" of unproven therapies and their proponents without having the therapy investigated – the therapy is guilty of quackery until proven otherwise. I am convinced that **ALL** therapies, unproven or otherwise, should be put through the same rigors of science to the degree that they can, and then evaluate the findings.

TREATMENT: EFFECTIVE OR NOT EFFECTIVE, DOES IT WORK? Rather than classify treatment as conventional, or unproven, or alternative, treatments should have only two broad classifications: **EFFECTIVE** or **NONEFFECTIVE** therapy. Does the treatment prolong survival and improve the quality of life? **Is the treatment effective? Does it work?** And at the same time, does the treatment do little or no harm?

For example, breast-conserving surgery with radiation therapy, modified radical mastectomy, and radical mastectomy all produce the same survival. Likewise, chemotherapy, hormonal therapy, and unproven therapy in the example above produce the same survival. Survival is the same for both examples, but which modality produces the fewer side effects – which one would you pick? The **EFFECTIVE** choices are obvious.

If there were a cure for cancer somewhere, in someone's hideaway clinic, it would not remain secret, and all the fuss about the correct cancer treatment would be over. A cure for cancer could never be kept a secret.

Patients considering any treatment must always ask, "What are the risks and what are the benefits?" If the risks are minimal and the benefit is great, then there is no question that the treatment should be entertained. However, if the risks are great and the benefit is minimal, reject that treatment.

CONCLUSION

Hormonal therapy and chemotherapy afford the same the average duration of response, disease-free interval, and survival. Chemotherapy is no more curative than hormonal therapy, and it is much more toxic. So, why is chemotherapy still used?

Patients with cancer have grown up listening to organized cancer groups, physicians, and media extolling the virtues of chemotherapy. The more often you hear it, the more you believe that if you have cancer, you must have chemotherapy. And patients want hope. For instance, over half of a group of patients receiving chemotherapy for metastatic disease (incurable) believed that they would be cured, and all of these patients believed that chances of "cure" were greater than 50% when they were told the opposite.[73] And even when they were told what the cure rates were for their stage of disease, patients discounted them.

American oncologists are more likely to advise chemotherapy over hormonal therapy than their counterpart oncologists in Europe.[74] Most oncologists advise chemotherapy believing it will improve survival when it actually does not.[74] And patients want their physicians to make the major decisions.[75]

The *Lancet* editorial staff wrote on February 6, 1993, "Breast cancer: Have we lost our way?"[76] The editorial stated, "... we acknowledge the failures of primary therapy and secondary prevention." The *Lancet* convened a conference in 1994 to review new issues to help breast cancer patients and acknowledge the failure of existing treatment. The *Lancet* staff concluded:[77]

"CHEMOTHERAPY IN THE MANAGEMENT OF BREAST CANCER HAS A DIM FUTURE."

Survival for breast cancer patients has changed little since 1930 using conventional treatment. However, I am convinced, based on the Japanese and other data already reviewed, that women who follow an optimal lifestyle (Ten Point Plan) coupled to effective treatment using non-immunosuppressing agents when possible, will fare better and live longer (Figure 24.1). They will be more competent immunologically, and their cancers will not be fed by lifestyle factors that we know perpetuate cancer growth.

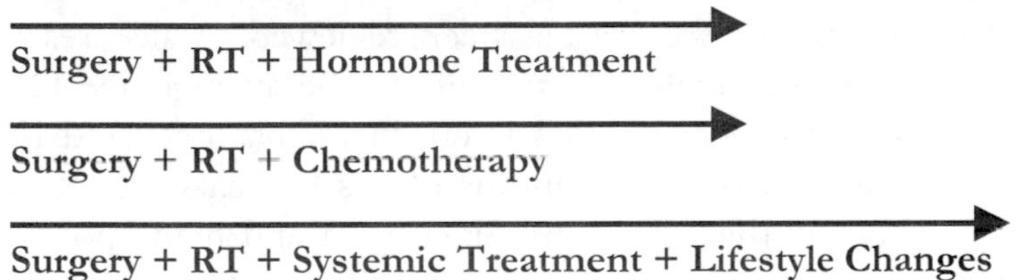

Figure 24.1 Survival (Lifespan) for Breast Cancer Patients

Elizabeth decided to have her ovaries removed and strictly adhere to the Simone Ten point Plan for lifestyle modification to extend her life.

25

Male Breast Cancer

John's History

Two years ago when John was 46, he noted a hard lump just behind his left nipple. He didn't think too much about it until it got bigger. He saw his physician who suggested watching it for a while. Finally a biopsy proved it to be a breast cancer.

Every year in the United States, about 1500 men develop breast cancer and 400 men die of the disease. Male breast cancer was first recorded in 3000 B.C., and in recent years, information about large numbers of cases has been reviewed.[1] Male breast cancer is similar to female breast cancer. The average age for developing breast cancer in men is 60, but it has occurred in males as young as 5 years old and as old as 93 years old. It is rare in men below the age of 30. Since men and many physicians tend to ignore symptoms or masses in the breast, men with breast cancer often come to see a physician at a very late stage in the disease as compared to women. Often, there is an 18 to 24 months delay in seeing a physician from the onset of symptoms.

RISK FACTORS

- **Diet:** High-fat, low-fiber and lack of vitamins and minerals.
- **Family History**: About one-third have a female family member with breast cancer, but many have male family members with breast cancer.[2]
- **Genetics**: 3% of those with Klinefelter's syndrome (extra X chromosome, obese, and gynecomastia) develop breast cancer.

• **Radiation** before age 20 for benign conditions (gynecomastia, enlarged thymus, eczema of the chest, chest burns, tuberculosis) increases breast cancer risk.[3]

• **Estrogens** administered in large amounts increase risk in male transsexuals, as well as in male heart and ulcer patients.[4-6]

• **Liver Disease** increases risk (infections of the liver in Africa, alcohol abuse, cirrhosis, or chronic malnutrition). Estrogens rise in these conditions because the dysfunctional liver cannot metabolize them. Male breast cancers account for 15% of all breast cancers in Zambia, 6.4% in Egypt, and 4.6% in India but only 0.8% in the United States.[7]

• **Other Risk Factors:** History of mumps orchitis (testicular inflammation) or mumps as an adult; testicular injury, undescended testes, and obesity.[8]

DETECTION

When a mass is palpated and detected, it must be differentiated from benign gynecomastia. The physician must take a history of drug use, hormone use, excess alcohol consumption, and all the other risk factors already mentioned, and also obtain a mammogram. As with any other breast mass, it must be removed for pathological examination, estrogen receptor status, etc.

DIAGNOSIS

Men with breast cancer often initially report a painless mass in the center of the breast region around the nipple. It is usually only on one side. The second most common presentation is in the upper outer quadrant. A bloody nipple discharge, with or without nipple inversion, is commonly seen in about 80% of all male breast cancers.

PATHOLOGY

Infiltrating ductal cancer is the most common type in men just as for women. Ductal carcinoma *in situ* is rarely found because screening mammograms are not done. Paget's disease of the nipple and inflammatory breast carcinoma are less common.

STAGING is identical to that described on page 201: size of the cancer, lymph node status, and the other laboratory and X-ray studies that define whether the disease has spread from the breast to other parts of the body.

Because of the small size of the male breast, it is common for the cancer to be fixed to the chest wall measuring about 4 centimeters. The nodes are positive in over half the cases.

Remember, men usually come to the doctor at more advanced stages than women. If a breast mass is palpated by a man, he generally ignores it; the physician generally does not routinely examine male breasts for breast masses, and older men generally have a higher mortality from other causes.

CONVENTIONAL LOCAL TREATMENT is as described for women, Chapter 23. Primary radiation therapy with breast-conserving surgery can be an option and is equal in terms of both survival and local tumor control compared to modified radical mastectomy.[9,10] More men are conscious of their appearance and desire the breast conserving surgery.

CONVENTIONAL SYSTEMIC TREATMENT is hormonal because 80% of male breast cancers are estrogen receptor positive. Hormonal treatment is more effective than chemotherapy and produce more durable responses.

The main objective in hormonal therapy is simply to alter the current hormonal milieu that is feeding the tumor. So if estrogens feed the tumor, take it away; if testosterone feeds the tumor, take it away. The Hormonal Therapy guidelines set forth in Chapter 24 apply to male breast cancer. Orchiectomy, tamoxifen, or other hormonal maneuvers have produced tumor regressions in about 85% of the men.[11-13] Psychological and cultural issues limit the routine performance of orchiectomy in these patients. Tamoxifen, DES, progesterone, megestrol, and antiandrogens (cyproterone and flutamide) produce tumor regressions. And as we learned in women using high doses of estrogen to treat female breast cancer, high doses of testosterone have been effective in causing tumor regression in as many as 60% of cases.[14-16] And even cortisone has been beneficial in about 40% of the cases.

Management of recurrences or metastatic disease is handled in an identical manner as for women. Almost half of the patients who receive tamoxifen for treatment of metastatic disease have a complete or partial response. When diethylstilbestrol (DES) is used, a response rate of about 40% is obtained. If tamoxifen was used first and disease progressed, orchiectomy was effective thereafter.

Because the number of patients in various studies is so small, there is a wide range of survival statistics for each stage. Table 25.1 shows the range for five-year survival by stage.[17,18]

Table 25.1 Five Year Survival by Stage for Male Breast Cancer

Stage	Range of Five Year Survival
I	75%-85%
II	44%-75%
III	16%-43%
IV	0%-8%

CONCLUSION

Male breast cancer behaves similarly to female breast cancer including risk factors; natural history; response rates to various treatment modalities such as surgery, radiation, and systemic therapies; as well as survival. As with women, survival is probably much improved if lifestyle factors are modified. It behooves all people with breast cancer, regardless of sex, to modify lifestyle factors in an attempt to improve their survival and quality of life as well as general well-being.

John started "effective" conventional therapy and dramatically modified his lifestyle to optimize his lifespan.

26
Quality of Life and Ethics

Miriam's History
Miriam is 36 with three young children. She has metastatic breast cancer and until recently her quality of life was alright according to her. Now she is faced with disease that is not responding to treatment. What should she be told and what should she do?

Since 1930, overall survival (life span) has not changed for patients with breast cancer. In the ensuing years, treatments have become increasingly toxic. Issues concerning quality of life and ethics have, therefore, become quite important.

QUALITY OF LIFE is very important and should measure physical symptoms, psychological well-being, social functioning, daily activity levels, cognitive abilities, sexual dysfunction, and overall general life satisfaction. Quality of life assessments have been used for many illnesses including cardiovascular disease, strokes, and now cancer.

The National Cancer Institute has recommended that clinical trials include quality of life assessments and the U.S. Food and Drug Administration recognizes the benefit to quality of life as a basis for approval of new anticancer drugs.[1]

When two treatments yield similar disease-free survival and/or survival, the treatment that affords a better quality of life should be recommended. Conversely, if one treatment is effective but diminishes the quality of life so much that its use is unacceptable, that treatment is not worth undertaking.

Cancer treatments affect the quality of life. We demonstrated a better quality of life for 50 consecutive breast cancer patients receiving radiation therapy and/or chemotherapy who followed the Ten Point Plan (Chapter 6) that included certain vitamins and minerals. An international study showed substantial differences in quality of life scores between national groups. English-speaking patients in Europe were best able to cope with their cancer. German and Swedish patients, however, coped moderately well with their cancers. And the Italians were least able to cope.[2] This pattern fits with the conception that Northern Europeans are more reserved and complain less than Southern Europeans.

Studies of quality of life for patients receiving marrow transplants have not had clear-cut results. Some patients have an excellent quality of life following bone marrow transplant, but others do not fare as well.[3]

SEXUALITY AND BODY IMAGE

Any illness brings about changes in feelings of well being. Although rarely dealt with by the physician, sexual function is an integral part of an individual's well being.[4] Sexuality is important for all ages. In fact, 60% of breast cancer patients want more information on the impact of cancer on sexuality, and 55% want to discuss sexuality openly with their physicians which rarely occurs.

Psychosexual dysfunction occurs in 20% to 50% of breast cancer patients.[5-7] Researchers comment that the breast is a symbol of womanhood and sexuality, and hypothesize that mastectomies usually devastate a woman's feelings of attractiveness and sexual desire. Women whose self-esteem or body image is connected to their breast as a source of attractiveness may be at particular risk after mastectomy or other alterations of the breast. However, studies don't bear that out.

• **LUMPECTOMY OR MASTECTOMY DOES NOT SIGNIFICANTLY INFLUENCE SEXUAL DYSFUNCTION.** In a review of 12 studies, women who had lumpectomy and radiation therapy had less sexual dysfunction than women who underwent mastectomy because they had less fear of recurrence and a more positive feelings about their bodies, particularly in the nude.[8-10] But when women with mastectomies were compared with women who underwent breast biopsies for benign disease or to other women who underwent gall bladder removal, no increased rate of psychological or sexual dysfunction was found in any of these groups.[11,12] Only about 25% of women have significant anxiety, depression, and sexual problems after having had modified radical mastectomy.

A woman's overall psychological health, depression and anxiety, loss of energy and libido, loss of control, altered body image, isolation and fear, satisfaction with the relationship to her partner, current sexual life are important predictors of sexual satisfaction after a diagnosis of breast cancer. It appears women who have problems with sexuality and body image in a relationship, generally have these problems long before a diagnosis of cancer is made. And although the diagnosis of cancer heightens these anxieties, breast cancer *per se* has a minimal impact on sexuality.

- **BREAST RECONSTRUCTION IMPROVES BODY IMAGE** for women who have mastectomy.[13-15] Women who undergo reconstruction feel "whole again." They can wear a variety of clothing and feel comfortable with all the styles. There seems to be equal satisfaction for women who have immediate reconstruction and women who have reconstruction at a later time.
- **SYSTEMIC TREATMENT MOST COMMON CAUSE OF SEXUAL DYSFUNCTION** in breast cancer patients because it causes premature or severe menopausal symptoms. Also, other side effects like fatigue, nausea, vomiting, low white blood count, infections, etc., all lower libido. Postmenopausal symptoms rapidly develop in young women undergoing chemotherapy, particularly in those between the ages of 35 and 40. Body image also changes in women undergoing chemotherapy due to the loss of their hair, change in skin texture, and weight changes. Even when hair does grow back after chemotherapy is stopped, it does not re-grow identically to what it was. The use of tamoxifen or bilateral ovarian ablation will bring on postmenopausal symptoms or slightly intensify those already existing. Tamoxifen, however, will provide enough vaginal lubrication.

Table 26.1 reviews the female sexual response cycle for women as described in Masters and Johnson.[16] Systemic treatment, chemotherapy or hormonal treatment, decreases the sexual responses for both young and older women.

Table 26.1 Female Sexual Response Cycle

	Young Women	Older Women
Excitement	Vaginal Lubrication Expansion of inner 2/3 vagina Elevation cervix/uterus Mild increase in breast size Clitoral, labial swelling	Reduced lubrication Reduced vagina expansion Slowed response No increase in breast size
Plateau	Increased uterine elevation leading to tenting and clitoral retraction Outer 1/3 vagina swells called "orgasmic platform" Sex flush Areolar swelling, nipple erection Increased labial color	Reduced uterine elevation Reduced vaginal elasticity Reduced sex flush Less muscle tension
Orgasm	Uterine contractions Contractions of outer 1/3 of vagina and anal sphincters Increased sex flush	Weaker/spastic contraction Shorter duration
Resolution	Orgasmic platform disappears Labial color fades Breasts, clitoris decrease in size Uterus moves back to resting Multi-orgasmic capacity	Multi-orgasmic capacity retained Faster return to prearousal state

QUESTIONS REGARDING SEXUALITY are rarely asked. However, one investigator is convinced that the following questions should be made part of any breast cancer questionnaire to determine the woman's quality of life with regard to sexuality.[17]

- How often does the woman have sex with her partner?
- How often does she feel desire for sex?
- How often does she masturbate?
- Is there enough vaginal lubrication for comfortable activity?
- What kinds of stimulation help her reach orgasm?
- What range of sexual practices is comfortable for her?

- Have her breast cancer diagnosis and treatment changed her sexual frequency, function, or the types of touch used?
- Has she had a loss of pleasure from breast caressing?

HOME CARE should be the principal setting for breast cancer patients in the terminal stages because they will feel less anxious and more at ease at home than in a hospital or nursing-home setting. The older patient has more concerns regarding transportation, finances, and symptoms from other chronic illnesses in addition to the cancer. All the creature comforts that the patient is used to are there at hand. And truly the ideal setting for such a patient is in the home because a hospital setting can offer little that home care can't offer.

Family members must assume responsibility for physical and psychosocial demands of the patient with cancer. Everyone in the family has a new set of physical and psychosocial demands as care providers. The quality of life for both the patient and the family is a major issue and concern. A patient needs physical comforts and information. A care provider needs household management skills and information. When both groups are considered, the priority need is psychological. But the following must be addressed when caring for the terminal breast cancer patient at home:[18]

- Pain control and symptom management
- Communication with the physician
- Preparation for death
- Opportunity to achieve a sense of completion

QUALITY OF LIFE SUMMARY. Each of the qualities of life must be addressed and may determine the choice of treatment: physical symptoms, performance, general well-being, cognitive abilities, sexual dysfunction, and overall life satisfaction. Quality of life issues are now on equal footing with efficacy when the FDA considers a new drug.

ETHICS

Do patients with cancer really want to know the exact day they are going to die? And if a doctor does give them a range of time for life, how many patients then go home, mark the calendar, and proceed to die on that day? Most people who grow up in an industrialized society with multimedia communications are aware that patients who have cancer generally will die of it. This is not a revelation.

In my experience, all cancer patients who receive treatment, and, hence, interact with physicians and other patients in treatment areas, know their situation. Even very young people know. A six-year-old boy who I was treating for leukemia at the National Cancer Institute, asked me what it was like in heaven. A national survey found that 96% of Americans wanted to be told if they had cancer and 85% wanted to know how long they would live if their cancer usually led to death in less than a year.[19]

Moreover, a legal case involving ethical informed consent (*Arato v. Avedon*)[20] asked whether the law should force physicians to report statistical life expectancy information to patients. Mr. Arato had pancreas cancer that was treated surgically, then with experimental chemotherapy and radiation because there "is no effective treatment." The surgeon and oncologist never told Mr. Arato and his wife that only 5% survive for 5 years, nor did they give a prognosis or estimate of his life expectancy, nor were they asked. A recurrence occurred and the physicians knew he would die within a few months, but did not tell the patient about life expectancy.

The patient died and his wife sued the physicians claiming that the doctors were obligated under California's informed consent law to tell the patient about survival figures before asking him to consent to chemotherapy. The court decided Mr. Arato should have been informed. The physicians said if the patient knew of the high mortality rate, he would have no hope. And during the 70 visits, the patient did not ask questions about his life expectancy indicating to the physicians that he did not want to know. The patient's wife said had the patient known the facts, he would have declined all treatment and attended to his business affairs. His wife incurred tax losses due to poor business planning.

The lower court favored the physicians. The appeal court reversed the decision. The California Supreme Court upheld the decision in favor of the wife because of the doctrine of informed consent based on four tenets:

1. Patients are generally ignorant of medicine.
2. Patients have a right to control their own bodies and thus to decide about medical treatment.
3. To be effective, consent to medical treatment must be informed.
4. Patients are dependent upon their physicians for truthful information and must trust them (making the doctor-patient relationship a "fiduciary" or trust relationship rather that an arm's length business relationship).

The court concluded "the physician is under a legal duty to disclose all material information – information regarded as significant by a reasonable person in the person's position when deciding to accept or reject a recommended medical procedure – needed to make an informed decision regarding a proposed treatment."

The practice of medicine is an art as well as a science. It involves compassion and honesty. A good physician will always give a ray of hope as well as discuss the implications of a grave situation.

It is often easier to give another round of ineffective chemotherapy than to tell patients that there is nothing left in the anti-cancer arsenal.[21] The clinician should sit with patients and families, hold their hands and tell them there is no way to control their cancer, but they will not be abandoned and will be made as comfortable as possible.

Physicians are required to tell the patient about the probability that a proposed treatment will be successful and specifically define what the word "successful" means. A reasonable person should understand the probability of success from a particular treatment and then decide whether to accept that treatment or not. The poor results with conventional medicine are, of course, the whole basis for the ground swell concerning alternative medicine in the United States. Our culture emphasizes life and youth and vitality. We tend to shy away from talking about death and dying. Hope should always be given, but not false hope. We must inform patients of studies regarding particular treatments and life expectancy and/or benefits from those treatments.

Sometimes there are financial conflicts that arise when one treatment is considered over another treatment. It has been said that the chief beneficiaries of cancer treatments that don't change survival and cause harm are often the oncology community and pharmaceutical companies and their stockholders.[22]

We really need to start thinking in terms of **EFFECTIVE** or **NONEFFECTIVE** treatment and tell patients about treatments in those terms. For instance, chemotherapy is noneffective for pancreas cancer. And perhaps, as I have said in the past, aggressive treatment to keep a person alive in the last several weeks of his or her life would stop if the patient and the family were truly informed about the futility of such efforts. The costs of health care provided to a patient in terminal stages in a hospital are enormous and consume anywhere from 20 to 30 percent of all the health-care dollars. The patient and the family may be responsible for this because they "want everything done." The physician is partly responsible because "our technology should help these patients." And the legal profession may, in part, be responsible as well; if everything is not done, will the family sue the physician?

Miriam appreciated that she was told the truth about her terminal situation. This gave her "special time" with her family in her own home.

27

Untreated Breast Cancer: Its Natural History

Carol's History

Carol is 53 with advanced stage breast cancer but refuses any treatment because of religious beliefs. Her family understands but all would like to know if she will live as long as a patient who has had all treatments possible.

The natural history of a disease is defined as that which happens to a person who has that disease and is unable or unwilling to receive any treatment for it. In many instances, there were no treatments for a particular disease in the 1800s. In other cases, patients may not accept treatments for religious or other beliefs, or may have another medical condition that precludes the use of certain treatments. Hence, these patients can be studied and followed and compared to patients who have had various treatments.

One of the first studies of the natural history of breast cancer was published in 1962.[1] In a hospital cancer ward in England between the years 1805 and 1933, 250 patients were seen with advanced breast cancer – stages III and IV. Close to 70% had ulcerations when first seen and none were treated with surgery, radiation, hormone therapy, or any other intervention. These patients were admitted only for terminal care and, in every instance, a postmortem examination was performed. Only about 35% of the cases had histological documentation, but the records at the hospital were meticulous and well documented. Quite interestingly, 20% of this group was still alive after five years and 5% survived ten years. These figures are relatively comparable to those of other studies and for those patients who have been treated with various modern conventional modalities (Chapter 24).

A study conducted by the End Results Section of the Biometry Branch of the National Cancer Institute of patients treated with modern conventional treatment showed outcomes almost identical to the untreated English study outcomes. About 40% of all breast cancer patients die at the same rate as in the English study – about 25% per year. The other 60% die at a rate of 2.5% per year, which is again similar to the rate for the second group in the English study. This has obvious implications:

Treatment or no treatment, 60% of breast cancer patients have a protracted course, no matter what, and 40% die at a high rate, no matter what.

Analysis of what is called tumor doubling times provides another piece of evidence regarding the natural history of breast cancer. Most cancers are detected when the diameter is about 1 cm; this size contains about 1 billion cells, or 1×10^9 cells. To accumulate that number of cells, and assuming no other factors are involved in the process of cellular division (but there are many), it takes about 20 divisions from the initial single cancer cell. One study states an average doubling time is about 109 days, and if one assumes that no other factors are involved it would take about 8 to 9 years to reach 1 billion cells.[2] Cancers metastasize before we can detect them. If a cancer is discovered between annual mammogram screening, the doubling time is about 30 to 70 days.[3] The slowest doubling time recorded is 944 days[2] by one investigator, and as long as 5 years by another investigator.[4] The natural history data are also supplemented by reviewing autopsy findings. About 6% of all women dying of other causes have breast carcinoma *in situ*, and 20% have dysplasia (abnormally cells).[5] About 25% of women had invasive cancer or premalignant lesions.[6]

BREAST CANCER IS NOT CURABLE THE WAY IT IS TREATED TODAY. However, that is a difficult issue to resolve given that breast cancer has a late age of onset, generally, and a long natural history, which means death occurs long after the initial diagnosis is made. Hence, claims of "cure" in studies having only a short follow-up time – less than twenty to forty years – are unjustified.[7-11] Long survival of a particular breast cancer patient who has had "conventional treatment" may actually be due to the natural history of the disease and have nothing to do with the treatment.

"Cure" is largely elusive and statistically disguised. The oncology community defines "cure" to mean 5 years after treatment. If death occurs one day after 5 years, the "cure" is unaltered in the statistical record – that patient is nonetheless dead. The word "cure" should only be applied when a patient is given a treatment (e.g., antibiotics for a sore throat) and the patient then lives an uninterrupted life having the same life expectancy as a person who never got that sore throat.

The controversy of whether breast cancer is curable or not stems back for over one hundred years. A ***belief system*** has been operational for this period of time and longer. Most surgeons believed the more disease removed, the better the chance to effect a cure. And the mentality for years has been: "If we cannot conquer cancer, at least let us give it the full works."[12]

Even in the late 1800s, it was known that less was as effective as more. A surgeon in 1888 said there was no evidence to suggest that a simple mastectomy was inferior to the very radical operations that were being done in his time, which included removal of all axillary lymph nodes, clearance of the entire axilla, removal of the lymph nodes above the collar bone, total mastectomy, or even removal of the entire upper limb at the shoulder joint.[13] Jackson commented that these radical operations were unscientific and needlessly "cruel" to many women. And he said that clinicians should not ignore the clinical experience that had shown radical surgery did not decrease recurrence: "I hope we shall not. . . wander on the strength of a delusion as to the local nature of the disease." Lewison, in his textbook for breast cancer stated, "we must now be born again believers and anticipate the golden age of cancer surgery, complemented by radiotherapy, hormone therapy, chemotherapy, and immunotherapy."[14]

Breast cancer is a systemic disease. It metastasizes early before it is detectable by current screening methods.[15,16] Time of diagnosis will have little effect on the development of metastases; therefore, delay in diagnosis does not unfavorably influence survival for those with breast cancer.[17]

Survival is more closely related to the actual biology of the breast cancer than to early detection, diagnosis, and treatment. Because of our limited technology, we are unable to detect cancer masses less than 1 cm in diameter. So if there is 1/2 cm of disease in a particular organ, we will never see it. If there are 100,000 cells or 1,000,000 cells or 10 million cells in an organ or site other than the breast, we cannot find it with our current technology. Generally, cancers less than 1 cm in diameter will be demonstrated clinically after about 10 years.[17] And, as reviewed in earlier chapters, early treatment intervention after a breast cancer has been "detected early" has not changed survival. For instance, surgical removal of breast cancers less than 1 cm in diameter should not have been treated at all. Patients with these lesions will do quite well. We are simply detecting breast cancer earlier along its natural history of growth than we would without our current mammogram technology and most of them are *in situ* carcinomas.

Desperate people do desperate things. And the belief system in medicine is no different. In 1977, about 50% of all breast cancer surgeries in the United States were radical mastectomies, and in 1981, about 77% of all operations were modified radical mastectomies. Today, little has changed. Modified radical mastectomies are still performed even though we know that conservative surgical procedure (i.e., lumpectomy and node sampling) with radiation yields identical survival rates. Our zeal also to find the right combination of chemotherapeutic agents, the correct high dose, and to subject breast cancer patients to more and more aggressive treatment in hopes of finding the "cure" is no different. The truth is that if we employ only current conventional techniques, we will obtain the same survival figures for patients with breast cancer that were obtained over one hundred years ago. If we apply the same current conventional techniques, we will obtain the same survival curves as obtained for women who never had treatment at all. Take a look again at the graph on page 4. We must rethink what we are doing, what we are administering, and shift to a brand new paradigm.

We must recommend that patients with breast cancer radically change their lifestyles. The data in earlier chapters demonstrate that lifestyle modification as per our Ten Point Plan (Chapter 28) will increase survival. We must integrate lifestyle modification with the ***judicious*** use of techniques and treatments, and then and only then will we add years to the survival curve.

Carol refused conventional treatment and modified her lifestyle knowing she would help herself greatly.

Part 5

Simone Ten-Point Plan for Integrative Breast Care

28
The Simone Ten-Point Plan for Integrative Breast Care

You can do many things to control the destiny of your life and the lives of your loved ones. Eighty percent of women experience benign breast disease causing pain and other symptoms that simply do not have to be. You can decrease the severity of these symptoms and the risk of developing breast cancer from benign breast disease. Breast cancer affects one in eight women, and those odds are getting worse. Eighty to ninety percent of all cancers are related to lifestyle factors: nutrition (high-fat, low-fiber diet, and lack of nutrients), tobacco smoke, alcohol, chemical carcinogens, ozone, air pollution, industrial exposure, some hormones and drugs, sedentary lifestyle, and lack of spirituality, etc. As we have learned, many of these cancer risk factors also put you at risk for developing and worsening cardiovascular diseases. Since we can now identify many of these factors, we should modify them to lessen our risks.

The likelihood of drastically increasing the number of cancer cures by conventional cancer therapies in the foreseeable future is not great, even though some of the very best minds and technologies are involved in cancer research. Cancer is the most complex group of diseases known, and there are many different causes. We must all do our part to *prevent* cancer in order to substantially reduce the number of new cancer cases. Americans need to know the risk factors for cancer and cardiovascular diseases. Adults who become aware of these risk factors and then modify their diets and lifestyles accordingly will reduce their risk of developing the diseases. Table 27.1 provides a check list of the risk factors for cancer and heart disease that you can control and those you cannot control. As you now know, you have direct control over virtually all of them except one – age.

Table 27.1 Risk Factors for Cancer and Heart Disease

Risk Factor	Controllable
• **Nutritional** – Fat Intake, Fiber Intake, Vitamin/Mineral Intake, Food Additives, Caffeine Intake	Yes
• **Obesity**	Yes
• **Tobacco Use**	Yes
• **Alcohol Use**	Yes
• **Drug Use**	Yes
• **Pesticides**	Yes
• **Environmental Factors** – Air Pollution (Outdoor, Ozone Depletion, Acid Rain), Indoor Pollution, Water Pollution and Treatment, Electromagnetic Fields	Yes
• **Radiation** – Sun exposure, Suntan Booths, Unneeded X-ray	Yes
• **Sexual-Social** – Female and Male Promiscuity, AIDS spread	Yes
• **Hormonal Factors** – Menarche*, First Pregnancy, Abortion or Miscarriage First Trimester of First Pregnancy, Benign Breast Disease, Failure to Repair Undescended Testicle, DES, Oral Contraceptive Use, Hormone Replacement Therapy, Androgen Use	Yes
• **Sedentary Lifestyle**	Yes
• **Stress**	Yes
• **Occupational Exposure Factors**	Yes
• **High Blood Pressure**	Yes
• **Lack of Comprehensive Physical Examination**	Yes
• **Age**	No

* A high-fat diet triggers early menarche.

Children will benefit the most from properly modified nutritional factors and daily habits. Information on nutrition should be part of a child's education throughout the school years, because nutritional practices and habits are easily modified in youth. If parents and teachers set the example of healthy lifestyle factors, children will continue these practices throughout their lives. There will be a consequent decrease in the incidence of cancer, cardiovascular and other diseases.

What can you do to help yourself?

Simply, I have presented the current body of scientific information concerning benign breast disease, breast cancer, and the factors that promote an existing breast cancer. I now will discuss how those risk factors can be modified. Whether you have a benign breast problem or breast cancer, you will be better off when you closely adhere to my recommendations. As you have read, survival – lifespan – is positively affected mainly by proper lifestyle and not by existing conventional treatments. The preponderance of scientific information suggests that breast health can be achieved by following our Ten-Point Plan. **Our Ten Point Plan can decrease the risk for breast disease and increase the possibility of survival for those who have breast cancer.**

THE SIMONE TEN POINT PLAN FOR BREAST HEALTH

POINT 1. NUTRITION.

• **MAINTAIN AN IDEAL WEIGHT.** Decrease calories. Repeated fluctuations in your weight can increase the risk for heart attack and death.

• **LOW-FAT, LOW-CHOLESTEROL FOODS.** No four-legged animals, shellfish, or dairy products unless skim or non-fat products – not whole, 1%, or 2%.

To reduce cholesterol, avoid:	To reduce triglycerides, avoid:
• Four-legged Animals	• Alcohol
• Dairy, except skim or non-fat	• Fruit, fruit juices
• Shellfish	• Cookie, candy, cake

Triglycerides are sugar-fats and are increased by anything that tastes sweet to your tongue. Triglycerides thicken the bloodstream and makes the LDL-cholesterol small, dense, and better able to block arteries.[1] Cholesterol takes about 6 months to come down, but triglycerides take only about 6 weeks. Remember, there are no fairies that sprinkle cholesterol or triglycerides into your blood while you are sleeping!

If your total dietary fats are less than 20 percent of your total calories, you will attain breast health and decrease your risk of cancer and other health risks. It is also virtually impossible to gain weight on such a low-fat diet.

o *Poultry* cooked without the skin. White meat is best. Goose and duck are too fatty.

o *Fish* – all are fine except shellfish, sardines, mackerel, and fish canned in oil, all of which are high in fat or cholesterol.

o *Egg whites* are alright, not the yolk.

o *Eliminate saturated and polyunsaturated fats* – butter, margarine, meat fat, lard, and all oils.

o *Limit garnishes and sauces.* Ketchup and vinegar are fine. Unless they are fat-free, don't use salad dressings, prepared gravies and sauces, mayonnaise, sandwich spreads, or other products containing fats, oils, or egg yolks.

o *Food Labels* – you need to know how to read them to determine the percentage of fat calories from it. You need to know two numbers from the label: the total number of calories per ounce, and the number of fat grams per ounce, then add an imaginary zero to that number. Let's look at specific examples:

	Light Potato Chips	**Pretzel**
Total calories	120 per serving	100 per serving
Total fat grams	6	1
Imaginary zero to fat	60	10
Ratio	60 divided by 120	10 divided by 100
Percentage Fat	50%	10%
Eating these, you will:		
Gain weight	YES	NO
Decrease breast health	YES	NO
Increase risk for disease	YES	NO
Promote existing disease	YES	NO

What if there is no food label to read? Well, you already know which foods are good and which are not – look at Table 27.2.

Table 27.2 Percent Fat Calories in Foods

Good		Bad	
Vegetables/Fruit	<10%	Beef and Lamb	50-80%
Breads	10-20%	Pork (the "white meat")	80%
Fish	10-20%	Dairy – non-skim	60-90%
Pasta, Grains, Cereals	10-20%	Eggs	70%
Poultry (no skin)	20-35%	Diet Margarine	100%

• **CONSUME *SOLUBLE* AND *INSOLUBLE* FIBER** (25-35 grams/day). Fruits, vegetables, cereals are mainly *insoluble* fibers. Pectins, gums, and mucilages have *soluble* fibers that can decrease cholesterol, trigylcerides, sugars, and carcinogens. Both increase fecal bulk and bowel movement frequency, slow an irritable bowel, or speed up a constipated bowel. Use a supplement of *soluble* fiber to insure a consistent amount each day.

Taken with water, soluble fiber supplements make you feel full due to longer time in stomach and, hence, can be used effectively to decrease your appetite so that you lose weight.

You can eat whole or lightly milled grains like rice, barley, and buckwheat. Whole-wheat bread and whole-wheat pasta, cereals, crackers, and other grain products can also be eaten as can unsweetened fruit juices and unsweetened cooked, canned, or frozen fruit.

• **AVOID BUTTER ROLLS, COMMERCIAL BISCUITS, MUFFINS, DOUGHNUTS, SWEET ROLLS, CAKES, EGG BREAD, CHEESE BREAD,** and commercial mixes containing dried eggs and whole milk.

• **SUPPLEMENT YOUR DIET WITH THE CORRECT NUTRIENTS, IN THE CORRECT DOSES, IN THE CORRECT CHEMICAL FORM, AND THE CORRECT RATIO OF ONE TO ANOTHER BASED ON YOUR LIFESTYLE.** Take high doses of all antioxidants (the carotenoids, vitamins C and E, selenium, cysteine, bioflavonoids, copper, zinc), and the B vitamins with food; calcium and its enhancing agents, at bedtime.

Simone Antioxidant – Nutrient Supplementation			
Carotene	30 mg	**Selenium**	200 mcg
Lutein	20 mcg	**Copper**	3 mg
Lycopene	20 mcg	**Zinc**	30 mg
Vitamin A	5500 IU	Iodine	150 mcg
Vitamin D	400 IU	Potassium	30 mg
Vitamin E	400 IU	Chromium	125 mcg
Vitamin C	350 mg	Manganese	2.5 mg
Folic Acid	400 mcg	Molybdenum	50 mg
Vitamin B1	10 mg	Inositol	10 mg
Vitamin B2	10 mg	PABA	10 mg
Niacinamide	40 mg	**Bioflavonoids**	10 mg
Vitamin B6	10 mg	Choline	10 mg
Vitamin B12	18 mcg	**L-Cysteine**	20 mg
Biotin	150 mcg	**L-Arginine**	5 mg
Pantothenic acid	20 mg		

*Antioxidants are bolded

Simone Calcium Formula	
Calcium carbonate	1000 mg
Magnesium	280 mg
Potassium bicarbonate	200 mg
Boron	4 mg
L-Lysine	4 mg
Silicon	4 mg
Threonine	4 mg

Simone Fiber Formula	
Soluble Fiber	800 mg
Pectin, Gums (Guar, oat)	
Mucilages (kelp, psyllium)	
Insoluble Fiber	200 mg

Simone Essential Fatty Acids	
Linolenic Acid	2 to 8 grams
Linoleic Acid	3 to 9 grams

o Most nutrients should be taken with food. However, calcium and nutrients that enhance its metabolism should be taken at bedtime or on an empty stomach because most foods (fiber) will bind calcium and render it useless. Most supplements have calcium in the same tablet with the other nutrients, and, in effect, you get little or none of it when taken with food.

o Do not take supplements that contain iron because iron is associated with cancer promotion. There are many causes of anemia so unless you have a true iron deficiency anemia, there is no reason to take any supplemental iron, and this applies to menstruating women, too. If you do have a documented iron deficiency anemia, then you should be treated by a physician with therapeutic doses of iron in a thirty-day period. Patients who have a cancer and/or receive chemotherapy or radiation therapy usually have an anemia related to chronic disease and/or to therapy. No amount of iron will correct this anemia because it is not due to an iron deficiency.

• **ELIMINATE TABLE SALT.** Add only a minimal amount of salt while cooking. Most condiments, pickles, dressings, prepared sauces, canned vegetables, bouillon cubes, pot pies, popcorn, sauerkraut, and caviar have high amounts of salt in them.

• **AVOID FOOD ADDITIVES.** Avoid all foods containing nitrates, nitrites, or other harmful additives, or that were processed using a harmful technique (see Chapter 10). No pickled relish.

• **LIMIT SNACKS AND DESSERTS.** Healthy snacks or desserts include fresh fruit and canned fruit without added sugar, water ices, gelatin, and puddings made with skim milk. Do not eat commercially prepared cakes, pies, cookies, doughnuts, and mixes; coconut or coconut oil; frozen cream pies; potato chips and other deep-fried snacks; whole-milk puddings; ice cream; candy; chocolate; or gum with sugar.

• **BEVERAGES.** Distilled water, unsweetened fruit juices, and vegetable juices are great. Avoid caffeine-containing beverages – coffee, tea, cola, etc. Skim milk or non-fat products are OK – but remember dairy causes mucus production.

• **REMEMBER GOOD NUTRITION WHEN DINING OUT.** Call the restaurant to see if your needs as outlined here can be accommodated. Airlines and ocean liners will also help you. Request that your food be prepared without any salt products (Chinese food is high in sodium). Use lemon juice or vinegar on your salad.

• **TAKE 325 MG ASPIRIN EVERY OTHER DAY WITH FOOD IF YOU ARE ABLE.** Aspirin can decrease the risk of cardiovascular disease and also decrease the risk of cancer spread.

POINT 2. TOBACCO.

DO NOT SMOKE, CHEW, SNUFF, OR INHALE OTHER PEOPLE'S SMOKE. There is no easy, painless way to quit. The best way is simply to go "cold turkey" without tapering off or using any expensive smoke-ending courses. Remember, tobacco smoke also endangers the health of nonsmokers. As a nonsmoker, demand that smokers not smoke in your presence, especially in public or work-related areas.

POINT 3. ALCOHOL and CAFFEINE.

AVOID ALL ALCOHOL, OR HAVE ONE DRINK OR LESS PER WEEK. AVOID CAFFEINE (COFFEE, TEA, CHOCOLATE).

POINT 4. RADIATION.

X-RAYS ONLY WHEN NEEDED. USE SUNSCREENS AND SUNGLASSES. AVOID ELECTROMAGNETIC FIELDS from home appliances, office equipment, and outside electric fields. All radiation is cumulative.

POINT 5. ENVIRONMENT.

KEEP AIR, WATER, AND WORKPLACE CLEAN, ESPECIALLY IN YOUR OWN HOUSEHOLD. Avoid prolonged exposure to household cleaning fluids, solvents, and paint thinners. Some may be hazardous if inhaled in high concentrations. Pesticides, fungicides, and other home garden and lawn chemicals are also dangerous. Environmental protection standards should be rigorously observed. For instance, a person working with asbestos (insulation, brake lining, etc.) should wear a mask to protect the respiratory and gastrointestinal systems.

POINT 6. SEXUAL-SOCIAL FACTORS, HORMONES, DRUGS.

AVOID PROMISCUITY, HORMONES, AND ANY UNNECESSARY DRUGS.

POINT 7. LEARN THE SEVEN EARLY WARNING SIGNS

- Lump in breast
- Nonhealing sore
- Change in wart/mole
- Unusual bleeding
- Persistent cough/hoarseness
- Change in bowel/bladder habits
- Indigestion/trouble swallowing

POINT 8. EXERCISE

Brisk walking for 20 minutes four times a week or household chores, or weekend warrior activities are good forms of exercise. Exercise can enhance the immune system, decrease the risk of cancer, cardiovascular disease, and osteoporosis. Everyone should start a program of exercise, but see a physician before doing so if you are at risk for cardiovascular disease. Initially the exercising should start out slowly, then increase to a comfortable level. I stress fast walking because it is easier to do than other forms of exercise – no equipment to buy, no change of clothing, no one to rely on except yourself. You can walk in a shopping mall in inclement weather. Calisthenics should also be done to firm up abdominal-wall muscles and decrease that "spare tire." Five to ten sit-ups, with knees bent, can readily be done at home every day. Lower back pain is one of the most common pains in America. Simple stretching and flexing exercises will prevent and treat lower back pain.

Remember, the data show that some amount of exercise is better than none. Just a little exercise every day will benefit you enormously. Choose an exercise program that you are likely to follow, and stick with your exercise routine.

POINT 9. STRESS MODIFICATION, SPIRITUALITY, SEXUALITY

Stress is a risk factor for the development and promotion of breast disease. To promote breast health, you must modify your stress. Control stress by whatever means you can: meditation, self-hypnosis, spirituality, intimacy, or self-love, biofeedback, music, hot-water showers, or other methods you find relaxing. Stress is a killer! So find out what will help you relax.

Spirituality, or the Life Force, is what gives people hope and produces a calming and peaceful effect. Spirituality is often ignored by many people until they get into trouble with an illness or other aspects of life. Spirituality is comprised of many components. The scientific connection between the mind and body is inescapable. The mind has great control over the body and the immune system. So your attitude in dealing with any crisis is critical. Good spiritual attitude is important for good health and the proper functioning of the immune system. Having a good spiritual life is important for wellness and health. Lack of spirituality is a risk factor for illness. Remember the words of the Bible:

> "Pleasant words are like a honeycomb, sweetness to the soul and health to the body" – Book of Proverbs (16:24)
>
> "A man's spirit will endure sickness; but a broken spirit who can bear?" – Book of Proverbs (1.08:14)

Seek the psychological and emotional comfort of other people as well. Avoid loneliness.

Sexuality is also important. Re-read the section in Chapter 25 on Sexuality and Body Image. Do what makes you feel good; this will further relieve stress.

POINT 10. COMPREHENSIVE PHYSICAL EXAM.

EARLY DIAGNOSIS IS IMPORTANT. PREVENTION IS THE KEY TO WELLNESS.

All women who have lumpy breasts should have a comprehensive physical examination (combines a thorough history and a scalp-to-toe examination) with appropriate counseling and laboratory studies in order to prevent or detect early cancer or heart disease. If a physician is looking for early cancer and it is present, it then can probably be found.

A thorough history should include questions about all the risk factors for cancer listed in Chapter 3, as well as the questions at the end of this plan. The physical examination is important and should be complete, starting at the scalp and finishing at the toes. One capable, highly trained specialist should perform the entire examination, rather than your gynecologist doing the Pap smear and breast exam, your cardiologist checking the heart, your dentist looking in your mouth, and so on. The examining physician must be thorough in examining your breasts. All the examination techniques outlined in Chapter 20 should be followed for a complete breast examination.

Laboratory tests are another part of an asymptomatic noncancerous person's work-up. Little more than one ounce of blood and urine is taken and assayed. Table 27.3 lists the laboratory tests, the normal range of the tests, and the functions tested.

Table 27.3 Laboratory Tests for a Comprehensive Physical

Laboratory Test	Normal Range
Stool for Occult Blood	Negative
Blood Counts: Hemoglobin	Female: 11.5-15 Male: 12.5-17
White Cell Count	3,700-10,500
Platelet Count	155,000-385,000
Cholesterol	130-200
Triglycerides	50-200
Glucose – blood sugar	65-115
Kidney Function: Creatinine	0.6-1.5
Blood Urea Nitrogen	5-25
Electrolytes: Calcium	8.5-10.8
Phosphate	2.4-4.5
Magnesium	1.3-2.1
Sodium	135-147
Chloride	96-109
Potassium	3.5-5.3
CO_2	23-33
Uric Acid	3.0-9.0
Liver Function : Total Protein	6.0-8.5
Albumin	3.5-5.5
Alkaline phosphatase	25-140
SGPT	0-45
SGOT	0-40
LDH	0-240
Total Bilirubin	0.1-1.2

Since breast cancer patients have a higher incidence of colon cancer, testing the stool for trace amounts of blood is another important laboratory examination. Trace amounts of blood in the stool can result from some lesion(s) in the gastrointestinal tract, which can be a gastrointestinal cancer. Prior to and during the collection of the stool specimens, it is important to completely avoid red meat for three entire days, because red meat contains animal blood that will produce a positive result in the test. All other instructions must also be followed.

Certain fiberoptic procedures should be done when indicated. By using a fiberoptic laryngoscope, we have found many lesions of the nasopharynx and larynx when examining patients who have been exposed to passive smoke for several hours a day, patients who have been hoarse for two weeks or more, or other high-risk patients.

A colonoscopy is an examination of the colon with a fiberoptic flexible instrument, looking for abnormalities like lesions that may bleed. Indications for doing a fiberoptic colonoscopy are:

1. To evaluate the colon when an abnormality was found with a barium enema.
2. To discover and excise polyps.
3. To evaluate unexplained bleeding: A positive occult blood stool test (detection of blood in the stool that could not be seen by the eye); Bleeding from the rectum.
4. To investigate an unexplained iron deficiency anemia.
5. To survey for colon cancer: A strong family history of colon cancer; To check the entire colon in a patient with a treatable cancer or polyp; A follow-up after resection of polyp or cancer at eighteen to thirty-six month intervals, depending on the clinical circumstances; In a patient with ulcerative colitis.
6. To investigate chronic inflammatory bowel disease.
7. To control bleeding.

An annual chest X-ray should be done in high-risk asymptomatic patients. If a cancer mass is found in the periphery of the lung, it can be surgically removed thereby affording the patient an excellent chance for cure. A person's lung function can be readily assessed by pulmonary function testing – a series of tests that determine the quantity and speed of the air moving in and out of the lungs, the volumes of the lungs, etc.

You will feel better and stay well by following this Simone Ten Point Plan

BREAST SURVEILLANCE: ASYMPTOMATIC WOMEN.

1. Physical Exam by Physician – all women starting at age 35.

SURVEILLANCE FOLLOW-UP: ASYMPTOMATIC BREAST CANCER PATIENTS (looking for recurrence or metastases)

Current Convention	Sufficient
Physical exam by physician	Physical exam by physician
First 2 years: every 3months	First 3 years: every 3-6 months
Years 2 to 4: every 4 months	Years 4 to 5: every 6-12 months
Years 5 to 6: every 6 months	6+ years: annually
6+ years: annually	
Laboratory tests	Laboratory tests – not needed except
Mammogram, chest X-ray, liver function tests	Mammogram annually

With these "routine" tests, an abnormality is found in less than 2 percent of all asymptomatic breast cancer patients.

THE CANCER QUESTIONNAIRE below will help you work with your physician. If, after answering the questions, you find you have three or more of the possible "yes" answers in any one category, consult your physician.

CANCER QUESTIONNAIRE

	NO	YES
General		
1. Have you been told by a doctor that you had cancer? If yes, what kind?_______	___	___
2. Have any of your blood relatives had cancer? If yes, what kind?_______	___	___
3. Have you lost 10-15 pounds over the past 6 months without knowing why?	___	___
Lungs		
4. Have you coughed up blood in the past several weeks?	___	___
5. Have you had a chronic cough daily?	___	___
6. Have you been told that you have emphysema?	___	___
7. Have you had pneumonia twice or more in the past year?	___	___
8. Have you ever smoked?	___	___
9. Did you quit smoking less than 15 years ago?	___	___
10. Do you smoke now?	___	___
Cigarettes: Number packs/day ___ Number of years___		

	NO	YES
Cigars Number cigars/day ___		
Pipe Number bowls/day ___		
11. Do you inhale others' smoke for one or more hours/day?	___	___
Larynx (voice box)		
12. Have you had persistent hoarseness?	___	___
Mouth and Throat		
13. Have you had the following lasting more than 1 month?		
Pain or difficulty swallowing	___	___
Pain or tenderness in the mouth	___	___
A sore or white spot in your mouth	___	___
14. Do you drink more than 4 oz of wine, 12 oz beer, or 1.5 oz whiskey every day?	___	___
Stomach		
15. Have you vomited blood in the past month?	___	___
16. Have you had black stools in the past 6 months?	___	___
Does this happen when you are not taking iron?	___	___
17. Have you had stomach pains several times a week?	___	___
18. Has a doctor said that you had an ulcer or stomach polyps?	___	___
Large Intestine and Rectum		
19. Have you had a change in your usual bowel habits?	___	___
20. Has your stool become narrow in diameter?	___	___
21. Does this happen with every bowel movement?	___	___
22. Have you had bleeding from the rectum?	___	___
23. Have you had mucus in your stool every time?	___	___
24. Have you been told that you have a polyp in the colon?	___	___
25. Have you had ulcerative colitis?	___	___
Breasts		
26. Do you self-examine your breasts each month?	___	___
27. Do you have a lump in either breast?	___	___
28. Have you had breast pain recently?	___	___
Does this pain occur when you are not menstruating?	___	___
29. Has there been discharge or bleeding from your nipples, or have they begun to pull in (retract)?	___	___
30. Are there any changes in the skin of your breasts?	___	___
31. Have you ever had a breast biopsy?	___	___
Cervix, Uterus, and Vagina		
32. Do you have vaginal bleeding or spotting?	___	___
If Yes: Is it between periods?	___	___
Is it after sexual intercourse?	___	___
Is it after menopause?	___	___
33. Have you stopped having your periods?	___	___
At what age? ___		
Since then, have you ever had hormone therapy?	___	___
Have you had a hysterectomy?	___	___

	NO	YES
34. Have you ever had sexual intercourse?	___	___
Did you first have intercourse before age 16?	___	___
35. Did your mother take DES when pregnant with you?	___	___
Skin		
36. Has there been bleeding or change in a mole on you?	___	___
37. Do you have a mole on your body where it may be irritated by underwear, a belt, etc?	___	___
38. Do you have a sore that does not heal?	___	___
39. Do you have a severe scar from a burn?	___	___
40. Do you have fair skin and sunburn easily?	___	___
41. Do you sunbathe for hours or use a suntanning booth?	___	___
Thyroid		
42. Can you see or feel a lump in the lower front of your neck?	___	___
43. Have you had X-ray treatment to your face for acne, tonsil enlargement, or other reasons?	___	___
Kidney and Urinary Bladder		
44. Have you had blood in your urine?	___	___

CONCLUSION

The Cancer Questionnaire is only good if you take the time to answer the questions. Similarly, the points in my plan are only good if *you* follow them. The decision is yours.

Now after reading **The Truth About Breast Health – Breast Cancer** you already understand some of the ways in which you can attain breast health, and reduce your risk for breast cancer and risk of breast cancer recurrence. Start by following the Ten-Point Plan presented here. And turn the page to find out what comes next.

29
Now What?

This may be the ending of my book, but it should be just a beginning for you. I hope the book has given you the information you need to understand what breast health is all about. Armed with this information, there are things you can and ***should*** do.

The responsibility for breast health does not lie with other people. It falls directly in your hands. It's up to you to do something. Start by taking care of yourself. Modify your lifestyle with your optimum health in mind. And if you should feel a lump, don't let fear immobilize you. See your health-care practitioner.

Next, take care of those close to you. Tell them to do something. If you want to take it one step further, join an organization or group. Work with others in support groups that aid and educate cancer patients and their families. Join with others to lobby against such cancer risks as second-hand smoke, air pollution, and toxic wastes. Anything can be accomplished if we work together.

Afterword

You have read quite a bit of information. But you should come away with a single important thought: **You have almost total control over the destiny of your health.** More and more people realize that by controlling risk factors – especially the major ones like nutrition, tobacco use, and alcohol consumption – you can control your well-being.

You now have the knowledge and the tools to modify your lifestyle to optimize your health and the health of your loved ones. You have the chance for a rendezvous with your well-being. Determine your own health's destiny. Seize this opportunity! Do it now!

For more information, please write to:

Charles B. Simone, M.D.
Simone Protective Cancer Institute
123 Franklin Corner Road
Lawrenceville, NJ 08648
DrSimone.com

Other Books by Charles B. Simone, M.D.

- **Cancer and Nutrition** (1981, updated multiple times)
- **How To Save Yourself From a Terrorist Attack** (2002)
- **Shark Cartilage and Cancer** (1994)

Medical and Scientific References

Introduction

1. U.S. Department of Health and Human Services, Public Health Service. 1990. The Surgeon General's Report on Nutrition and Health. Wash, D.C., US Gov Print Office.
2. Greenlee RT, Hill-Harmon M, Murray T, et al. Cancer statistics, 2001. *CA - Cancer J Clin.* 2001; 51: 15-36.
3. Bailar J, E Smith. Progress against cancer? *NEJM.* 1986; 314:1226-32.
4. Boyd J, ed. NCAB approves year 2000 report. *The Cancer Letter.* 2000; 11(28):1-6.
5. Kolata G. Is the war on cancer being won? *Science* 1985; 29:543-44.
6. Boffey P. Cancer progress: Are the statistics telling the truth? *New York Times* Sept 18 1984; C1.
7. Bush H. Cancer cure. *Science.* 1984; 84:34-35.
8. Blonston G. Cancer prevention. *Science.* 1984; 84:36-39.
9. Marshall E. Experts clash over cancer data. *Science.* 1990;250:900-902.
10. Simone, CB. Cancer and Nutrition. McGraw-Hill.1983; revised 1995. Pages 1-237.
11. National Academy of Sciences, National Research Council, Food and Nutrition Board. 1989. *Diet and health: Implications for reducing chronic disease risk.* Washington, D.C.: National Academy Press.
12. The Surgeon General's Report on Nutrition and Health. 1988.
13. Butrum, et al. NCI dietary guidelines: Rationale. *Am J Clin Nutrition.* 1988; 48:888-95.
14. U.S. Bureau of Vital Statistics from 1900 to present.
15. *CA- A Cancer J for Clinicians.* 1962 – present.
16. Perception of cancer risks. *JNCI.* Sept 1,1993.

Chapter 1
The Scope of Breast Disease

1. Greenlee RT, Hill-Harmon MB, Murray T, Thun M. Cancer statistics, 2001. *CA Cancer J Clin.* 2001; 51: 15-36.
2. Cohen P, et al. Seasonality in the occurrence of breast cancer. *Canc Res.* 1983; 43:892-893.
3. Parkin DN, et al. Estimates of the worldwide frequency of 12 major cancers. *Bull WHO.* 1984; 62:163182.
4. Mittra I, et al. Early detection of breast cancer in developing countries. *Lancet.* 1989; April1:719-720.
5. Boyle R, et al. Trends in diet related cancers in Japan: A conundrum? *Lancet.* 1993; 342:752.

Chapter 2
Benign Breast Syndromes

1. Boyd, et al. Effects of a low fat, high carbohydrate diet on symptoms of cyclical mastopathy. *Lancet.* 1988; ii:128-132.
2. Facchinetti F, et al. Oral magnesium successfully relieves premenstrual mood changes. *Obstet Gynecol.* 1991; 78:178-181.
3. Minton, et al. Response of fibrocystic disease to caffeine withdrawal and correlation of cyclic nucleotides with breast disease. *Am J Obstot Gynocol.* 1979; 135:157-158.
4. Ernster, et al. Effects of caffeine free diet on benign breast disease: A randomized trial. *Surgery.* 1982; 91(3):263-267.
5. Javitt NB, Budai, Miller, et al. Breast-gut connection: origin of chenodeoxycholic acid in breast cyst fluid. *Lancet.* 1994; 343:633-35.
6. Dixon JM, et al. Risk of breast cancer in women with palpable breast cysts – a prospective study. *Lancet.* 1999; 353: 1742-45.
7. Dupont W, et al. Long term risk of breast cancer in women with fibroadenoma. *NEJM.* 1994; 331:10-15.
8. Jacobs TW, Byrne C, Colditz G, et al. Radial scars in benign breast biopsy specimens and the risk of breast cancer. *NEJM.* 1999; 340:430-6.
9. McBride G. Revised Consensus on Benign Breast Conditions. *Oncology Times.* December 1992, 22.
10. Kapdi CC, Parekh. The male breast. *Radiol Clin North Am.* 1983; 21:137.
11. Nuttal FQ. Gynecomastia as a physical finding in normal men. *J Clin Endocrinol Metab.* 1979; 48:338.
12. Carlson HE. Current concepts: Gynecomastia. *NEJM.* 1980; 303:671.
13. Fletcher S, et al. Physician's abilities to detect lumps in silicone breast models. *JAMA.* 1985; 253(15):2224-2228.
14. National Cancer Institute. Breast Cancer Prevention Trial shows major benefit, some risk [web site news release]. Available: http://cancertrials.nci.nih.gov (accessed May 28, 1998.
15. Powles T, Eeles R, Ashley S, et al. Interim analysis of the incidence of breast cancer in the Royal Marsden Hospital tamoxifen randomized chemoprevention trial. *Lancet.* 1998; 352: 98-101.
16. Veronesi U, Maisonneeuve P, Costa A, et al. Prevention of breast cancer with tamoxifen: preliminary findings from the Italian randomized trial among hysterectomised women. *Lancet.* 1998; 352:93-97.

17. Special report: Breast Cancer Prevention Trial. *Oncology Bulletin.* June 4-19, 1992.
18. Fornander, et al. Long term adjuvant tamoxifen in early breast cancer. *JNCI.* 1990; 83:1450-1459.
19. Love, et al. Bone mineral density in women with breast cancer treated with adjuvant tamoxifen for at least two years. *Breast Cancer Res Treat.* 1988; 12:279-302.
20. Gotfredson, et al. The effect of tamoxifen on bone mineral content in premenopausal women with breast cancer. *Cancer.* 1984; 53:853-857.
21. Fentiman, et al. Bone mineral content of women receiving tamoxifen for mastalgia. *Br J Cancer.* 1989;60:262-264.
22. Powles, et al. A pilot trial to evaluate the acute toxicity and feasibility of tamoxifen for prevention of breast cancer. *Br J Cancer.* 1989; 60:126-131.
23. Costantino J, Kuller L, Ives D, et al. Coronary heart disease mortality and adjuvant tamoxifen therapy. *J Natl Cancer Inst.* 1997; 89(11):776-82.

Chapter 3

An Overview of Risk Factors

1. The National Academy of Sciences. 1982. Nutrition, diet, and cancer.
2. Wynder EL, GB Gori. Contribution of the environment to cancer incidence: An epidemiologic exercise. *JNCI.* 1977; 58:825.
3. Workshop on Fat and Cancer. September Supplement to *Cancer Res.* 1981; 41(9):3677.
4. Mulvihill J. Genetic repertory of human neoplasia. In Genetics of human cancer. 1977 Ed. JJ Mulvihill, RW, Miller, and JF Fraumeni. New York: Raven Press, 137.
5. Armstrong B, R Doll. Environmental factors and cancer incidence and mortality in different countries, with special reference to dietary practices. *Intl J Cancer.* 1975; 15:617.
6. Bjarnason O, N Day, G Snaedal, Tilinuis. The effect of year of birth on the breast cancer age incidence curve in Iceland. *Intl J Cancer.* 1974; 13:689.
7. Miller AB. Nutrition and cancer. *Prev Med* 1980; 9:189.
8. Eskin BA. Iodine and mammary cancer. In: Inorganic and nutrition aspects of cancer, ed. G.H. Schrauzer. 1978; New York: Plenum Press, 293-304.
9. Upton AC. Future directions in cancer prevention. *Prev Med* 1980; 9:309.
10. Shank RC, GN Wogan, JB Gibson, et al. Dietary aflatoxins and human liver cancer.II. Aflatoxins in market foods and foodstuffs of Thailand and Hong Kong. *Food Cosmet Toxicol.* 1972; 10:61.
11. Tomatis L, C Agthe, H Bartsch, et al. Evaluation of the carcinogenicity of chemicals: A review of the monograph program of the International Agency for Research on Cancer. *Cancer Res.* 1982; 38:877.
12. Dargie H. Calcium channel blockers and the clinician. *Lancet.* 1996; 348:488.
13. Horton R. Do calcium antagonists cause cancer? *Lancet.* 1996; 348:49.
14. Correa A, Jackson L, Mohan A, et al. Use of hair dyes, hematopoietic neoplasms, and lymphomas: A literature review. *Cancer Investigation.* 2000; 18(5): 467-479.
15. Wattenberg LW. Inhibitors of chemical carcinogenesis. *Adv Cancer Res* 1978; 26:197.
16. Pierce RC, M Katz. Dependency of polynuclear aromatic hydrocarbons on size distribution of atmospheric aerosols. *Environ Sci Technol* 1975; 9:347.
17. U.S. Environmental Protection Agency. Preliminary assessment of suspected carcinogens in drinking water. Report to Congress. Environmental Protection Agency, Washington, D.C.1975.
18. Harris RH, Page, Reiches. Carcinogenic hazards of organic chemicals in drinking water. In: Incidence of cancer in humans, ed. H.H. Hiatt, et al. Cold Spring Harbor Lab, 1977.
19. Dixon AK, Dendy P. Spiral CT: how much does radiation dose matter? *Lancet.* 1998; 352:1082-83.
20. Boice J, Mandel J, Doody M. Breast cancer among radiologic technologists. *JAMA.* 1995; 274: 394-401.
21. Gardner MJ, et al. Results of case-control study of leukemia and lymphoma among young people near Sellafield nuclear plant in West Cumbria. *BMJ.* 1990; 300:423-29.
22. Wing S, et al. 1991. Mortality among workers at Oak Ridge National Laboratory: Evidence of radiation effects in follow-up through 1984. *JAMA.* 1991; 265:1397-1408.
23. Jablon S, et al. Cancer in populations living near nuclear facilities. *JAMA.* 1991; 265:1403-8.
24. Mawson AR. Breast cancer in female flight attendants. *Lancet.* 1998; 352:626.
25. Stewart T, N Stewart. Breast cancer in female flight attendants. *Lancet.* 1995; 346:1379.
26. Gundestrup M, Storm HH. Radiation-induced acute myeloid leukaemia and other cancers in commercial jet cockpit crew: a

population-based cohort study. *Lancet.* 1999; 354:2029-31.

27. International Agency for Research on Cancer. 1980. Annual Report. World Health Organization. Lyon, France.
28. Miller, D.G. On the nature of susceptibility to cancer. *Cancer* 1980; 46:1307.
29. Walford, R.L. The immunological theory of aging. Munksgaard, Copenhagen, 1969.
30. Kahn, HA. The Dorn study of smoking and mortality among US veterans: Report on eight years of observation. In: Epidemiological study of cancer and other chronic diseases. NCI Mono. 19. Washington, D.C. US Gov Printing Office. 1966.
31. Lichtenstein P, Holm N, et al. Environmental and heritable factors in the causation of cancer. *NEJM.* 2000; 343:78-85.
32. Weber GL, Garber JE. Family history and breast cancer: probabilities and possibilities. *JAMA;* 1993; 270:1602-1603.
33. Benditt EP, JM Benditt. Evidence for a monoclonal origin of human atherosclerotic plaques. *Proc Natl Acad Sci.* 1973; 70:1753.
34. Pero RW, C Bryngelsson, F Mitelman, et al. High blood pressure related to carcinogen induced unscheduled DNA synthesis, DNA carcinogen binding, and chromosomal aberrations in human lymphocytes. *Proc Natl Acad Sci* 1976; 73:2496.32.
35. de Waard F, EA Banders-van Halewijn, J Huizinga. 1964. The bimodal age distribution of patients with mammary cancer. *Cancer.* 1964; 17:141
36. Dyer AR, J Stamler, AM Berkson, et al. High blood pressure: A risk factor for cancer mortality. *Lancet.* 1975; i:1051.
37. Cotton T, et al. Breast cancer in mothers prescribed DES in pregnancy. *JAMA.* 1993; 269(16):2096-2100.
38. Wobbes T, Koops, Oldhoff. The relation between testicular tumors, undescended testes, and inguinal hernias. *J Surg Onc.* 1980; 14:45
39. IARC monographs on the evaluation of carcinogenic risks to humans 1994-1999. Geneva: WHO Publications.
40. Sharp DW. Gastric cancer: A new role for *Helicobacter pylori Science Watch.* 1993; 4:5.
41. Morgan RA, Dornsife RE, et al. In vitro infections of human bone marrow by feline leukemia viruses. *Virology.* 1993; 193:439-42.
42. Collinge J, Palmer M, et al. Transmission of fatal familial insomnia to laboratory animals. *Lancet.* 1995; 346:569-70.
43. Diringer H. Proposed link between transmissible spongiform encephalopathies of man and animals. *Lancet.* 1995; 346:1208-10.

Chapter 4

Nutrition, Immunity, and Cancer

1. Cannon PR. Antibodies and protein reserves. *J Immunol.* 1942; 44:107.
2. Chandra R. Nutrition and immunology. New York: Alan R. Liss, Inc. Press. 1989; 3.
3. Rous P. The influence of diet on transplanted and spontaneous mouse tumors. *J Exp Med.* 1914; 20:433.4.
4. Tannenbaum A. The initiation and growth of tumors. Introduction I. Effects of underfeeding. *Am J Cancer.* 1940; 38:335.
5. Simone CB, Henkart. Permeability changes induced in erythrocyte ghost targets by antibody-dependent cytotoxic effector cells: Evidence for membrane pores. *J Immunol.* 1980; 124:954.
6. Burnet FM. Immunological surveillance. Oxford: Pergamon Press.1970.
7. Kersey JH, Spector, and R.A. Good. Primary immunodeficiency diseases and cancer: The immunodeficiency-cancer registry. *Intl J Cancer.* 1973; 12:333.
8. Spector G, Perry III, Good RA, Kersey. Immunodeficiency diseases and malignancy. The immunopathology of lymphoreticular neoplasms. 1978. ed. JJ Twomey, and RA Good. New York: Plenum Publishing, 203.
9. Penn. Malignant tumors in organ transplant recipients. New York: Springer-Verlag.
10. Birkeland SA, Kemp E, Hauge M. Renal transplantation and cancer. The Scandia transplant material. *Tissue Antigens.* 1975; 6:28.
11. Chandra R. Nutrition and immunology.
12. Delafuente, Panush. Potential of drug-related immunoenhancement of the geriatric patient. *Geriatric Med* 1990; 9:32-40.
13. Jeevan A, Kripke. Ozone depletion and the immune system. *Lancet.* 1993; 342:1159-1160.
14. Cooper KD, et al.UV exposure reduces immunization rate and promotes tolerance to epicutaneous antigens in humans. *Proc Natl Acad Sci.* 1992; 89:8497-8501.
15. Vermeer M, et al. Effects of ultraviolet B light on cutaneous immune responses of humans with deeply pigmented skin. *J Invest Dermatol.* 1991; 97:729-734.
16. Yoshikawa T, et al. Susceptibility to effects of UVB radiation on induction of contact hypersensitivity as a risk factor for skin cancer in man. *J Invest Dermatol.* 1990; 95:530-536.
17. Peters E, et al. Vitamin C supplementation reduces post-race symptoms of upper respiratory tract infection in ultramarathon runners. *Am J Clin Nutr.* 1993; 57:170-171.

18. Heath GW. Exercise and incidence of upper respiratory tract infections. *Med Sci Sports Exerc.* 1991; 23:152-157.
19. Aschekenasy A. Dietary protein and amino acids in leucopoiesis. *World Rev Nutri Diet.* 1975; 21:152.
20. Jose DG, Good RA. Absence of enhancing antibody in cell-mediated immunity to tumor homografts in protein deficient rats. *Nature.* 1971; 231:807.
21. Passwell JH, Steward, Soothill. The effects of protein malnutrition on macrophage function and the amount and affinity of antibody response. *Clin Exp Immunol.* 1974; 17:491.
22. Van Oss CJ. Influence of glucose levels on the *in vitro* phagocytosis of bacteria by human neutrophils. *Infect Immunol.* 1971; 4:54.
23. Perille PE, Nolan, Finch. Studies of the resistance to infection in diabetes mellitus: Local exudative cellular response. *J Lab Clin Med.* 1972; 59:1008.
24. Bagdade JD, Root, Bulger. Impaired leukocyte function in patients with poorly controlled diabetes. *Diabetes.* 1974; 23:9.
25. Stuart AE, Davidson. Effect of simple lipids on antibody formation after ingestion of foreign red cells. *J Pathol Bacteriol.* 1976; 87:305.
26. Santiago-Delpin E, Szepsenwol. Prolonged survival of skin and tumor allografts in mice on high fat diets. *JNCI.* 1977; 59:459.
27. DiLuzio N, Wooles. Depression of phagocytic activity and immune response by methyl palmitate. *Am J Physiol.* 1964; 206:939.

Chapter 5

Antioxidants and Other Cancer-Fighting Nutrients

1. Pietrzik, K. Concept of borderline vitamin deficiencies. *Int J Vit Nutr Res* 1985; 27:61-73.
2. Brin M. Dilemma of marginal vitamin deficiency. *Proc 9th Int Cong Nutrition*, Mexico 1972; 4:102-115.
3. Werback MR. Marginal nutrient deficiencies. In: Textbook of Nutritional Medicine. Third Line Press. Tarzana, CA. 1999; Pp:32-41.
4. US Depart of HEW. HANES: Health and Nutrition Examination Survey 1974. Pub No. 74-1219-1. Rockville, MD.
5. Baker H, Frank O. Sub-clinical vitamin deficits in various age groups. *Int J Vit Nutr Res.* 1985; 27:47-59.
6. US Dept. of Agriculture, Human Nutrition Information Service, 1985. Continuing Survey of Food Intakes by Individuals. CSFII Report No. 85-4.
7. Popkin B, Siega-Riz A, Haines P. A comparison of dietary trends among racial and socioeconomic groups in the US. *NEJM.* 1996; 335:716-20.
8. Ideas for better eating. Menus and recipes to make use of the dietary guidelines. Sci and Ed Admin/Human Nutrition. U.S. Dept. of Agriculture January 1981.
9. Dietary intake source data: US 1976-80. National Health Survey: 11, No. 231, DHHS Pub (PHS) 83-1681.March '83.
10. US Dept. of Agriculture. Nationwide Food Survey. 1980
11. Kant, et al. National Health and Nutrient Examination Survey II. *JADA.* 1991; 91:1526-32.
12. Pao E, Mickle. 1981. Problem nutrients in the United States. *Food Technology* September.
13. Krehl WA. The role of nutrition in preventing disease. Davidson Conference USC School of Dentistry. Feb. 29, 1981
14. Roe D. Drug-induced nutritional deficiencies. 1976.Connecticut: The AVI Publishing, Co.
15. Lieber C. Alcohol and malnutrition in the pathogenesis of liver disease and nutrition. VA Hospital. Mt. Sinai School of Medicine. New York, Bronx, NY. Sept.1975.
16. Baker H, Frank, Zetterman, et al. Inability of chronic alcoholics with liver disease to use food as a source of folates, thiamine and vitamin B6. *Amer J Clin Nutr* 1975; 28:1377-80.
17. Payne I, Lu G, Meyer K. Relationships of dietary tryptophan and niacin to tryptophan metabolism in alcoholics and non-alcoholics. *Am J Clin Nutr* 1974; 27:572-579.
18. Lumeng L, Li TK. Vitamin B6 metabolism in chronic alcohol abuse. *J Clin Invest.* 1974; 53:57-61.
19. Lieber C, Baraona, Leo, and Garro A. Metabolism and metabolic effects of ethanol, including interaction with drugs, carcinogens and nutrition. *Mutat Res* 1987;186:201-233.
20. Halsted C, Heise C. Ethanol and vitamin metabolism. *Pharmac Ther.* 1987; 34:453-64.
21. Aoki K, Ito Y, Sasaki, et al. Smoking, alcohol drinking and serum carotenoids levels. *Jpn J Cancer Res Gann.* 1987; 78:1049-56.
22. Fazio V, Flint D, Wahlqvist M. Acute effects of alcohol on plasma ascorbic acid in healthy subjects. *Am J Clin Nutr.* 1981; 34:2394-96.
23. Pelletier O. Vitamin C and cigarette smokers. *Ann NY Acad Sci.* 1975; 258:156-166.
24. US Department of Health, Education and Welfare. The health consequences of smoking. January 1973.

25. Hornig D, Glatthaar B. Vitamin C and smoking: Increased requirement of smokers. *Int J Vit Nutr Res.*1985; 27:139-155.
26. Menkes M, Constock G, Vuilleumier J, et al. Vitamin C is lower in smokers. *NEJM.* 1986; 315:1250-4.
27. Chow C, Thacker R, Changchit C, et al. Lower levels of vitamin C and carotenes in plasma of cigarette smokers. *J Am Coll Nutr.* 1986; 5:305-312.
28. Witter F, Blake D, Baumgardner R, et al. Folate, carotene, and smoking. *Am J Obstet Gynecol.* 1982; 144:857.
29. Gerster H. Beta-carotene and smoking. *J Nutr Growth Cancer.* 1987; 4:45-49.
30. Pacht E, Kaseki H, Mohammed J, et al. Deficiency of vitamin E in the alveolar fluid of cigarette smokers. *J Clin Invest* 1986; 77:789-96.
31. Serfontein W, Ubbink J, DeVilliers J, and Becker. Depressed plasma pyridoxal-5'-phosphate levels in tobacco-smoking men. *Atherosclerosis.* 1986; 59:341-346.
32. Who's dieting and why. 1978. A.C. Nielsen Co.
33. Welsh S, Marston R. Review of trends in food used in the United States, 1909 to 1980. *J A Dietetic Assn.* 1982; August.
34. Kasper H. Vitamins in prevention and therapy: Recent findings in vitamin research. *Fortschritte der Medizin* 1964; 82:22.
35. Horo E, Brin M, Faloon W. Fasting in obesity: Thiamine depletion as measured by erythrocyte activity changes. *Arch Int Med.* 1983; 117:175-81.
36. Fisher M, Lachance P. Nutrition evaluation of published weight-reducing diets. *J Am Diet Assoc.*1985; 85:450-454.
37. Leevy C, Cardi L, Frank O, et al. Incidence and significance of hypovitaminemia in a randomly selected municipal hospital population. *Am J Clin Nutr* 1965;17: 259.
38. Bristrian, Bruce, et al. Prevalence of malnutrition in general medical patients. *JAMA.* 1976; 235:15-18.
39. Lemoine, et al. Vitamin B1, B2, B6 and status in hospital inpatients. *Am J Clin Nutr.* 1980; Dec 33-37.
40. Driezen S. Nutrition and the immune response – a review. *Internat J Vit Nur Res.* 1979; 49.
41. Beisel, et al. Single-nutrient effects on immunologic functions. JAMA. 1981; 245.
42. Pollack SV. Nutritional factors affecting wound healing. *J Dermatol Surg Oncol.* 1979; 5:8.
43. Kaminsky M, Windborn A.1978. Nutritional assessment guide. Midwest Nutrition, Ed and Res Foundation, Inc.
44. Nationwide Food Consumption Survey, Spring 1980. U.S. Dept of Agriculture, Science and Education Administration, Beltsville, MD.
45. Dietary intake source data. United States 1976-80.
46. Kirsch A, Bidlack W. Nutrition and the elderly: Vitamin status and efficacy of supplementation. *Nutr* 1987; 3:305-314.
47. Baker H, Jaslow S, Frank O. Severe impairment of dietary folate utilization in the elderly. *J Am Geriatrics Soc.* 1978; 26:218-221.
48. First Health and Nutrition Examination Survey. 1971. U.S. Public Health Service. Vol. 72.
49. Connelly TJ, Becker A, McDonald J. Bachelor scurvy. *Intl J Dermatol.* 1982; 21:209-211.
50. Schorah CJ. Inappropriate vitamin C reserves: Their frequency and significance in an urban population. In: The importance of vitamins to health. Ed. T.G. Taylor. 1978. Lancaster, England: MTP Press, 61-72.
51. Garry PJ, Goodwin J, Hunt, et al. Nutritional status in a healthy elderly population: Dietary and supplemental intakes. *Am J Clin Nutr.* 1982; 36:319-331.
52. Roe DA. Drug-Induced Nutritional Deficiencies, 2nd ed. 1985. Westport, CT: AVI Publishing Co. 1-87.
53. Brin, M. Drugs and environmental chemicals in relation to vitamin needs. In: Nutrition and Drug Interrelations. 1978. Ed. JN Hathcock and J. Coon. NY: Academic Press, 131-50.
54. Driskell JA, Geders J, Urban M. Vitamin B6 status of young men, women, and women using oral contraceptives. *J Lab Clin Med* 1976; 87:813-821.
55. Prasad A, Lei K, Oberleas, et al.Effect of oral contraceptive agents on nutrients. *Am J Clin Nutr* 1975; 28:385-91.
56. Rivers JM, Devine M. Plasma ascorbic acid concentrations and oral contraceptives. *Am J Clin Nutr.*1972; 25:684-89.
57. Truswell AS. Drugs affecting nutritional state. *Br Med J.* 1985; 291:1333-37.
58. Clark A, Mossholder, Gates R. Folacin status in adolescent females. *Am J Clin Nutr.* 1987; 46:302-306.
59. Sumner SK, Liebman M, Wakefield. Vitamin A status of adolescent girls. *Nutr Rep Intl.* 1987; 35:423-431.
60. Saito N, Kimura M, Kuchiba, Itokawa. Blood thiamine levels in outpatients with diabetes mellitus. J Nutr Sci Vitaminol. 1987; 33:421-430.

61. Mooradian AD, Morley J. Micronutrient status in diabetes mellitus. *Am J Clin Nutr.* 1987; 45:877-895.

62. Vobecky JS, Vobecky J. Vitamin status of women during pregnancy. In: Vitamins and minerals in pregnancy and lactation. Ed. H. Berger. Nestle Nutrition Workshop Series, Vol. 16. NY: Vevey/Raven Press, Ltd., 1988; 109-111.

63. Peterkin BB, Kerr R, Hama M. Nutritional adequacy of diets of low-income households. *J Nut Ed.* 1987;14(3):102.

64. Shenai JP, Chytil F, Jhaveri, Stahlman. Plasma vitamin A and retinol-binding protein in premature and term neonates. *J Pediatr.* 1981; 99:302-305.

65. Heinonen K, Mononen I, Mononen T, et al. Plasma vitamin C levels are low in premature infants fed human milk. *Am J Clin Nutr.* 1986; 43:923-924.

66. Vitamin E status of premature infants. *Nutr Rev.* 1986; 44:166-167.

67. Dietary intake source data. United States 1976-80.

68. First Health and Nutrition Examination Survey. U.S. Public Health Service.

69. Schoenthaler SJ, Bier ID. Vitamin-mineral intake and intelligence: A macrolevel analysis of randomized controlled trials. *J Alternative Complementary Med: Research on Paradigm, Practice, Policy.* 1999; 5:125-134.

70. Schoenthaler SJ, Bier ID. The effect of vitamin-mineral supplementation on the intelligence of American school children in grades one to six: A randomized double-blind placebo-controlled trial. *J Alternative Complementary Med: Research on Paradigm, Practice, Policy.* 1999; 6:19-30.

71. Eysenck HJ Schoenthaler SJ. Raising IQ level by vitamin mineral supplementation. In: Sternberg R, Grigorenko E, eds. *Intelligence, Heredity and Environment.*Cambridge, UK. Cambridge Univ Press. 1997; 363-392.

72. Schoenthaler SJ, Bier ID. The impact of enhancing nutrition using vitamin-mineral tablets on academic performance among school children: A randomized double-blind placebo-controlled trial. Paper submitted

73. Schoenthaler SJ, Doraz WE, Wakefield. The impact of a low food additive and sucrose diet on academic performance in 803 New York City public schools. *Intl J Biosocial Res.* 1986; 8:185-195.

74. Schoenthaler SJ, Amos SP, Doraz WE, et al. Controlled trial of vitamin mineral supplementation on intelligence and brain function. *Personality Individual Differences.* 1991; 112:343-350.

75. Benton and Roberts. Effect of vitamin and mineral supplementation on intelligence of a sample of school children. *Lancet.* 1988; Jan.:140-144.

76. Campbell, et al. Vitamins, minerals, and I.Q. *Lancet.* 1988; Sept:744-745.

77. Letter to the Editor. Vitamin/mineral supplementation and non-verbal intelligence. *Lancet.* 1988; Feb:407-409.

78. Grantham-McGregor SM, et al. Nutritional supplementation, psychosocial stimulation, and mental development of stunted children: The Jamaican study. *Lancet.* 1991; 338:1-5.

79. Brown, et al. J Pediatrics. 1972; 81:714.

80. Webb and Oski. Iron deficiency and IQ. *J Pediatr.* 1973; 82:827-30.

81. Benton, et al. Glucose improves attention and reaction. Biol Psychol. 1972; 24:95-100.

82. Benton. Influence of vitamin C on psychological testing. *Psychopharmacology.* 1982; 75:98-99.

83. Pfeiffer C, Braverman E. Zinc, the brain and behavior. *Biol Psychiat.*1982; 17:513-31.

84. Godfrey P, et al. Enhancement of recovery from psychiatric illness by methylfolate. *Lancet.* 1990; 336:392-394.

85. Schoenthaler SJ, Bier ID. The effect of vitamin-mineral supplementation on juvenile delinquency among American school children: A randomized double-blind placebo-controlled trial. *J Alternative Complementary Med: Research on Paradigm, Practice, Policy.* 2000; 6:7-18.

86. Schoenthaler SJ, Amos SP, Hudes. A randomized trial of the effect of vitamin mineral supplementation on serious institutional rule violations. Submitted 2001.

87. Schoenthaler SJ, Bier ID. The effect of randomized vitamin-mineral supplementation on violent and non-violent antisocial behavior among incarcerated juveniles. *J Nutr Environmental Med.* 1997; 7:343-352.

88. Schoenthaler SJ. Diet and crime: An empirical examinatin of the value of nutrition in the control and treatment of incarcerated juvenile offenders. *Intl J Biosocial Res.* 1983; 1:25-39.

89. Schoenthaler SJ. Diet and delinquency: A multi state replication. *Intl J Biosocial Res.* 1983; 5:70-78.

90. Schoenthaler SJ. Diet and delinquency: Empirical testing of seven theories. *Intl J Biosocial Res.* 1986; 7:108-131.

91. *Vitamin C in Health and Disease.* Packer L, Fuchs J, Eds. 1997. Marcel Dekker, Inc. New York.

92. *Natural Antioxidants in Human Health and Disease.* Frei B, Ed. 1994. Academic Press, San Diego, CA..

93. *Vitamin E in Health and Disease.* Packer L, Fuchs J, Eds. 1993. Marcel Dekker, Inc. New York.

94. *Beyond Deficiency: New Views on the Function and Health Effects of Vitamins.* Sauberlich HE, Machlin LJ, Eds. 1992. New York Academy of Sciences, New York, NY.

95. Newberne PM, Locniskar M. Roles of micronutrients in cancer prevention: recent evidence from the laboratory. *Prog Clin Biol Res.* 1990; 346: 119-134.

96. Beckman KB, Ames BN. Oxidative decay of DNA. *J Biol Chem.* 1997; 272:19633-36.

97. Ames BN, Shigenaga MK, Park EM. DNA damage by endogenous oxidants as a cause of aging and cancer. In: *Oxidative Damage and Repair: Chemical, Biological, and Medical Aspects.* Davies KJA, Ed. 1991. pp 181-187. Pergamon Press, NY.

98. *Oncology Overview: Free Radicals and Peroxides in the Etiology of Cancer.* Pryor WA and National Cancer Institute, Eds. 1987. Government Printing Office, Washington, DC.

99. *Free Radicals in Biology and Medicine. Third Edition.* Halliwell B, Gutteridge JM, Eds. 1999; Oxford University Press. Oxford.

100. Kaul A, Khanduja KL. Polyphenols inhibit promotional phase of tumorigenesis: Relevance of superoxide radicals. *Nutr Cancer.* 1998; 32:81-85.

101. Cerutti P. Oxy-radicals and cancer. *Lancet.* 1994; 344:862-3.

102. Cerutti PA, Ghosh R, et al. The role of the cellular antioxidant defense in oxidant carcinogenesis. *Environ Health Perspect.* 1994; 102:123-30.

103. Marnett LJ. Peroxyl free radicals: potential mediators of tumor initiation and promotion. *Carcinogenesis.* 1987; 8:1365-73.

104. Shigenaga MK, Park JW, et al. *In vivo* oxidative DNA damage: measurement of 8-hydroxy-2-deoxyguanosine in DNA and urine by high-performance liquid chromatography with electrochemical detection. *Methods Enzymol.* 1990; 186:521-30.

105. Ames BN. Dietary carcinogens and anticarcinogens. *Science.* 1983; 221:1256-64.

106. Cooney RV, Kappock TJ et al. Solubilization, cellular uptake, and activity of beta-carotene and other carotenoids as inhibitors of neoplastic transformation in cultured cells. *Methods Enzymol.* 1996; 214: 55-68.

107. *Antimutagenesis and Anticarcinogenesis Mechanisms II.* Kuroda Y, et al. Eds. 1990. Plenum Press. New York.

108. Block G, Schwarz R. Ascorbic acid and cancer: animal and cell culture data. In: *Natural Antioxidants in Human Health and Disease.* Frei B, Ed. 1994; pp129-155. Academic Press, San Diego, CA.

109. Block G. The data support a role for antioxidants in reducing cancer risk. *Nutr Rev.* 1992; 50:207-213.

110. Krinsky NI. Carotenoids and cancer: basic research studies. In: *Natural Antioxidants in Human Health and Disease.* Frei B, Ed. 1994; pp239-261. Academic Press, San Diego, CA.

111. Onogi N, Okuno M, et al. Antiproliferative effect of carotenoids on human colon cancer cells without conversion to retinoic acid. *Nutrition and Cancer.* 1998; 32: 20-24.

112. Rock CL, Flatt SW, Wright, et al. Responsiveness of serum carotenoids to a high-vegetable diet intervention designed to prevent breast cancer recurrence. *Cancer Epid Biomarkers Prev.* 1997; 6: 617-23.

113. Menkes MS, Comstock GW, et al. Serum beta-carotene, vitamins A and E, selenium and the risk of lung cancer. *NEJM.* 1986; 315:1250-54.

114. Wattenberg LW. Inhibition of carcinogenesis by minor nutrient constituents of the diet. *Proc Nutr Soc.* 1990; 49:173-83.

115. Knekt P. Vitamin E and cancer prevention. In: *Natural Antioxidants in Human Health and Disease.* Frei B, Ed. 1994; pp199-238. Academic Press, San Diego, CA.

116. Fontham ETH. Vitamin C, vitamin C rich foods, and cancer: epidemiologic studies. In: *Natural Antioxidants in Human Health and Disease.* Frei B, Ed. 1994; pp 157-197. Academic Press, San Diego, CA.

117. Patterson RE, White E, Kristal AR, et al. Vitamin supplementation and cancer risk: the epidemiological evidence. *Cancer Causes Control.* 1997; 8: 786-802.

118. Bostick RM, Potter JD, et al. Reduced risk of colon cancer with high intakes of vitamin E: the Iowa women's health study. *Cancer Res.* 1993; 53:4230-37.

119. Hunter DJ, et al. 1993. A prospective study of the intake of vitamins C, E, A and the risk of breast cancer. *NEJM.* 1993; 329:234-240.

120. Ennever FK, Pasket. 1993. Vitamins and breast cancer. *NEJM.* 1993; 329:1579-1580.

121. Jumann A, Holmberg L, et al. Carotene intake and the risk of postmenopausal breast cancer. *Epidemiology.* 1999; 10:49-53.

122. Bohlke K, Spiegelman D, et al. Vitamins A, C, and E and the risk of breast cancer. *Br J Cancer.* 1999; 79:23-29.

123. Verhoeven DTH, Asses N, et al. Vitamin C and E, retinal, carotene, and dietary fibre in relation to breast cancer risk. *Br J Cancer.* 1997; 75: 149-55.

124. Negri E, LaVecchio C, et al. Intake of selected micronutrients and the risk of breast cancer. *Int J Cancer.* 1996; 65: 140-44.

125. Punnonen R, et al. Activities of antioxidant enzymes and lipid peroxidation in endometrial cancer. *Eur J Cancer.* 1993; 29:266-269.

126. Palan PR, et al. Beta-carotene levels in exfoliated cervical vaginal epithelial cells in cervical intra-epithelial neoplasia and cervical cancer. *Am J Obstet-Gynecol.* 1992; 167:1899-1903.

127. Gridley G, et al. Vitamin supplement use and reduced risk of oral and pharyngeal cancer. *Am J Epidemiol.* 1992; 135:1083-092.

128. Zheng W, et al. Serum micronutrients and subsequent risk of oral and pharyngeal cancer. *Cancer Res.* 1993; 53:795-98.

129. Barone J, et al. Vitamin supplement use and risk for oral and esophageal cancer. *Nutr Cancer.* 1992; 18(1):31-41.

130. Shibata A, et al. Intake of vegetables, fruits, beta-carotene, vitamin C, and vitamin supplements and cancer incidence among the elderly: A prospective study. *Br J Cancer.* 1992; 66:673-679.

131. LeMarchand L, et al. Intake of specific carotenoids and lung cancer risk. *Cancer Epidemiol Biomarkers Prevent.* 1993; 2:183-187.

132. Knekt P, et al. Dietary antioxidants and the risk of lung cancer. *Am J Epidemiol.* 1991; 134(5): 471-479.

133. Stahelin HB, et al. Plasma antioxidant vitamins and subsequent cancer mortality in the 12-year follow up of the prospective Basel Study. *Am J Epidemiol.* 1994; 133(8):766-775.

134. Comstock GW, Alberg AJ, et al. The risk of developing lung cancer associated with antioxidants in the blood: Ascorbic acid, carotenoids, tocopherol, selenium, and total peroxyl radical absorbing capacity. *Cancer Epidemiol Biomarkers Prev.* 1997; 6: 907-16.

135. Prestin-Martin S, Pogoda JM, et al. Prenatal vitamin supplementation and risk of childhood brain tumors. *Int J Cancer.* 1998; 11:17-22.

136. Eichholzer M, Stahelin HB, et al. Prediction of male cancer mortality by plasma levels of interacting vitamins: 17 year follow-up of the prospective Basel study. *Int J Cancer.* 1996; 66:145-50.

137. Gann PH, Ma J, et al. Lower prostate cancer risk in men with elevated plasma lycopene levels: results of a prospective analysis. *Cancer Res.* 1999; 59:1225-30.

138. Maramag C, Menon M, et al. Effect of vitamin C on prostate cancer cells *in vitro. The Prostate.* 1997; 32:188-95.

139. Chen J, et al. Antioxidant status and cancer mortality in China. *Int J Epidemiol.* 1992; 21(4):625-635.

140. Blot WJ, et al. Nutrition intervention trials in Linxian, China: Supplementation with specific vitamin-mineral combinations, cancer incidence, and disease specific mortality in the general population. *JNCI.* 1993; 85(18):1483-1492.

141. Smigel K. Dietary supplements reduce cancer deaths in China. *JNCI.* 1993; 85(18):1448-1450.

142. Jaakkola, et al. Treatment with antioxidant and other nutrients in combination with chemotherapy and irradiation therapy in patients with small cell lung cancer. *Anticancer Research.* 1992; 12(3):599-606.

143. Li JY, et al. Nutrition intervention trials in Linxian, China: Multiple vitamin and mineral supplementation, cancer incidence, and disease-specific mortality among adults with esophageal dysplasia. *JNCI.* 1993; 85:1492-1498.

144. Lippman S, et al. Comparison of low dose isotretinoin with beta-carotene to prevent oral carcinogenesis. *NEJM.* 1993; 328:15-20.

145. Toma S, et al. GI Treatment of oral leukoplakia with beta-carotene. *Oncology.* 1992; 49:77-81.

146. Benner S, et al. Regression of oral leukoplakia with alpha-tocopherol. *JNCI.* 1993; 85:44-47.

147. Benner and Hong. Clinical chemoprevention: developing a cancer prevention strategy. *JNCI.* 1993; 85:1446-47.

148. Paganelli, et al. Effect of vitamin A, C, and E supplementation on rectal cell proliferation in patients with colorectal adenomas. *JNCI.* 1992; 84:47-51.

149. Riemersma, et al. Risk of angina pectoris and concentrations of vitamins A, C, E, and carotene. *Lancet.* 1991; 337:1-5.

150. Fairburn K, et al. Alpha-Tocopherol, lipids, and lipoproteins in knee joint fluid and serum from patients with inflammatory joint disease. *Clinical Science.* 1992; 83:657-664.

151. Scheen AJ. Antioxidant vitamins in the prevention of cardiovascular diseases. First

part: epidemiologic studies. *Rev Med Liege* 2000;55:11-8.

152. Scheen AJ. Antioxidant vitamins in the prevention of cardiovascular diseases. 2nd part: results of clinical trials. *Rev Med Liege* 2000;55:105-9.
153. Boaz M, Smetana S, et al. Secondary prevention with antioxidants of cardiovascular disease in endstage renal disease (SPACE): randomized trial. *Lancet.* 2000; 356:1213-18.
154. Giugliano D. Dietary antioxidants for cardiovascular prevention. *Nutr Metab Cardiovasc Dis* 2000;10:38-44
155. Marchioli R, Negri M, et al. Antioxidant vitamins and prevention of cardiovascular disease: laboratory, epidemiological and clinical trial data. *Pharmacol Res* 1999; 40:227-38.
156. Nappo F, et al. Impairment of endothelial function by hyperhomocystein and reversal by antioxidants. *JAMA.* 1999; 281:2113-18.
157. Monnier L , Avignon A , Colette C , Piperno M. Primary nutritional and drug prevention of atherosclerosis. *Rev Med Interne* 1999; 3:360-370.
158. Faggiotto A, Paoletti R. State-of-the-Art lecture. Statins and blockers of the renin-angiotensin system: vascular protection beyond their primary mode of action. *Hypertension* 1999; 34:987-96.
159. Yla-Herttuala S. Oxidized LDL and atherogenesis. *Ann N Y Acad Sci* 1999; 874:134-7.
160. Carrasquedo F, Glanc M, Fraga C. Tissue damage in acute myocardial infarction: selective protection by vitamin E. *Free Radic Biol Med* 1999; 26:1587-90.
161. Navarro-Alarcon M, Serrana H, et al. Serum and urine selenium concentrations in patients with cardiovascular diseases and relationship to other nutritional indexes. *Ann Nutr Metab* 1999;43:30-6.
162. Stampher M, et al. Vitamin E consumption and the risk of coronary disease in women. *NEJM* 1993; 328:1444-49.
163. Rimm E, et al. Vitamin E consumption and the risk of coronary heart disease in men. *NEJM.* 1993; 328:1450-56.
164. Steinberg D. Antioxidant vitamins and coronary heart disease. *NEJM.* 1993; 328:1487-1489.
165. Dieber-Rotheneder, et al. Effect of oral supplementation with D-alpha-tocopherol on the vitamin E content of human low-density lipoproteins and its oxidation resistance. *J Lipid Res.* 1991; 32:1325-32.
166. Graziano, et al. Beta-carotene therapy for chronic stable angina. *Circulation.* 1990; 82:201.
167. Gey, et al. Plasma levels of antioxidant vitamins in relation to ischemic heart disease and cancer. *Am J Clin Nutr.* 1987; 45:1368-77.
168. Gey, et al. Poor plasma status of carotene and vitamin C is associated with higher mortality from ischemic heart disease and stroke: Basel Study. *Clin Investig.* 1993; 71:3-6.
169. Mialal and Grundy. Effect of dietary supplementation with alpha-tocopherol on the oxidative modification of low density lipoprotein. *J Lipid Res.* 1992; 33:899-906.
170. Kok, et al. Serum selenium, vitamin antioxidants, and cardiovascular mortality: A 9 year follow-up study in the Netherlands. *Am J Clin Nutr.* 1987; 45:462-468.
171. Kardinal, et al. Antioxidants in adipose tissue and risk of myocardial infarction: the EURAMIC study. *Lancet.* 1993; 342:1379-82.
172. Hertog, et al. Dietary antioxidant flavonoids and risk of coronary heart disease: the Zutphen Elderly Study. *Lancet.* 1993; 342:1007-11.
173. Enstrom, et al. Vitamin C intake and mortality among a sample of the U.S. population. *Epidemiology.* 1992; 3:194-202.
174. Block, G. Vitamin C and reduced mortality. *Epidemiology.* 1992; 3:189-191.
175. Princen, et al. Supplementation with vitamin E but not beta-carotene *in vivo* protects low-density lipoprotein from lipid peroxidation *in vitro. Arteriosclerosis & Thrombosis.* 1992; 12:554-562.
176. Reaven, et al. Effect of dietary antioxidant combinations in humans. Protection of LDL by vitamin E but not by beta-carotene. *Arteriosclerosis & Thrombosis.* 1993; 13: 590-600.
177. Riemersma, et al. Risk of angina pectoris and plasma concentrations of vitamins A, C, and E and carotene. *Lancet.* 1991; 337:1-5.
178. Trout. Vitamin C and cardiovascular risk factors. *Am J Clin Nutr.* 1991; 53:322S-325S.
179. Salonen, et al. Relationship of serum selenium and antioxidants to plasma lipoproteins, platelet aggregability, and prevalent ischaemic heart disease in eastern Finnish men. *Atherosclerosis.* 1988; 70:155-160.
180. Murphy, et al. Antioxidant depletion in aortic cross clamping ischemia. *Free Rad Biol Med.* 1992; 13:95-100.
181. Christen W, Gaziano J, Hennekens CH, et al. Design of Physicians' Health Study II--a randomized trial of beta-carotene, vitamins E and C, and multivitamins, in prevention of cancer, cardiovascular disease, and eye disease, and review of results of completed trials. *Ann Epidemiol* 2000;10:125-34.

182. Cumming R, Mitchell P, Smith W. Diet and cataract: the Blue Mountains Eye Study. *Ophthalmology* 2000;107:450-6.

183. The age-related eye disease study: a clinical trial of zinc and antioxidants-age-related eye disease study report no. 2. *J Nutr.* 2000;130(5S Suppl):1516S-9S

184. Christen WG. Antioxidant vitamins and age-related eye disease. *Proc Assoc Am Physicians.*1999;111:16-21.

185. Brown L, Rimm EB, Seddon JM, et al. A prospective study of carotenoid intake and risk of cataract extraction in US men. *Am J Clin Nutr* 1999;70:517-24.

186. Chasan-Taber L, Willett WC, Seddon JM, et al. A prospective study of carotenoid and vitamin A intakes and risk of cataract extraction in US women. *Am J Clin Nutr* 1999; 70:509-16.

187. Garrett S, McNeil J, Silagy C, et al. Methodology of the VECAT study: vitamin E intervention in cataract and age-related maculopathy. *Ophthalmic Epidemiol* 1999; 6:195-208.

188. Stahelin HB. The impact of antioxidants on chronic disease in ageing and in old age. *Int J Vitam Nutr Res* 1999; 69:146-9.

189. Lyle BJ, Mares-Perlman JA, Klein BE, et al. Antioxidant intake and risk of incident age-related nuclear cataracts in the Beaver Dam Eye Study. *Am J Epidemiol* 1999;149:801-9.

190. Delcourt C, Cristol J, Leger C, et al. Associations of antioxidant enzymes with cataract and age-related macular degeneration. The POLA Study. Pathologies Oculaires Liees a l'Age. *Ophthalmology.* 1999;106:215-22.

191. The Age-Related Eye Disease Study (AREDS): design implications AREDS report no. 1. The Age-Related Eye Disease Study Research Group. *Control Clin Trials* 1999; 20:573-600.

192. Sperduto R, et al. Linxian cataract studies. Two nutritional intervention trials. *Arch Ophthalmol.* 1993; 111:1246-1253.

193. Hankinson S, et al. Nutrient intake and cataract extraction in women: A prospective study. *BMJ.* 1992 305:335<196>339.

194. Taylor, A. Cataract: Relationships between nutrition and oxidation. *J Am Coll Nutr.* 1993; 12:138-146.

195. Jacques and Chylack. Vitamin C plasma level inversely related to cataract incidence. Am J Clin Nutr. 1991; 53:352-55.

196. Seddon J.M., et al. The use of vitamin supplements and the risk of cataract among U.S. male physicians. *Am J Public Health.* 1994; 84:788-792.

197. Vitale S, et al. Plasma antioxidants and risk of cortical and nuclear cataract. *Epidemiology.* 1993; 4:195-203.

198. Robertson, et al. Ann NY Acad Sci. 1989; 570:372-382.

199. Knekt, et al. Serum antioxidant vitamins and risk of cataract. *BMJ.* 1992; 305:1392-1394.

200. Berkson BM. A conservative triple antioxidant approach to treatment of hepatitis C. *Med Kiln.* 1999; 94:Supp III:84-89.

201. Hemila. Vitamin C and lowering of blood pressure. *J Hypertension.*1991; 9:1076-78.

202. Guilliano T. Ed. Free Radicals, Antioxidants, and Eye Disease. 1999; The Standard Publishing Co. Plover, WI.

203. Snow KK, Seddon JM. Do age-related macular degeneration and cardiovascular disease share common antecedents? *Ophthalmic Epidemiol* 1999; 6:125-43.

204. West S, et al. Are antioxidants or supplements protective for age-related macular degeneration? *Arch Opthalmol.* 1994; 112:222-227.

205. Seddon JM, et al. Vitamins, minerals, and macular degeneration. *Arch Opthalmol.* 1994; 112:176-179.

206. Seddon JM, et al. Dietary carotenoids, vitamins A, C, and E, and advanced age-related macular degeneration. *JAMA* 1994; 272:1413-1420.

207. Sano M, Ernesto C, et al. Controlled trial of selegiline, vitamin C, or both for Alzheimer's. *NEJM.* 1997; 336:1216-22.

208. Sano M, et al. Retinoids and design of multicenter study of selegiline and vitamin E for Alzheimer's. *Alzheimers Dis Assoc Disorders.* 1996; 10:132-140.

209. Lethem R, Orrell M. Antioxidants and dementia. *Lancet.* 1997; 349:1189-91.

210. Levy, S., et al. The anticonvulsant effects of vitamin E. *Can J Neurol Sci.* 1992; 19:201-203.

211. Mutations in the copper-zinc containing superoxide dismutase gene are associated with Lou Gehrig's Disease. *Nutr Rev.* 1993; 51:243-245.

212. Yapa S. Detection of subclinical ascorbic deficiency in early Parkinson's disease. *Public Health.* 1993;106:393-395.

213. Fahn S. A pilot trial of high dose alpha-Tocopherol and ascorbate in early Parkinson's disease. *Ann Neurol.* 1992; 32:S128-S132.

214. The Parkinson's Study Group. Effects of Tocopherol and Deprenyl on the progression of disability in early Parkinson's Disease. *NEJM.* 1993; 328:176-183.

215. Shriqui C, et al. Vitamin E in the treatment of Tardive Dyskinesia: A double blind placebo controlled study. *Am J Psychiatry*. 1992; 149:391-393.
216. Bower B. Vitamin E may ease movement disorder. *Science News*. 1992; 141:351.
217. Adler L, et al. Vitamin E treatment of tardive dyskinesia. *Am J Psychiatry*. 1994.
218. Perrig W, Perrig P, Stahelin. Antioxidants enhance memory in the old and very old. *J Am Geriatr Soc*. 1997; 45:718-24.
219. Cooper DA, Eldridge AL, Peters JC. Dietary carotenoids and certain cancers, heart disease, and age-related macular degeneration: a review of recent research. *Nutr Rev*. 1999; 57:201-14.
220. Faure H, Fayol V, Galabert C, et al. Carotenoids: 2. Diseases and supplementation studies. *Ann Biol Clin*. 1999; 57:273-82.
221. Ascherio A, Rimm EB, Hernan MA, et al. Relation of consumption of vitamin E, vitamin C, and carotenoids to risk for stroke among men in the United States. *Ann Intern Med*. 1999;130:963-70.
222. Bendich, A. Antioxidant vitamins and their function in immune responses. 1989. New York: Plenum Publishing Corp.
223. Brown L, Rimm ER, et al. A prospective study of carotene intake and cataracts. *Am J Clin Nutr*. 1999; 70:509-24.
224. Bendich A. Safety of beta-carotene. Review. *Nutr Cancer*. 1988; 11:207-214.
225. Pryor WA. Letter to Editor. Beta-carotene, vitamin E and lung cancer. *NEJM*. 1994; 612.
226. Pryor WA, Stahl W, Rock CL. Beta-carotene: From biochemistry to clinical trials. *Nutr Rev*. 2000;
227. Riboli E, Gonzalez CA, Lopez-Abente G, Errezola M Diet and bladder cancer in Spain: A multi-centre case-control study. *Intl J Cancer* 1991;49:214-219.
228. Bohlke K, Spiegelman D, Trichopoulou A, et al. Vitamins A, C and E and the risk of breast cancer: results from a case-control study in Greece. *Br J Cancer*. 1999;79:23-9.
229. Zhang S, Hunter DJ, Forman MR, et al. Dietary carotenoids and vitamins A, C, and E and risk of breast cancer. *JNCI*. 1999;91:547-556.
230. Torun M, Akgul S, Sargin H. Serum vitamin E level in patients with breast cancer. *J Clin PharmTherapeutics* 1995;20:173-178.
231. Favero A, Parpinel M, Franceschi S. Diet and risk of breast cancer: Major findings from an Italian case-control study. *Biomed Pharm* 1998;52:109-115.
232. Mezzetti M, La Vecchia C, Decarli A, et al. Population attributable risk for breast cancer: Diet, nutrition, and exercise. *JNCI* 1998;90:389-394.
233. Mannisto S, Pietinen P, Virtanen M. Diet and risk of breast cancer in a case-control study: Does the threat of disease have an influence on recall bias? *J Clin Epidem* 1999;52:429-439.
234. Cuzick J, Destavola BL, Russell MJ. Vitamin A, vitamin E, and the risk of cervical intraepithelial neoplasia. *BritJCanc* 1990;62:651-652.
235. Ho GYF, Palan PR, Basu J, et al. Viral characteristics of human papillomavirus infection and antioxidant levels as risk factors for cervical dysplasia. *Intl J Cancer* 1998; 78:594-599.
236. Verrault R, Chu J, Mandelson M. A case-control study of diet and invasive cervical cancer. *Intl J Cancer* 1989; 43:1050-1054.
237. Roncucci L, Di Donato P, Carati L, et al. Antioxidant vitamins or lactulose for the prevention of the recurrence of colorectal adenomas. *Diseases Colon Rectum* 1993; 36:227-234.
238. Whelan RL, Horvath KD, Gleason NR, et al. Vitamin and calcium supplement use is associated with decreased adenoma recurrence in patients with a previous history of neoplasia. *Diseases Colon Rectum* 1999; 42:212-217.
239. Bostick RM, Poter JD, McKenzie DR, et al. Reduced risk of colon cancer with high intake of vitamin E: The Iowa Women's Health Study. *Cancer Res* 1993;53:4230-4237.
240. La Vecchia C, Braga C, Negri E, et al. Intake of selected micronutrients and risk of colorectal cancer. *Intl JCancer* 1997; 73:525-530.
241. White E, et al. Vitamin E lowers colon cancer risk. *Cancer Epidemiology Biomarker Prev.* 1997; 6:769-74.
242. Knekt P, Jarvinen R, Seppanen R, et al. Dietary antioxidants and the risk of lung cancer. *Am J Epidem* 1991; 134:471-479.
243. Yong L-C, Brown CC, Schatzkin A, et al. Intake of vitamins E, C, and A and risk of lung cancer. The NHANES I epidemiologic followup study. *Am J Epidem* 1997; 146:231-243.
244. Knekt P. Vitamin E and smoking and the risk of lung cancer. *Ann NY Acad Sci* 1993; 686:280-288.
245. Woodson K, Tangrea J, Barrett M ,et al. Serum alpha-tocopherol and subsequent risk of lung cancer among male smokers. *JNCI*. 1999; 91:1738-1743.

246. Le Gardeur B, Lopez S, Johnson WD. A case-control study of serum vitamins A, E, and C in lung cancer patients. *Nutr and Cancer* 1990; 14:133-140.

247. Harris R, Key T, Silcocks P, et al. A case-control study of dietary carotene in men with lung cancer and in men with other epithelial cancers. *Nutr and Cancer* 1991;15:63-68.

248. Barone J, Taioli E, Herbert JR, Wynder EL. Vitamin supplement use and risk for oral and esophageal cancer. *Nutr and Cancer* 1992;18:31-41.

249. Gridley G, McLaughlin JK, Block G,et al. Vitamin supplement use and reduced risk of oral and pharyngeal cancer. *Am JEpidem* 1992;135:1083-1092.

250. Negri E, Franceschi S, Bosetti C, et al. Selected micronutrients and oral and pharyngeal cancer. *Intl J Cancer* 2000; 86:122-127.

251. Heinonen OP, et al. Vitamin E supplements lower prostate cancer risk by one third. *JNCI.* 1998; 90:440-46.

252. Stryker WS, Stampfer MJ, Stein EA, et al. Diet, plasma levels of beta-carotene and alpha-tocopherol, and risk of malignant melanoma. *Am JEpidem* 1990; 131:597-611.

253. Blot WJ, Li J-Y, Taylor PR, et al. Nutrition intervention trials in Linxian, China: Supplementation with specific vitamin/mineral combinations, cancer incidence and disease-specific mortality in the general population. *JNCI.* 1993; 85:1483-1492.

254. Buiatti E, Palli D, Decarli A,et al. A case-control study of gastric cancer and diet in Italy. *Intl J Cancer* 1989; 44:611-616.

255. Charpiot P, Calaf R, DiCostanzo J, et al. Vitamin A, vitamin E, retinal binding protein (RBP) and prealbumin in digestive cancers. *Intl J Vitamin Nutri Res.* 1989; 59:323-328.

256. Shklar G, Oh S. Basis for cancer prevention by vitamin E. *Cancer Invest.* 2000; 18:214-22.

257. Gonzalez M, Mora E, et al. Vitamins C and E and cancer: An update on nutritional oncology. *Cancer Prev Intl.* 1998; 3:215-24.

258. Rimm E, Stampfer M, et al. Vitamin E consumption and the risk of coronary heart disease in men and women. *NEJM.* 1993; 328:1444-56.

259. Takamatsu S, et al. Effects on health of dietary supplementatin with 100 mg of d-alpha-tocopheryl daily for 6 years. *J Intl Med Res.* 1995; 23:342-57.

260. Stephans N, et al. Randomized controlled trial of vitamin E in patient with coronary disease: CHAOS Study. *Lancet.* 1996; 347:781-86.

261. Rapola J, et al. Effect of vitamin E and carotene on incidence of angina pectoris. *JAMA.* 1996; 275:693-98.

262. Hodis H, Mack W, et al. Serial coronary angiographic evidence that antioxidant vitamin intake reduces progression of coronary artery disease. *JAMA.* 1995; 273:1849-54.

263. Pryor W. Can vitamin E protect humans against the pathological effects of ozone in smog? *Am J Clin Nutr.* 1991; 53:702-722.

264. London R, Sundaram G, et al. Alpha-tocopherol, mammary dysplasia and steroid hormones. *Cancer Res.* 1981; 4:249-253.

265. Ceriello, et al. Vitamin E reduction of protein glycosylation in diabetics. *Diabetes Care.* 1992; 14:68-72.

266. Fogarty A, et al. Vitamin E, IgE, and atopy. *Lancet.* 2000; 356:573-74.

267. Kappus H, Diplock A. Tolerance and safety of vitamin E. *Free Rad Biol Med.* 1992; 13:55-74.

268. Bendich and Machlin. Safety of oral intake of vitamin E: A Review. *Am J Clin Nutr.* 1988; 48:612-19.

269. Vitamin E. 1989. Tenth Edition of Recommended Dietary Allowances. National Research Council. National Academy Press. Washington D.C.

270. Henning S, et al. Glutathione blood levels and other oxidant defense indices in men fed diets low in vitamin C. *J Nutr.* 1991; 121:1969-75.

271. Kamat AM, Lamm DL. Chemoprevention of urological cancer. *J Urol* 1999;161:1748-60.

272. Young KJ, Lee PN. Intervention studies on cancer. *Eur J Cancer Prev* 1999;8:91-103.

273. Shibata A, Paganini-Hill A. Intake of vegetables, fruit, beta-carotene, vitamin C and vitamin supplements and cancer incidence among the elderly: A prospective study. *Brit Journal Canc* 1992; 66:673-679.

274. Zhang S, Hunter DJ, Forman MR, et al. Dietary carotenoids and vitamins A, C, and E and risk of breast cancer. *JNCI.*1999;91:547-556.

275. Zaridze D, Evstifeeva T, Boyle P. Chemoprevention of oral leukoplakia and chronic esophagitis in an area of high incidence of oral and esophageal cancer. *Annals of Epidemiology* 1993;3:225-234.

276. Landa M-C, Frago N, Tres A. Diet and the risk of breast cancer in Spain. *Europ J Cancer Prevent* 1994;3:313 320.

277. Yuan J-M, Wang Q-S, Ross RK. Diet and breast cancer in Shangai and Tianjin, China. *Brit J Cancer* 1995; 71:1353-1358.

278. Ronco A, De Stefani E, Boffetta P,et al. Vegetables, fruits, and related nutrients and risk of breast cancer: A case-control study in Uruguay. *Nutri and Cancer* 1999; 35:111-119.

279. Verrault R, Chu J, Mandelson M, Shy K. A case-control study of diet and invasive cervical cancer. *Intl J Cancer* 1989; 43:1050-1054.

280. Herrero R, Potischman N, Brinton LA,et al. A case-control study of nutrient status and invasive cervical cancer. I. Dietary indicators. *Am J Epidem* 1991; 134:1335-1346.

281. Van Eenwyk J, Davis FG, Bowen PE. Dietary and serum carotenoids and cervical intraepithelial neoplasia. *Intl J Cancer* 1991; 48:34-38.

282. Shibata A, Paganini-Hill A. Intake of vegetables, fruit, beta-carotene, vitamin C and vitamin supplements and cancer incidence among the elderly: A prospective study. *Brit J Cancer* 1992;66:673-679.

283. La Vecchia C, Negri E, Decarli A,et al. A case-control study of diet and colorectal cancer in northern Italy. *Intl J Cancer* 1988; 41:492-498.

284. Freudenheim JL, Graham S, Marshall JR. A case-control study of diet and rectal cancer in Western New York. *Am J Epidem* 1990; 131:612-624.

285. Ferraroni M, et al. Selected micronutrient intake and the risk of colorectal cancer. *Br J Cancer.*1994; 70:1150-1155.

286. La Vecchia C, et al. Intake of selected micronutrients and risk of colorectal cancer. *Intl J Cancer* 1997; 73:525-530.

287. Knekt P, Jarvinen R, et al. Dietary antioxidants and the risk of lung cancer. *Am J Epidem* 1991; 134:471-479.

288. Bandera EV, Freudenheim JL, et al. Diet and alcohol consumption and lung cancer risk in the New York State Cohort (United States). *Cancer Causes and Control* 1997; 8:828-840.

289. Ocke MC, Bueno-de-Mesquita HB, et al. Repeated measurements of vegetables, fruits, beta-carotene, and vitamins C and E in relation to lung cancer. The Zutphen Study. *Am J Epidem* 1997;145:358-365.

290. Yong L-C, Brown CC, et al. Intake of vitamins E, C, and A and risk of lung cancer. The NHANES I epidemiologic followup study. *Am J Epidem* 1997;146:231-243.

291. Voorrips LE, Goldbohm RA, et al. A prospective cohort study on antioxidant and folate intake and male lung cancer risk. *Cancer Epidem, Biomarkers Prevent* 2000;9:357-365.

292. Fontham ETH, Pickle LW, et al. Dietary vitamins A and C and lung cancer risk in Louisiana. *Cancer* 1988; 62:2267-2273.

293. Le Marchand L, et al. Vegetable consumption and lung cancer risk: A population-based case-control study in Hawaii. *JNCI.* 1989; 81:1158-1164.

294. McLaughlin JK, Gridley G, et al. Dietary factors in oral and pharyngeal cancer. *JNCI* 1988;80:1237-1243.

295. De Stefani E, et al. Diet and risk of cancer of the aerodigestive tract - II. Nutrients. *Oral Oncology* 1999;35:22-26.

296. Negri E, Franceschi S, et al. Selected micronutrients and oral and pharyngeal cancer. *Intl J Cancer* 2000; 86:122-127.

297. Eichholzer M, Stahelin HB, et al. Prediction of male cancer mortality by plasma levels of interacting vitamins: 17-year follow-up of the prospective Basel study. *Intl J Cancer* 1996; 66:145-150.

298. Deneo-Pellegrini H, et al. Foods, nutrients and prostate cancer: A case-control study in Uruguay. *Br J Cancer* 1999; 80:591-597.

299. Correa P, et al. Chemoprevention of gastric dysplasia: Randomized trial of antioxidant supplements and anti-*Helicobacter pylori* therapy. *JNCI* 2000; 92:1881-1888.

300. Botterweck AM, van den Brant PA, Goldbohm. Vitamins, carotenoids, dietary fiber, and the risk of gastric carcinoma. *Cancer* 2000; 88:737-748.

301. You W-C, Blot WJ, et al.. Diet and high risk of stomach cancer in Shandong, China. *Cancer Res* 1988; 48:3518-3523.

302. Buiatti E, Palli D, et al.. A case-control study of gastric cancer and diet in Italy. *Intl J Cancer* 1989; 44:611-616.

303. Boeing H, Frentzel-Beyme R, Berger M, et al. Case-control study on stomach cancer in Germany. *Intl J Cancer* 1991; 47:858-864.

304. La Vecchia C, Ferraroni M, et al. Selected micronutrient intake and the risk of gastric cancer. *Cancer Epidem, Biomark Prevent* 1994; 3:393-398.

305. Kaaks R, Tuyns AJ, et al. Nutrient intake patterns and gastric cancer risk: A case-control study in Belgium. *Intl J Cancer* 1998; 78:415-420.

306. Ekstrom AM, et al. Dietary antioxidant intake and the risk of cardia cancer and non-cardia cancer of the intestinal and diffuse types: A population-based case-control study in Sweden. *Intl J Cancer* 2000; 87:133-140.

307. You W-C, Zhang L, et al. Gastric dysplasia and gastric cancer: Helicobacter pylori, serum vitamin C, and other risk factors. *JNCI* 2000; 92:1607-1612.

308. Cameron E. In: Hyaluronidase and cancer. 1966; New York: Pergamon Press.

309. Pauling L. Preventive nutrition. *Medicine on the Midway*. 1972; 27:15.

310. Duffy S, Gokce, et al. Treatment of hypertension with ascorbic acid. *Lancet*. 1999; 354:2048-49.

311. Hall and Greendale. The relation of dietary vitamin C to bone mineral density. *Calcif Tissue Intl*. 1998;63:183-89.

312. US NHANES III. *Arch Int Med*. 2000; 160:931-36.

313. Bendich. Antioxidant vitamins and their function in immune response.

314. Hoffer A. Ascorbic acid and toxicity. *NEJM*. 1971; 285:635.

315. Klenner FR. Vitamin C and toxicity. *J Appl Nutr*. 1971; 23:61.

316. Hollman PC, Feskens EJ, Katan MB. Tea flavonols in cardiovascular disease and cancer epidemiology. *Proc Soc Exp Biol Med* 1999;220:198-202.

317. Hertog M, Feskens et al. Dietary antioxidant flavonoids and risk of heart disease. *Lancet*. 1993; 342:1007-11.

318. Rayman MP. The importance of selenium to human health. *Lancet*. 2000; 356:233-41.

319. Young VR, Richardson. Nutrients, vitamins, and minerals in cancer prevention. Facts and fallacies. *Cancer*. 1979; 43:2125.

320. Sakurai H, Tsuchiya K. A tentative recommendation for the maximum daily intake of selenium. *Environ Physiol Biochem*. 1975; 5:107.

321. Magalova T, Bella V, Brtkova A, et al. Copper, zinc and superoxide dismutase in precancerous, benign diseases and gastric, colorectal and breast cancer. *Neoplasma* 1999;46:100-4.

322. Frost,P, Chen JC, Rabbini I, et al. The effects of zinc deficiency on immune response. *Proc Clin Biol Res*. 1977; 14:143.

323. Ziegler D, Reljanovic M, et al. Alpha-lipoic acid in the treatment of diabetic polyneuropathy in Germany: current evidence from clinical trials. *Exp Clin Endocrin Diabetes*. 1999; 107:421-30.

324. Ziegler D, Hanefeld M, et al. Treatment of symptomatic diabetic peripheral neuropathy with antioxidant lipoic acid. A three week multicenter randomized controlled trial (ALADIN Study). *Diabetologia*. 1995; 38: 1425-33.

325. Reljanovic M, Reichel C, et al. Treatment of diabetic peripheral neuropathy with alpha-lipoic acid. A two tier randomized multicenter double-blind placebo-controlled trial. (ALADIN II). *Free Radical Res*. 1999; 31:171-79.

326. Ziegler D, Hanefeld M, et al. Treatment of symptomatic diabetic peripheral neuropathy with antioxidant lipoic acid. A 7 month multicenter randomized controlled trial (ALADIN III Study). *Diabetes Care*. 1999; 22:1296-1301.

327. Ruhnau KJ, Meissner HP, et al. Effects of three weeks oral treatment with the antioxidant alpha lipoic acid in symptomatic diabetic polyneuropathy. *Diabetes Med*. 1999; 16:1040-43.

328. Ou P, Nourooz ZJ, et al. Activation of aldose reductase in rat lens and metal-ion chelation by alpha lipoic acid. *Free Radical Res*. 1996; 25:337-46.

329. Filina AA, Davydova N, et al. Lipoic acid as a means of metabolic therapy of open angle glaucoma. *Vestn Oftalmol*. 1995; 111:6-8. Prehn JH, Karkoutly C, et al. Lipoic acid reduces neuronal injury after cerebral ischemia. *J Cereb Blood Flow Metabol*. 1992; 12:78-87.

330. Prehn JH, Karkoutly C, et al. Lipoic acid reduces neuronal injury after cerebral ischemia. *J Cereb Blood Flow Metabol*. 1992; 12:78-87.

331. Speizer FE, Colditz GA, Hunter DJ, et al. Prospective study of smoking, antioxidant intake, and lung cancer in middle-aged women (USA). *Cancer Causes Control*. 1999;10:475-82.

332. Virtamo J. Vitamins and lung cancer. *Proc Nutr Soc* 1999; 58:329-33.

333. Young KJ, Lee PN. Intervention studies on cancer. *Eur J Cancer Prev*. 1999;8:91-103.

334. Watkins ML, Erickson JD, Thun MJ, et al. Multivitamin use and mortality in a large prospective study. *Am J Epidemiol*. 2000;152:149-62.

335. Ohno Y, Wakai K, Dillon DS, et al. Dietary macro/micro-nutrients as a breast cancer risk: findings from nutritional case-control study in Jakarta, Indonesia. *Gan To Kagaku Ryoho*. 2000; 2:412-9.

336. Bogden JD, Louria DB. Aging and the immune system: the role of micronutrient nutrition. *Nutrition* 1999;15:593-5.

337. Chasan-Taber L, Willett WC, Seddon JM, et al. A prospective study of carotenoid and vitamin A intakes and risk of cataract extraction in US women. *Am J Clin Nutr* 1999; 70:509-16.

338. Lefebvre P, et al. Retinoic acid stimulates regeneration of mammalian auditory hair cells. *Science*. 1993; 260:692-95.

339. Rosenberg H, Felzman AN. In: The Book of Vitamin Therapy. 1974. New York: Berkley Publishing Corp.

340. Goodman LS, Gilman A, eds. A Pharmacological Basis of Therapeutics. 1977. 5th ed. New York: Macmillan.

341. Bendich and Langseth. Safety of vitamin A. *Am J Clin Nutr.* 1989; 49:358-371.
342. Lipkin M, Newmark HL. Vitamin D, calcium and prevention of breast cancer: a review. *J Am Coll Nutr* 1999;18:392S-397S.
343. Janowsky EC, Lester GE, Weinberg CR. Association between low levels of 1,25-dihydroxyvitamin D and breast cancer risk. *Public Health Nutr.* 1999;2:283-91.
344. Garland, et al. Serum vitamin D and colon cancer- 8 year prospective study. *Lancet.* 1989;18:1176-78.
345. Reitsma, et al. Regulation of myc gene expression. *Nature.* 1983; 306:492-495.
346. Mariani E, Ravaglia G, Forti P, et al. Vitamin D, thyroid hormones and muscle mass influence natural killer (NK) innate immunity in healthy nonagenarians and centenarians. *Clin Exp Immunol.* 1999;116:19-27.
347. Ross JA, Davies SM. Vitamin K prophylaxis and childhood cancer. *Med Pediatr Oncol.* 2000;34:434-7.
348. Boros LG. Population thiamine status and varying cancer rates between western, Asian and African countries. *Anticancer Res* 2000;20:2245-8.
349. Rosenblatt KA, Thomas DB, Jimenez LM. The relationship between diet and breast cancer in US men. *Cancer Causes Control* 1999;10:107-13.
350. Elam M, Henninghake, et al. Effect of niacin on lipids and glycemic control. *JAMA.* 2000; 284:1263-70.
351. Wu K, Helzlsouer KJ, Comstock GW, et al. A prospective study on folate, B12, and pyridoxal 5'-phosphate (B6) and breast cancer. Cancer *Epidemiol Biomarkers Prev* 1999;8:209-17.
352. Zhang S, Hunter DJ, Hankinson SE, et al. A prospective study of folate intake and the risk of breast cancer. *JAMA* 1999; 281:1632-7.
353. Giovannucci, et al. Multiple vitamins reduce cancer risk. *JNCI.* 1993; 85:875-84.
354. Lipkin M, Newmark HL. Vitamin D, calcium and prevention of breast cancer: a review. *J Am Coll Nutr* 1999;18:392S-397S.
355. Cascienu S, et al. Effects of calcium and vitamin supplementation on colon cancer. *Cancer Invest.* 2000; 18:411-16.
356. Garland, et al. Dietary vitamin D and calcium and risk of colorectal cancer: A 19 year prospective study in men. *Lancet.* 1985; i:307.
357. Newmark H. Teens' low-calcium diets may increase breast cancer risk. *Oncology News Intl.* 1993; 2(11):2.
358. Baron JA, Beach, et al. Calcium supplementation for the prevention of colorectal adenomas. *NEJM.* 1999; 340:101-7.
359. V Matkovic, JZ Ilich, et al.Urinary calcium, sodium, and bone mass of young females. *Am J Clin Nutr* 1995; 62: 417-425.
360. Weaver CM, Peacock M, et al. Adolescent nutrition in the prevention of postmenopausal osteoporosis. *J Clin Endocrinol Metab.* 1999; 84: 1839-43.
361. Rodan GA. Therapeutic approaches to Bone Diseases. *Science.* 2000; 289:1508-14.
362. Bonjour et al. Gain in bone mass in pre pubertal girls 3-5 years after discontinuation of calcium supplementation. *Lancet.* 2001; 358:1208-12.
363. Bendich A, Leader S, Muhuri P. Supplemental calcium for the prevention of hip fracture: potential health-economic benefits. *Clin Ther.* 1999;21:1058-72.
364. Ullom-Minnich P. Prevention of osteoporosis and fractures. *Am Fam Physician* 1999;60:194-202.
365. Marci CD, Viechnicki MB, et al. Bone mineral densitometry substantially influences health-related behaviors of postmenopausal women. *Calcif Tissue Int* 2000;66:113-8.
366. Cohen AJ, Roe FJ. Review of risk factors for osteoporosis with particular reference to a possible aetiological role of dietary salt. *Food Chem Toxicol* 2000;38:237-53.
367. Swaminathan R Nutritional factors in osteoporosis. *Int J Clin Pract* 1999;53:540-8.
368. O'Connell MB. Prevention and treatment of osteoporosis in the elderly. *Pharmacotherapy* 1999;19:7S-20S.
369. Hernandez-Avila M, et al. Caffeine, moderate alcohol intake and risk of fractures of the hip. *Am J Clin Nut.* 1991; 54:157-63.
370. Wong CA, Walsh L, et al. Inhaled corticosteroid use and bone-mineral density in patients with asthma. *Lancet.* 2000; 355:1399-403.
371. Liu B, et al. Use of selective serotonin-reuptake inhibitors or tricyclic antidepressants and risk of hip fractures in elderly people. *Lancet.* 1998; 351:1303-07.
372. Staessen JA, et al. Environmental exposure to cadmium, forearm bone density and risk of fractures: prospective population study. *Lancet.* 1999; 353:1140-44.
373. Bucher HC, Cook R, et al. Effects of dietary calcium supplementation on blood pressure. *JAMA.* 1996; 275:1016-1022.
374. Deary, et al. Calcium and Alzheimer's disease. *Lancet.*1986; (May 24):1219.
375. Pak, CY. Kidney stones. *Lancet.* 1998; 351:1797-801.

376. Curhan, G., et al. A prospective study of dietary calcium and the risk of symptomatic kidney stones. *NEJM*. 1993; 328:833-838.

377. NIH Consensus Development Panel on Optimal Calcium Intake. Optimal calcium intake. *JAMA*. 1994; 272:1942-1948.

378. Dawson-Hughes B, et al. Effect of calcium and vitamin D supplementation on bone density in men and women 65 years or older. *NEJM*. 1997; 337:670-6.

379. Khosla S, Riggs L. Treatment options for osteoporosis. *Mayo Clinic Proc.* 1995; 70:978-82.

380. Recommended Dietary Allowances. 1989. 10th Edition. National Research Council. National Academy Press. Washington, D.C.

381. Bigg, et al. Magnesium deficiency: Role in arrhythmias complicating acute myocardial infarction. *Med J Aust.* 1981; i:346-48.

382. Heptinstall, et al. Letters to the Editor. Lancet. 1986; 8:551-552.

383. Witteman J, et al. Reduction of hypertension with oral magnesium supplementation in women. *Am J Clin Nutr.* 1994; 60:124-31.

384. Britton J, et al. Dietary magnesium, lung function, wheezing in a randomized population. *Lancet.* 1994; 344:357-62.

385. Myers, Gianni, Simone. Oxidative destruction of membranes by doxorubicin-iron complex. *Biochemistry.* 1982; 21:1707-13.

386. Stevens R, et al. Body iron stores and risk of cancer. *NEJM.* 1988; 319:1047-1052.

387. Nelson R, et al. Body iron stores and risk of colonic neoplasia. *JNCI.* 1994; 86:455-60.

388. Simone CB, Simone NL, Simone CB II. Fibre supplementation. *Lancet.* 2001; 357:393.

389. Simone CB II, Simone NL, Simone CB. Consumption of fiber reduce the risk of colorectal cancer: A review. *J Ortho Mol Med.* 2000; 15:96-102.

390. Simone CB, Simone NL, Simone CB II. Fiber supplementation reduces the risk of colorectal cancer: A review. *Int J Integr Med.* 2000; 7:38-43.

391. Burkitt DP. Large-bowel cancer: An epidemiological jigsaw puzzle. *JNCI.* 1975; 54:3.

392. Stoll BA. Essential fatty acids, insulin resistance, and breast cancer risk. *Nutr Cancer.* 1998; 31:72-7.

393. Eynard AR. Does chronic essential fattyy acid deficiency constitute a pro-tumorigenic condition? *Med Hypotheses.* 1997; 48:55-62.

394. Stahl W, Sies H. Food sources of lycopene. *Arch Biochem Biophys.* 1996; 336:1-9.

395. Most don't take daily vitamins. *USA Today.* March 15, 2001.

396. Woods R. Nutrient intake patterns. VNIS Health Communications Conference. "Vitamins in Women's Health: New Roles, New Directions." March 1994. Page 16.

397. Greenwald P, Kelloff G, et al. Chemoprevention. *CA – A Cancer J Clin.* 1995; 45:31-49.

Chapter 6

Nutritional and Lifestyle Modification in Oncology Care

1. Basu TK. Significance of vitamins in cancer. *Oncology.* 1976; 33:183-186.
2. Bhuvarahamurthy V, et al. Effect of radiotherapy and chemoradiotherapy on the circulating antioxidant system of human uterine cervical carcinoma. *Mol Cell Biochem.* 1996; 158:17-23.
3. Clemens MR. Vitamins and therapy of malignancies. *Ther Umsch.* 1994; 51:483-488.
4. Erhola M, Kellokumpu et al. Effects of anthracyclin chemotherapy on plasma antioxidant capacity in small cell lung cancer patients. *Free Radic Biol Med.*1996; 21(3): 383-390.
5. Faber M, Coudray C, et al. Lipid peroxidation products, and vitamin and trace element status in patients with cancer before and after chemotherapy, including adriamycin. *Biol Trace Elem Res.* 1995; 47: 117-123.
6. Look MP, Musch E. Lipid peroxides in the polychemotherapy of cancer patients. *Chemotherapy.* 1994. 40:8-15.
7. Sangeetha P, Das UN, et al. Increase in free radical generation and lipid-peroxidation following chemotherapy for patients with cancer. *Free Radic Biol Med.* 1990; 8:15-19.
8. Myers C, Gianni L, Simone CB, et al. Oxidative destruction of erythrocyte ghost membranes catalysed by the doxorubicin-iron complex. *Biochemistry.* 1982; 21:1707-13.
9. Carmine TC, Evans P, Bruchelt G, et al. Presence of iron catalyst for free radical reactions in patients undergoing chemotherapy: implications for therapeutic management. *Cancer Lett.* 1995. 94:219-226.
10. Brody J. Vitamin Mania, Millions Take a Gamble on Health. *New York Times.* October 26, 1997. Front page.
11. Labriola D, Livingston R. Possible interactions between dietary antioxidants and chemotherapy. *Oncology.* 1999; 13:1003-11.

***In Vitro* cellular**

12. Anderson D, Basaran N, Blowers SD, Edwards AJ. The effect of antioxidants on bleomycin treatment in in vitro and in vivo genootoxicity assays. *Mutat Res.* 1995; 329:37-47.
13. Bump EA, Braunhut SJ, et al. Novel concepts in modification of radiation sensitivity. *Int J Radiat Oncol Biol Phys.* 1994; 29: 249-253.

14. Chiang CD, Song EJ, et al. Ascorbic acid increases accumulation and reverses vincristine resistance of human non-small cell lung cancer cells. *Biochem J.* 1994; 301:759-64.

15. DeLoecker W, et al. Effects of vitamin C treatment on human tumor cell growth in vitro. Synergism with combined chemotherapy action. *Anticancer Res* 1993; 13:103-106.

16. Miura T, Muraoka S, Ogiso T. Effect of ascorbate on adriamycin-Fe induced lipid peroxidation and DNA damage. *Pharmacol Toxicol.* 1994; 74:89-94.

17. Prasad KN, Hernandez C, et al. Modification of the effect of tamoxifen, cisplatin, DTIC, and interferon-alpha 2b on human melanoma cells in culture by a mixture of vitamins. *Nutrition and Cancer.* 1994; 22:233-45.

18. Prasad KN, Rama BN. Modification of the effect of pharmacological agents, ionizing radiation and hyperthermia on tumor cells by vitamin E. In: Vitamin, Nutrition and Cancer. Prasad KN ed. Karger, Basel. Pp 76. 1984.

19. Schwartz JL, Tanaka J, et al. Beta-carotene and/or vitamin E as modulators of alkylating agents in SCC-25 human squamous carcinoma cells. *Cancer Chemother Pharmacol* 1992; 29:207-13.

20. Zucali JR. Mechanisms of protection of hematopoietic stem cells from irradiation. *Leuk Lymphoma.* 1994; 13: 27-32.

Animal

21. Baldew GS, Mol JG, et al. The mechanism of interaction between cisplatin and selenite. *Biochem. Pharmacol.* 1991; 41:1429-37.

22. Ben-Amotz A, et al. Natural beta-carotene and whole body irradiation in rats. *Radiat Environ Biophys.* 1996; 35: 285-88.

23. Bogin E, Marom M, Levi. Changes in serum, liver and kidneys of cisplatin treated rats; effects of antioxidants. *Eur J Clin Chem Clin Biochem.* 1994; 32: 843-851.

24. Crary EJ, McCarty MF. Potential clinical applications for high-dose nutritional antioxidants. *Medical Hypothesis* 1984; 13:77-98.

25. El-Nahas SM, Mattar FE, Mohamed. Radioprotective effect of vitamins C and E. *Mutat Res.* 1993; 301:143-147.

26. Kilinc C, Ozcan O, et al. Vitamin E reduces bleomycin-induced lung fibrosis in mice. *J Basci Clin Physiol Pharmacol.* 1993; 4:249-269.

27. Nakamura T, Pinnell SR, et al. Vitamin C abrogates the deleterious effects of UVB radiation on cutaneous immunity by a mechanism that does not depend on TNF-alpha. *J Invest Dermatol.* 1997; 109:20-24.

28. Riabchenko NI, Ivannik BP, et al. The molecular, cellular and systemic mechanisms of the radioprotective action of multivitamin antioxidant complexes. *Radiats Biol Radioecol.* 1996; 36:895-99.

29. Sminia P, van der Kracht, et al. Hyperthermia, radiation carcinogenesis and the protective potential of vitamin A and N-acetylcysteine. *J Cancer Res Clin Oncol.* 1996; 122: 343-350.

30. Srinivasan V, Weiss JF. Radioprotection by vitamin E: injectable vitamin E administered alone or with WR-3689 enhances the survival of irradiated mice. *Int J Radiat Oncol Biol Phys.* 1992; 23: 841-845.

31. Vinitha R, et al. Effect of administering cyclophosphamide and vitamin E on the levels of tumor-marker enzymes in rats with experimentally induced fibrosarcoma. *Jpn J Med Sci Biol.* 1995; 48:145-156.

32. Wiseman JS, Senagore, Chaudry. Methods to prevent colonic injury in pelvic radiation. *Dis Colon Rectum.* 1994; 37:1090-94.

HUMAN

N-Acetyl Cysteine

33. Dorr RT. Cytoprotective agents for anthracyclines. *Seminars Oncol.* 1996. 23:23-34.

Dexrazoxane (ICRF-187)

34. Carlson R. Reducing the cardiotoxicity of the anthracyclincs. *Oncology* 1992; 6:95-108.

35. Klein P, Muggio FM. Cytoprotection: Shelter from the storm. *The Oncologist.* 1999; 4:112-121.

36. Lopez M, Vici, et al. Randomized prospective clinical trial of high-dose epirubicin and dexrazoxane in patients with advanced breast cancer and soft tissue sarcomas. *J Clin Oncol.* 1998. 16: 86-92.

Adriamycin - Human

37. Legha SS, Wang, et al. Clinical and pharmacological investigation of the effects of alpha-tocopherol on adriamycin cardiotoxicity. *Ann N Y Acad Sci.* 1982; 393:411-418.

38. Lenzhofer R, Ganzinger U, Rameis H, Moser K. Acute cardiac toxicity in patients after doxorubicin treatment and the effect of combined tocopherol and nifedipine pretreatment. *J Cancer Res Clin Oncol.* 1983; 106:143-147.

39. Myers CE, McGuire W. Adriamycin amelioration of toxicity by alpha-tocopherol. *Cancer Treat Rep.* 1976; 60:961-62.

40. Faure H, Coudray C, et al. 5-Hydroxymethyluracil excretion, plasma TBARS and plasma antioxidant vitamins in

adriamycin-treated patients. *Free Rad Biol Med.* 1996; 20: 979-83.

41. Pyrhonen S, Kuitunen T, Nyandoto P, Kouri M. Randomized comparison of fluorouracil, epidoxorubicin and methotrexate (FEMTX) plus supportive care with supportive care alone in patients with non-resectable gastric cancer. *Br J Cancer.* 1995; 71(3): 587-591.

42. Waltzman SA, Lorell, et al. Prospective study of tocopherol prophylaxis for anthracycline cardiac toxicity. *Curr Ther Res.* 1980; 28:682-86.

Human

43. Besa EC, Abraham IL, et al. Treatment with 13 cis-retinoic acid in transfusion-dependent patients with myelodysplastic syndromes and decreased toxicity with addition of alpha- tocopherol. *Am J Med* 1990; 89:739-747.

44. Cascinu S, Cordella L, et al. Neuroprotective effect of reduced glutathione on cisplatin based chemotherapy in advanced gastric cancer: a randomized double-blind placebo controled trial. *J Clin Oncol.* 1995; 13:26-32.

45. Clemens MR. Vitamins and therapy of malignancies. *Ther Umsch.* 1994; 51(7): 483-488.

46. DeRosa L, et al. Therapy of 'high risk' myelodysplastic syndromes with an association of low dose Ara-C, retinoic acid and 1,25 dihydroxyvitamin D3. *Biomed Pharmacother.* 1992; 46: 211-217.

47. Dimery I, Shirinian M, Heyne K, Lippman S, et al. Reduction in toxicity of high dose 13 cis-retinoic acid with alpha-tocopherol. *Proc Annu Meet Am Soc Clin Oncol.* 1992; 11:A399.

48. DiRe F, Bohm, et al. High dose cisplatin and cyclophosphamide with glutathione in the treatment of advanced ovarian cancer. *Ann. Oncol.* 1993: 4:55-61.

49. Faure H, Coudray C, et al. 5-Hydroxymethyluracil excretion, plasma TBARS and plasma antioxidant vitamins in adriamycin-treated patients. *Free Rad Biol Med.* 1996; 20: 979 983.

50. Ganser A, Mauer A, et al. Improved multi-lineage response of hematopoiesis in patients with myelodysplastic syndromes to a combination therapy with all-trans-retinoic acid, granulocyte colony-stimulating factor, erythropoietin and alpha-tocopherol. *Ann Hematol.* 1996; 72: 237-244.

51. Gottlober P, Krahn G, et al. The treatment of cutaneous radiation-induced fibrosis with pentoxifylline and vitamin E. *Strahlenther Onkol.* 1996; 172: 34-38.

52. Henriksson, Rogo, Grankvist. Interaction between cytostatics and nutrients. *Med Oncol Tumor Pharm* 1991; 8:79-86.

53. Iino Y, Takei H, Morishita Y. Adjuvant endocrine therapy for breast cancer. *Gan To Kagaku Ryoho.* 1995; 1:81-87.

54. Israel L, Hajji, et al. Vitamin A augmentation of the effects of chemotherapy in metastatic breast cancers after menopause. Randomized trial in 100 patients. *Annnles De Medecine Interne* 1985; 136:551-554.

55. Jaakkola K, Lahteenmaki et al. Treatment with antioxidant and other nutrients in combination with chemotherapy and irradiation in patients with small cell lung cancer. *Anticancer Res* 1992; 12:599-606.

56. Kim JH, *et al.* Use of vitamins as adjunct to conventional cancer therapy. In: Nutrients in Cancer Prevention and Treatment. Prasad KN, Santamaria L, Williams RM, eds. Pp 363-372. Humana Press, New Jersey. 1995.

57. Kim JH. Use of vitamins as adjunct to conventional cancer therapy. Second Denver Conference on Nutrition and Cancer, September 7, 1994.

58. Komiyama S, Kudoh S, et al. Synergistic combination of 5FU, vitamin A, and cobalt-60 radiation for head and neck tumors – antitumor combination therapy with vitamin A. *Auris, Nasus, Larynx* 1985; 12 S2:S239-S243.

59. Ladner HL, et al. In: Vitamins and Cancer, ed. F.L. Meyskens. Clifton, NJ: Humana Press, pp. 429. 1986.

60. Lee JS, Libshitz, et al. Edatrexate improves the antitumor effects of cyclophosphamide and cisplatin against non-small cell lung cancer. *Cancer.* 1991; 68: 959-964.

61. Lockwood K, et al. Apparent partial remission of breast cancer in 'high risk' patients supplemented with nutritional antioxidants, essential fatty acids and coenzyme Q10. *Mol Aspects Med.* 1994; 15: 231-240.

62. Lopez I, Goudou C, et al. Treatment of mucositis with vitamin E during administration of neutropenic antineoplastic agents. *Ann Med Interne.* 1994; 145: 405-408.

63. Lupulescu AP. Hormones, vitamins, and growth factors in cancer treatment and prevention. A critical appraisal. *Cancer.* 1996; 78: 2264-80.

64. Margolin KA, et al. Phase I study of mitomycin C and menadione in advanced solid tumors. *Cancer Chemother Pharmacol.* 1995; 36: 293-98.

65. Meyskens FL, Kopecky KJ. Phase III randomized trial of the treatment of chronic stage CML with pulse, intermittent busulfan

therapy (SWOG 7984): improved survival with the addition of oral vitamin A (50,000 IU/day). Seventh International Conference on the Adjuvant Therapy of Cancer. March 10, 1993. Tucson, AZ.

66. Mills E. The modifying effect of beta-carotene on radiation and chemotherapy induced oral mucositis. *Br J Cancer.* 1988; 57:416-17.

67. Nagoumey, et al. Menadiol with chemotherapies: feasibility for resistance modification. *Proc Ann Meet Am Soc Clin Oncol.* 1987; 6:A132.

68. Ojiro M, Takenoshita et al. Significance of vitamin K administration in patients under chemotherapy during postoperative fasting period. *Nippon Geka Gakkai Zasshi.* 1992; 93: 9-15.

69. Osaki T, Ueta E, et al. Prophylaxis of oral mucositis associated with chemoradiotherapy for oral carcinoma by Azelastine with other antioxidants. *Head Neck.* 1994;16: 331-339.

70. Parnis FX, Coleman, et al. A randomized double-blind placebo controlled clinical trial assessing the tolerability and efficacy of glutathione as an adjuvant to escalating doses of cisplatin in the treatment of advanced ovarian cancer. *Eur J Cancer.* 1995; 31A: 1721.

71. Pastorino U, Infante, et al. Adjuvant treatment of Stage I lung cancer with high-dose vitamins A. *J Clin Oncol.* 1993: 11:1216-22.

72. Plaxe S, Freddo J, et al. Phase I trial of cisplatin in combination with glutathione. *Gynecol Oncol.* 1994; 55:82-86.

73. Pyrhonen S, Kuitunen, et al. Randomized comparison of fluorouracil, epidoxorubicin and methotrexate (FEMTX) plus supportive care with supportive care alone in patients with non-resectable gastric cancer. *Br J Cancer.* 1995; 71: 587-91.

74. Recchia F, de Filippos S, et al. Cisplatin, vindesine, 5FU, beta-interferon and retinyl palmitate in advanced non-small cell lung cancer. *Proc Annu Meet Am Soc Clin Oncol.* 1993; 12: A1144.

75. Recchia F, Lelli S, et al. 5FU, cisplatin and retinol palmitate in the management of advanced cancer of the oral cavity. Phase II study. *Clin Ter.* 1993; 142:403-409.

76. Recchia F, Rea S, et al. Beta-interferon, retinoids and tamoxifen as maintenance therapy in metastatic breast cancer. *Clin Ter.* 1995; 146: 603-610.

77. Recchia F, Serafini F, et al. Phase II study of 5FU, folinic acid, epirubicin, mitomycin-C, beta-interferon and retinol palmitate in patients with unresectable pancreatic carcinoma. *Proc Annu Meet Am Assoc Cancer Res.* 1992; 33:A1296.

78. Recchia F, Sica G, et al. Interferon-beta, retinoids, and tamoxifen in the treatment of metastatic breast cancer: a phase II study. *J Interferon Cytokine Res.* 1995; 15: 605-610.

79. Rougereau A, Sallerin T, et al. Adjuvant treatment of patients with neoplastic lesions using the combination of a vitamin complex and an amino acid. Apropos of a series of 17 cases of epidermoid carcinoma of the upper aerodigestive tract. *Ann Gastroenterol Hepatol.* 1993; 29:99-102.

80. Sakamoto A, et al. In Medulation and Mediation of Cancer by Vitamins Karger, Basel, pp.330. 1983.

81. Santamaria, Benazzo, et al. First clinical case-report (1980-88) of cancer chemoprevention with beta-carotene plus canthaxanthin supplemented to patients after radical treatment. In: Nutrition, Growth and Cancer. Tryfiates GP, Prasad KN, eds. Alan R. Liss: New York. 1988.

82. Smyth Jf, Bowman A, et al. Glutathione reduces the toxicity and improves quality of life of women diagnosed with ovarian cancer treated with cisplatin: results of a double-blind, randomized trial. *Ann Oncol.* 1997; 8:569-573.

83. Stahelin HB. Critical reappraisal of vitamins and trace minerals in nutritional support of cancer patients. *Support Care Cancer.* 1993; 1: 295-297.

84. Tanaka N, Ochi K, et al. Clinical application of vitamin A, D, and E against malignant tumor in human. *Nippon Rinsho.* 1993; 51: 989-996.

85. Tedeschi M, et al. The role of glutathione in combination with cisplatin in the treatment of ovarian cancer. *Cancer Treatment Rev.* 1991; 18:253-259.

86. Tetef M, Margolin K, et al. Mitomycin C and menadione for the treatment of lung cancer: a Phase II trial. *Invest New Drugs.* 1995; 13:157-62.

87. Thiruvengadam R, Kaneshiro, et al. Effect of antioxidant vitamins and mineral on chemotherapy induced cytopenia. *Proc Annu Meet Am Soc Clin Oncol.* 1996; 15: A1793.

88. Wagdi P, Rouvinez G, et al. Cardioprotection in chemo- and radiotherapy for malignant diseases – an echocardiographic pilot. *Schweiz Rundsch Med Prax.* 1995; 84: 1220-23.

89. Wadleigh RG, Redman, et al. Vitamin E in the treatment of chemotherapy induced mucositis. *Am J Med.* 1992; 92: 481-84.

90. Wiernik PH, Yeap B, et al. Hexamethyl-melamine and low or moderate dose cisplatin with or without pyridoxine for the treatment of advanced ovarian carcinoma. *Cancer Invest.* 1992; 10:1-9.

91. Wood LA. Possible prevention of adriamycin-induced alopecia by tocopherol. NEJM 1985; 312(16):1060.

Amifostine (WR-2721) Antioxidant

92. Capizzi RL. Clinical status and optimal use of Amifostine. *Oncology.* 1999; 13(1):47-59.

93. Kligerman M, Glover D, Simone CB, et al. Toxicity of WR-2721 administered in single and multiple doses. *Int J Radiat Oncol Biol Phys.* 1984; 10:1773-76.

94. Schiller JH, Storer B, Berlin J, et al. Amifostine, cisplatin and vinblastine in metastatic non-small cell lung cancer: A report of high response rates and prolonged survival. *J Clin Oncol.* 1996; 14:1913-1921.

Folic Acid

95. Leeb BF. Folic acid and cyanocobalamin levels in serum and erythrocytes during low-dose methotrexate therapy of rheumatoid arthritis and psoriatic arthritis patients. *Clin Exp Rheum.* 1995; 13:459-463.

96. Morgan SL, Baggott JE, et al. Supplementation with folic acid during methotrexate therapy for rheumatoid arthritis. A double blind, placebo trial. *Ann Intern Med.*1994; 121: 833-41.

LIFESTYLE

97. Simone CB. Use of therapeutic levels of nutrients to augment oncology care. In: Adjuvant Nutrition in Cancer Treatment. Quillin P, and Williams M, eds. Academic Press, Tulsa, OK, p. 72. 1992.

98. Simone CB. Cancer and Nutrition, A Ten Point Plan to Decrease Your Risk of Getting Cancer. New York, McGraw-Hill 1981; revised, Garden City Park, Avery 1992.

99. Wynder E, Kajitani T, et al. A comparison of survival rates between American and Japanese patients with breast cancer. *Surg Gyn Obstet.* 1963;196-200.

100. Nemoto T, Tominago, et al. Differences in breast cancer between Japan and the U.S. *JNCI* 1977;58:193-197.

101. Sakamoto G, Sugano, Hartmann. Comparative clinicopathological study of breast cancer among Japanese and American females. *Jpn J Cancer Clin* 1979; 25:161-70.

102. Ward-Hinds M, Kolonel, Nomura, Lee. Stage-specific breast cancer incidence rates by age among Japanese and Caucasian women in Hawaii. *Br J Cancer* 1982; 45:118-123.

103. Kolonel L, Hankin, Lee, et al. Nutrient intakes in relation to cancer incidence in Hawaii. *Br J Cancer* 1981; 44:332-339.

104. Armstrong and Doll. Environmental factors and cancer incidenceand mortality in different countries with special reference to dietary practices. *Int J Cancer* 1975; 15:617-631.

105. Morrison AS, Lowe CR, et al. Some international differences in treatment and survival in breast cancer. *Int J Cancer.* 1976; 18:269-273.

106. Morrison AS, Lowe CR, MacMahon, et al. Incidence, risk factors and survival in breast cancer: report on five years of follow-up observation. *Europ J Cancer.*1977; 13:209-214.

107. Donegan WL, Hartz AJ, Rimm. The association of body weight with recurrent cancer of the breast. *Cancer* 1978; 41:1590-1594.

108. Abe R, Kumagai, et al. Biological characteristics of breast cancer in obesity. *Tohoku J Exp Med* 1976; 120:351-359.

109. Donegan WL, Rimm. The prognostic implications of obesity for surgical cure of breast cancer. *Breast* 1978; 4:14-17.

110. Sohrabi A, Sandoz J, et al. Recurrence of breast cancer. Obesity, tumor size, and axillary lymph node metatstases. *JAMA* 1980; 244:261-265.

111. Boyd NF, Campbell JE, et al. Body weight and prognosis in breast cancer. *JNCI* 1981; 67:785-789.

112. Tartter PI, Papatestas AE, et al. Cholesterol and obesity as prognostic factors in breast cancer. *Cancer.* 1981; 47:2222-27.

113. Buchwald, H. Cholesterol inhibition, cancer, and chemotherapy. *Lancet* 1992; 339:1154-1156.

114. Hoffer A and Pauling L. Hardin Jones biostatistical analysis of mortality data for cohorts of cancer patients with a large surviving fraction surviving at the termination of the study using vitamin C and other nutrients. *J Orthomolecular Med* 1990; 5:143.

115. Goodman MT, Kolonel LN, et al. Dietary factors in lung cancer prognosis. *European J Cancer* 1992; 28:495-501.

116. Foster, H.D. Lifestyle influences on spontaneous cancer regression. *Intl J Biosocial Research* 1988; 10:17-20.

117. Carter JP. Macrobiotic diet and cancer survival. *J Am College Nutr* 1993; 12:209-15.

118. Sakamoto G, Hartmann. et al. In: Modulation and Mediation of Cancer by Vitamins. Karger, Basel. 1983; p. 330.

119. Lamm DL. Megadose vitamins in bladder cancer: a double blind clinical trial. *J Urol.* 1994; 151:21-26.

120. Agus DB, Vera JC, Golde DW: Stromal cell oxidation: A mechanism by which tumors obtain vitamin C. *Cancer Res.*.1999; 59:4555-58.

121. Gopalakrishna R, Gundimeda, Chen. Vitamin E succinate inhibits protein kinase C: correlation with its unique inhibitory effects on cell growth and transformation. In: Nutrients in Cancer Prevention and Treatment. Prasad KN, Santamaria L, Williams, eds. Humana Press: NJ. Pp 21-37. 1995.

122. Prasad KN, Cohrs, Sharma. Decreased expression of c-myc and H-ras oncogenes in vitamin E succinate induced differentiation murine B-16 melanoma cells in culture. *Biochem Cell Biol.* 1990; 68:1250-55.

123. Cohrs RJ, Torelli S, *et al.* Effect of vitamin E succinate and a cAMP stimulating agent on the expression of c-myc and H-ras in murine neuroblastoma cell. *Int J Dev Biol Neurosci.* 1991; 9:187-194.

124. Kline K, Yu W, Zhao B. Vitamin E succinate: mechanisms of action as tumor cell growth inhibitor. In: Nutrients in Cancer Prevention and Treatment. Prasad KN, Santamaria L, Wiliams, eds. Humana Press: NJ. Pp 39-55. 1995.

Chapter 7

Free Radicals

1. Cross, et al. Oxygen radicals and human disease. *Ann Int Med.* 1987; 107:526-45.
2. Southorn P, Powis. Free radicals in medicine, chemical nature and biological reactions. *Mayo Clin Proc.* 1988; 63:381-389.
3. Aruoma Okezie I, et al. Oxygen free radicals and human diseases. *J Roy Soc Health.* 1991; 111:172-177.
4. Saul, et al. Free radicals, DNA damage, and aging. In Annals: Modern biological theories of aging. 1987. New York: Raven Press, 113-29.
5. Cerutti. Pro-oxidant states and tumor promotion. *Science.* 1985; 227:375-82.
6. Rubanyi. Vascular effects of oxygen-derived free radicals. *Free Rad Bio Med.* 1988; 4:107-20.
7. Hennig and Chow. Lipid peroxidation and endothelial cell injury: Implications in atherosclerosis. *Free Rad Bio Med.* 1988; 4:99-106.
8. Re-profusion injury after thrombolytic therapy for acute myocardial infarction. *Lancet.* 1989; Sept:655-57.
9. McCord. Oxygen derived free radicals in post ischemic tissue injury. *NEJM.* 1985; 312:159-63.

Chapter 8

Nutritional Factors

1. Wynder E, Gori P. Contribution of the environment to cancer incidence: An epidemiologic exercise. *JNCI.* 1977; 58:825.
2. The National Academy of Sciences. Nutrition, Diet, and Cancer. 1982.
3. Simone CB. Cancer and Nutrition: A Ten-Point Plan to Reduce Your Chances of Getting Cancer. 1983. New York: McGraw-Hill Book Co.
4. Moody. Aboriginal Health. 1983. Canberra, Australia: Australian National University Press, p. 92.
5. Truswell and Hansen. Medical research among the Kung. In Hunter-Gatherers. Lee and DeVore Ed S. Kalahari. Cambridge, Mass: Harvard University Press 1976.
6. Eaton, Konner. Paleolithic nutrition. *NEJM.*1985; 312:283-89.
7. Howe, et al. Dietary factors and risk of breast cancer; combined analysis of 12 case-control studies. *JNCI.* 1990; 82:561-569.
8. Graham S, et al. Diet in the epidemiology of breast cancer. *Am J Epidemiol.* 1982; 116:68-75.
9. Ewertz M,Caroline. Dietary factors and breast cancer risk in Denmark. *Inst J Epidemiol.* 1990; 46:779-784.
10. Van't Veer P, et al. Dietary fat and the risk of breast cancer. *Int J Epidemiol.* 1990; 19:12-18.
11. Graham S, et al. Nutritional epidemiology of postmenopausal breast cancer in Western New York. *Am J Epidemiol.* 1991; 34:552-566.
12. Frisch R. Dietary fat and the risk of breast cancer. *NEJM.* 1987; 317:165.
13. Lee H, et al. Dietary effects on breast cancer risk in Singapore. *Lancet.* 1991 337:1197-1200.
14. Kritchevsky D. Diet and cancer. *CA- Cancer J Clin.* 1991;41(6):328-33.
15. Weinhouse S, et al. ACS Guidelines on diet, nutrition, and cancer. *CA- Cancer J Clin.* 1991; 41:334-38.
16. Boyle P, et al. Trends in diet related cancers in Japan: A conundrum? *Lancet.* 1993; 342:752.
17. Golden B, et al. Estrogen excretion patterns and plasma levels in vegetarian and omnivorous women. *NEJM.* 1982; 307:1542-47.
18. Wydner EL, et al. Environmental factors of cancer of the colon and rectum. II. Japanese epidemiological data. *Cancer.* 1969; 32:1210.
19. Phillips R. Role of life-style and dietary habits in risk of cancer among Seventh-Day Adventists. *Cancer Res.* 1975; 35:3513.

20. Lyon J, Gardner, Klauber, Smart. Low cancer incidence and mortality in Utah. *Cancer.*1977; 39:2608.

21. Rosen P, Hellerstein, Horwitz. The low incidence of colorectal cancer in a high-risk population. *Cancer.* 1981; 48:2692.

22. Baptista J, Bruce, et al. On distribution of different fecapentaenes, the fecal mutagens, in the human population. *Cancer Letters.* 1984; 22:299.

23. Bruce W, Varghese, Farrer. A mutagen in the feces of normal humans. In:Origins of Human Cancer. ed. H Hiatt, Watson, Winsten, Cold Spring Harbor Lab, Cold Spring Harbor, NY. 1977; pps. 1641-44.

24. Jones D, et al. Dietary fat and breast cancer in the National Health and Nutrition Examination Survey I: epidemiologic follow-up study. *JNCI.* 1987; 79:465-471.

25. Knekt P, et al. Dietary fat and risk of breast cancer. *Am J Clin Nutr.* 1990; 52:903-908.

26. Howe G, et al. A cohort study of fat intake and risk of breast cancer. *JNCI.* 1991; 83:336-340.

27. Kushi L, et al. Dietary fat, breast cancer, adjustment for energy intake and categorization of risk. *Am J Epidemiol.* 1991; 134:714.

28. Ganz P, Schag. Nutrition and breast cancer. *Oncology.* 1993; 7:71-76.

29. Report of the Council on Scientific Affairs. Diet and Cancer: Where do matters stand? *Arch Intern Med.* 1993;153:50-56.

30. Toniolo P, et al. Calorie providing nutrients and risk of breast cancer. *JNCI.* 1989; 81:278.

31. LaVeccia C, et al. Comparative cancer epidemiology in the U.S. and Italy. *Cancer Res.* 1988; Dec 15: 1202-07.

32. Willett W, Hunter, et al. Dietary fat and fiber in relation to risk of breast cancer. *JAMA.* 1992; 268:203744.

33. Giovannucci E, et al. A comparison of prospective and retrospective assessments of diet in the study of breast cancer. *Am J Epidemiol.* 1991;134:714.

34. Marshall E. Search for a killer: focus shifts from fat to hormones. *Science.* 1993; 259:618-621.

35. Petrakis N, Gruenke, Craig. Cholesterol and cholesterol epoxide in nipple aspirate of human breast fluid. *Cancer Res.* 1981; 41:2563.

36. Wu AH, Ziegler RG, Nomura, et al. Soy intake and risk of breast cancer in Asians and Asian Americans. *Am J Clin Nutr.* 1998; 68:1437S-1443S.

37. Swain S, Santen R, Burger H, Pritchard K, eds. Treatment of Estrogen Deficiency Symptoms in Women Surviving Breast Cancer: Prevention of Osteoporosis and CV Effects of Estrogens and Antiestrogens. *Oncology.* 1999; 13:397-432.

38. Hsieh CY, Santell RC, et al. Estrogenic effects of genistein on the growth of estrogen receptor positive human breast cancer (MCF-7) cells *in vitro* and *in vivo*. *Cancer Res.* 1998; 58:3833-38.

39. McMichael-Phillips DF, Harding C, et al. Effects of soy protein supplementation on epithelial proliferation in the histologically normal human breast. *Am J Clin Nutr.* 1998; 68: 1431S-36S.

40. Eagon PK, Tress NB, Ayer, et al. Medicinal botanicals with hormonal activity. *Am Assoc for Cancer Res.* April 1999. 1073.

41. Tannenbaum A. The genesis and growth of tumors. Effects of a high-fat diet. *Cancer Res.*1942; 2:468.

42. Woutersen RA, Appel MJ, et al.Dietary fat and carcinogenesis: A Review. *Mutat Res.* 1999; 443:111-27.

43. Newman LA, Kuerer HM, et al. Special considerations in breast cancer risk and survival. *J Surg Oncol.* 1999;71:250-60.

44. Lewis CJ, Yetley EA. Health claims and observational human data: relation between dietary fat and cancer. *Am J Clin Nutr.* 1999;69:1357S-1364S.

45. Hilakivi CL, Clarke R. Influence of maternal diet on breast cancer risk among female offspring. *Nutrition.* 1999;15:392-401.

46. Wu AH, Pike MC, Stram. Meta-analysis: dietary fat intake, serum estrogen levels, and the risk of breast cancer. *JNCI.* 1999;91:529-34.

47. Eichholzer M. Nutrition and cancer. *Ther Umsch* 2000; 57:146-51.

48. Blair SN, Brodney S. Effects of physical inactivity and obesity on morbidity and mortality: current evidence and research issues. *Med Sci Sports Exerc* 1999;31:S646-62.

49. McCarty MF. Vegan proteins may reduce risk of cancer, obesity, and cardiovascular disease by promoting increased glucagon activity. *Med Hypotheses* 1999;53:459-85.

50. Saxe GA, Rock CL, Wicha MS. Diet and risk for breast cancer recurrence and survival. *Breast Cancer Res Treat* 1999; 53:241-53.

51. Bingham SA. High-meat diets and cancer risk. *Proc Nutr Soc* 1999; 58:243-8.

52. Bartsch H, Nair J, Owen RW. Dietary polyunsaturated fatty acids and cancers of the breast and colorectum: emerging evidence for their role as risk modifiers. *Carcinogenesis* 1999; 20:2209-18.

53. Kant AK, Schatzkin A, et al. A prospective study of diet quality and mortality in women. *JAMA* 2000;283:2109-15.
54. Wynder EL, Gori GB. Contribution of the environment to cancer incidence: An epidemiologic exercise. *JNCI.* 1977; 58:825.
55. Nutrition and Cancer, ed. W.D. DeWys. 1983. *Seminars in Oncol.* 1983; 10:1-367.
56. Workshop on Nutrition in Cancer Causation and Prevention. *Cancer Res.* 1983. 43:2386-2519.
57. Diet and Human Carcinogenesis Proceedings. *Nutrition and Cancer.* 1986; 8:1-71.
58. Executive Summary. Diet, Nutrition, and Cancer. *Cancer Res.* 1983; 43:3018-23.
59. Cohen L. Diet and cancer. *Scientific American.* 1987; 257:42-48.
60. Reddy B. Dietary fat and colon cancer. *Prev Med.* 1987; 16:460-467.
61. Proceeding of a Workshop. Dietary fat and fiber in carcinogenesis. *Prev Med.* 1987; 16:449-527.
62. National Research Council. Diet, Nutrition and Cancer. 1982. Washington, D.C.: National Academy Press.
63. Paptestas A, et al. Fecal steroid metabolites and breast cancer risk. *Cancer.* 1982;49:1201.
64. Brammer S, DeFelice. Dietary advice in regard to risk for colon and breast cancer. *Prev Med.* 1980; 9:544.
65. Vonderhaar BK. Prolactin involvement in breast cancer. *Endocr Relat Cancer.* 1999; Sep;6:389-404.
66. Alcantara E, Speckman. Diet, nutrition, and cancer. *Am J Clin Nutr.* 1976; 29:1035.
67. Carroll K. Experimental evidence of dietary factors and hormone dependent cancers. *Cancer Res.* 1975; 35:3374.
68. Carroll K, Gammel, Plunkett. Dietary fat and mammary cancer. *Can Med Assoc.* 1968; 98:590-594.
69. Drasar B, Irving. Environmental factors and cancer of the colon and breast. *Br J Cancer.* 1973; 27:167.
70. Kent S. Diet, hormones, and breast cancer. *Geriatrics.* 1979; 34:83.
71. Paptestas A, Panvelliwalla, et al. Fecal steroid metabolites and breast cancer risk. *Cancer.*1982; 49:1201.
72. Gregorio DI, Emrich, et al. Dietary fat consumption and survival among women with breast cancer. *JNCI.* 1985; 75:37-41.
73. Morrison A, Lowe, et al. Incidence, risk factors and survival in breast cancer: *Eur J Cancer.*1977; 13:209-214.
74. Wynder EL, Kajatani J, et al. A comparison of survival rates between American and Japanese patients with breast cancer. *Surg Gynecol Obstet.* 1963; 117:196-200.
75. Donegan WL, Hartz, Rimm. The association of body weight with recurrent cancer of the breast. *Cancer.* 1978; 41:1590-1594.
76. Morrison AS, Lowe, MacMahon, et al. Some international differences in treatment and survival in breast cancer. *Int J Cancer.* 1977; 18:269-273.
77. Tartter PI, Papatestas, Ioannovich, et al. Cholesterol and obesity as prognostic factors in breast cancer. *Cancer.* 1981;47:2222<196>2227.
78. Wynder EL, MacCornack, Hill, et al. Nutrition and the etiology and prevention of breast cancer. *Cancer Detection Prevent.* 1976; 1:293-310.
79. Kolonel L, Hankin, et al. Nutrient intakes in relation to cancer incidence in Hawaii. *Br J Cancer.* 1981; 44:332.
80. Nemoto T, Tominago, et al. Differences in breast cancer between Japan and the United States. *JNCI.* 1977;58:193-197.
81. Abe R, Kumagai, et al. Biological characteristics of breast cancer in obesity. *Tohoku J Exp Med.* 1976; 120:351-359.
82. Ward-Hines M, Kolonel, Nomura, Lee. Stage-specific breast cancer incidence rates by age among Japanese and Caucasian women in Hawaii, 1960-1979. *Br J Cancer.* 1982; 45:118-123.
83. Boyd NF, Campbell, et al. Body weight and prognosis in breast cancer. *JNCI.* 1981; 67:785-789.
84. Kwa HG, Bulbrook, Cleton, et al. 1978. An abnormal early evening peak of plasma prolactin in nulliparous and obese postmenopausal women.<MI> Int J Cancer<D> 22:691<196>693.
85. deWaard and Baanders-van Halewign. A prospective study in general practice on breast cancer risk in postmenopausal women.
86. McDonald R, Grodin, Sitteri. The utilization of plasma androstenedione for estrone production in women in endocrinology. *Excerpta Med Int Congr Ser.* 1969; 184:770-776.
87. O'Dea J, Wieland, Hallberg, et al. Effect of dietary weight loss on sex steriod binding, sex steroids and gonadotropins on obese postmenopausal women. *J Lab Clin Med.* 1979; 93:1004-1008.
88. Simone CB II, Simone N, Simone, CB. Consumption of fiber reduces the risk of cancer: A review. *J Orthomol Med.* 2000; 15:96-102.
89. Goldin, BR, Adlercreutz, et al. Estrogen excretion patterns and plasma levels in vege-

tarian and omnivorous women. *NEJM.* 1982; 307:1542-47

90. Knox EG. Foods and diseases. *Br J Prev Soc Med.* 1977; 31:71-80.
91. Armstrong and Doll. Environmental factors and cancer incidence and mortalities in different countries.
92. Jain, M., et al. A case control study of diet and colo-rectal cancer.
93. Hill MJ, Caygill CP. Sugar intake and the risk of colorectal cancer. *Eur J Cancer Prev* 1999;8:465-8.
94. Hems G. The contribution of diet and childbearing to breast cancer rates. *Br J Cancer.* 1978; 37:974-982.
95. DominoF, et al. The nicotine content of common vegetables. *NEJM.* 1993; 329:437.
96. Castro, Monji. Dietary nicotine and its significance in studies on tobacco smoking. *Biochem Arch.* 1986; 2:91-97.
97. Davis RA, et al. Dietary nicotine: a source of urinary cotinine. *J Food Chem Toxicol.* 1991; 29:821-827.
98. Domino EF, et al. Current experience with HPLC and GC-MS analyses of nicotine and cotinine. *Med Sci Res.* 1992; 20:859-860.
99. Ames BN. Dietary carcinogens and anticarcinogens: A Review. Science. 1983; 221:1256.
100. Browner WS, et al. What if Americans ate less fat? *JAMA.* 1998; 265:3285-3291.
101. Johnson C, et al. Declining serum cholesterol levels among U.S. adults. *JAMA.* 1993; 269:3002-08.
102. Burr, et al. Effects of changes in fat, fish, and fiber intakes on death and heart attack. *Lancet.* 1989;757-61.
103. Ferraro C. Why is high-fat food marketed? Customers demand it, that's why. *Investor's Daily* Sept 6, 1990:15.
104. Woodbury R. The great fast-food pig-out. *Time.* June 28, 1993:51.
105. O'Neill M. Fat, drink, and be merry' may be the next trend. *New York Times.* Jan. 2, 1994, front page.
106. Eating in America. Natural Foods. June 1994:20. (Survey conducted by MRCA information services for the National Livestock and Meat Board.)

Chapter 9
Obesity

1. Hannon BM, Lohman. The energy cost of overweight in the United States. *Am J Public Health.* 1978. 68:8.
2. Huang Z, Hankinson SE, et al. Dual effects of weight and weight gain on breast cancer risk. *JAMA.* 1997; 278:1407-11.
3. Kelsey JL, Baron J. Weight and risk for breast cancer. *JAMA.* 1997; 278:1448.
4. Cleary MP, Maihle NJ. The role of body mass index in the relative risk of developing premenopausal versus postmenopausal breast cancer. *Proc Society Exp Bio Med.* 1997; 216:28-43.
5. Bonn D. How weight gain affects breast cancer risk clarified. *Lancet.* 1997; 350:1371.
6. Armstrong B, Doll R. Environmental factors and cancer incidence and mortalities in different countries with special reference to dietary practices. *Int J Cancer.* 1975; 15:616.
7. Gaskill SP, et al. Breast cancer mortality and diet in the United States. *Cancer Res.* 1979; 39:3628.
8. de Waard F, Baanders-van Halewign EA. A prospective study in general practice on breast cancer risk in postmenopausal women. *J Cancer.* 1974; 14:153-160.
9. Hin TM, Chen KP, MacMahon B. Epidemiologic characteristics of cancer of the breast in Taiwan. *Cancer.* 1971; 27:1497-1504.
10. Mirra AP, Cole P, et al. Breast cancer in an area of high parity, Sao Paolo, Brazil. *Cancer Res* 1971; 31:77-83.
11. Kumar NB, Lyman, et al. Timing of weight gain and breast cancer risk. *Cancer* 1995 Jul 15;76:243-9.
12. Michels KB, Trichopoulos D, et al. Birthweight as a risk factor for breast cancer. *Lancet.* 1996; 348:1542-46.
13. London, et al. Prospective study of relative weight, height, and risk of breast cancer. *JAMA.* 1989; 262:2853-2858.
14. Schapira, et al. Abdominal obesity and breast cancer risk. *Ann Intern Med.* 1990; 112:182-186.
15. Ballard-Barbesh, et al. Body fat distribution and breast cancer in the Framingham study. *JNCI.* 1990; 82:286-290.
16. Folsom, et al. Increased incidence of breast cancer associated with abdominal adiposity in postmenopausal women. *Am J Epidemiol.* 1990; 131:794-803.
17. LeMarchand, et al. Body size at different periods of life and breast cancer risk. *Am J Epidemiol.* 1990;128:137-152.
18. Sellers, et al. Effect of family history, bodyfat distribution, and reproductive factors on the risk of postmenopausal breast cancer. *NEJM* 1992; 326:1323-1329.
19. Gaskill SP, McGuire WL, et al. Breast cancer mortality and diet in the United States. *Cancer Res.* 1979; 39:3628.45.
20. MacDonald PC, et al. Effect of obesity on conversion of plasma androstenedione to es-

trone in postmenopausal women with and without endometrial cancer. *Am J Obstet Gynecol.* 1978; 130:448-455.

21. Marshall E. Breast cancer. *Science.* 1993; 259:618-621.
22. Grodin, et al. Source of estrogen production in postmenopausal women. *J Clin Endocrinol Metab.* 1973; 36:207-214.
23. Sitteri, et al. Role of extraglandular estrogen in human endocrinology. In: Handbook of physiology, ed. Greep, Astwood. 1973; vol 2, pp. 15-629. Wash, DC: Am Physiol Soc.
24. Rose P, et al. Low fat diet in fibrocystic disease of the breast with cyclical mastalgia: a feasibility study. *Am J Clin Nutr.* 1985; 42:856.
25. Schapira, et al. Estimate of breast cancer risk reduction with weight loss. *Cancer.* 1991; 67:2622-2625.
26. Wynder and Hill. Prolactin, estrogens, and lipids in breast fluid. *Lancet.* 1977; 2:840..
27. Rose P, et al. Serum and breast duct fluid prolactin and estrogen levels in Finnish and American women and patients with fibrocystic breast disease. *Cancer.* 1986; 57:1550-54.
28. Lee-Han, et al. Compliance in a randomized clinical trial of dietary fat reduction in patients with breast dysplasia. *Am J Clin Nutr.* 1988; 48:575-586.
29. Insuli, et al. Results of a randomized feasibility study of a low fat diet. *Arch Intern Med.* 1990; 150:421-427.
30. Heber, et al. Reduction in serum estradiol in postmenopausal women given free access to a low fat high carbohydrate diet. *Nutrition.* 1991; 7:137-139.
31. Prentice, et al. Dietary fat reduction and plasma estradiol concentrations in healthy postmenopausal women. *JNCI.* 1990; 82:129-134.
32. Zhang S, Folsom AR, et al. Better breast cancer survival for postmenopausal women who are less overweight and eat less fat. The Iowa Women's Health Study. *Cancer* 1995; 15;76:275-83.
33. Zumoff B. Relationship of obesity to blood estrogens. *Cancer Res.* 1982; 42:3289-94.
34. Abe et al. Biological characteristics of breast cancer in obesity. *Tohoku J Exp Med.* 1976;120:351-359.
35. Kalish L. Relationship of body size with breast cancer. *J Clin Oncol.* 1984; 2:287-293.
36. Donegan et al. The association of body weight with recurrent cancer of the breast. *Cancer.* 1978; 41:1590-1594.
37. Howson et al. Body weight, serum cholesterol, and stage of primary breast cancer. *Cancer.* 1986; 58:2372-2381.
38. Kampert et al. Combined effects of childbearing, menstrual events, and body size on age-specific cancer risk. *Am J Epidemiol.* 1988; 128:962-979.
39. Albanes D. Caloric intake, body weight, and cancer: A review. *Nutr Cancer.* 1987; 9:199-217.
40. Manson, et al. Body weight and longevity: A review. *JAMA.* 1987; 257:353-358.

Chapter 10

Food Additives, Contaminants and Pesticides

1. Munro EC, Moodie C, et al. A carcinogenicity study of commercial saccharin in the rat. *Toxicol Appl Pharmacol.* 1975; 32:513.
2. Kessler I. Non-nutritive sweeteners and human bladder cancer: Preliminary findings. *J Urol.* 1976; 115:143.
3. Shubik P. Food additives. *Cancer.* 1979; 43:1982.
4. Sen NP. The evidence for the presence of dimethylnitrosamine in meat products. *Food Cosmet Toxicol.* 1972; 10:219.
5. Newberne PM. Nitrite promotes lymphoma incidence in rats. *Science.* 1979; 204:1079.
6. Toth B, Nagel D. Tumors induced in mice by N-methyl-N-formylhydrazine of the false moral *Gyromitra esculenta. J Nat Cancer Inst.* 1978; 60:201.
7. Lijinsky W, Shubik P. Benzo(a)pyrene and other polynuclear hydrocarbons in charcoal broiled meats. *Science.* 1964; 145:53.
8. Jeyaratnam J. Health problems of pesticide usage in the Third World. *Br J Indust Med.* 1985; 42:505-6.
9. Pimentel D, Perkins J. *Pest Control: Cultural and Environmental Aspects.* 1980; Boulder, Colorado: Westview Press.
10. Wong K., et al. Potent induction of human placental mono-oxygenase activity by previous dietary exposure to polychlorinated biphenyls and their thermal degradation products. *Lancet.* 1985 (March 30): 721-724.
11. Biscardi S. Pesticides linked to breast cancer? *Oncology Times.* 1991; (February):36.
12. Wolff M, et al. Blood levels of organochlorine residues and risk of breast cancer. *JNCI.* 1993; 85:648-652.
13. Longnecker M, et al. Blood levels of organochlorine residues and risk of breast cancer. *JNCI.* 1993; 85:1696-1697.
14. Milne D. Small study implicates PCBs in breast cancer. *JNCI.* 1992; 84:834-835.
15. Falck F, et al. Pesticides and polychlorinated biphenyl residues in human breast lipids and their relation to breast cancer. *Arch Environmental Health.* 1992; 47:143-146.

16. Mussalo-Rauhamaa H, et al. Occurrence of beta-hexachlorocyclohexane in breast cancer patients. *Cancer.* 1990; 6:2124-2128.
17. Westin JB. Carcinogens in Israeli milk: a study in regulatory failure. *International J Health Services.* 1993; 23:497-517.
18. Ramamoorthy K, Wang F, et al. Potency of combined estrogenic pesticides. *Science.* 1997; 275:405.
19. Borzsonyi M, et al. Agriculturally related carcinogen at risk. International Agency for Research on Cancer. *Science Publication.* 1984; 56:465-486.
20. National Toxicology Program. Fourth Annual Report on Carcinogens: Summary. U.S. Department of Health and Human Services. 1985; Publication NTP 85-002.
21. Vainio H, et al. Data on the carcinogenicity of chemicals in the IARC monographs programme. *Carcinogenesis.* 1985; 6:1653-1665.
22. Environmental Protection Agency. Carcinogens. Federal Register. 1986; (September 24).
23. Watterson A. Pesticide user's health and safety handbook: An international guide. 1988; New York: Van Nostrand Reinhold, 420.
24. Eriksson M, et al. Exposure to dioxins as a risk factor for soft tissue sarcoma.
25. Hardell L, et al. The association between soft tissue sarcomas and exposure to phenoxyacetic acids: A new case-referent study. *Cancer.* 1988; 62:652-56.
26. Hardell L., et al. Epidemiologic study of socioeconomic factors and clinical findings in Hodgkin's disease, and reanalysis of previous data regarding chemical exposure. *Br J Cancer.* 1983; 48:217-25.
27. Hardell L, et al. Malignant lymphoma and exposure to chemicals, especially organic solvents, chlorophenols and phenoxy acids: A case-control study. *Br J Cancer.* 1981; 43:169-76.
28. Woods JS, et al. Soft tissue sarcoma and non-Hodgkin's lymphoma in relation to phenoxyherbicide and chlorinated phenol exposure in western Washington. *JNCI.* 1987; 78:899-910.
29. Persson B, et al. Malignant lymphomas and occupational exposures. *Br J Ind Med.* 1989; 46:516-20.
30. Axelson O, et al. Herbicide exposure and tumor mortality: An updated epidemiologic investigation on Swedish railroad car workers. *Scand J Work Environ Health.* 1980; 6:73-9.
31. Thiess AM, et al. 1982. Mortality study of persons exposed to dioxin in a trichlorophenol-process accident that occurred in the BASF AG on Nov 17, 1953. *Am J Ind Med.* 1982; 3:179-89.
32. Hardell L, et al. Epidemiological study of nasal and nasopharyngeal cancer and their relation to phenoxy acid or chlorophenol exposure. *Am J Ind Med.* 1982; 3:247-57.
33. Kociba R, et al. Results of a two-year chronic toxicity and oncogenicity study of 2, 3, 7, 8-tetrachlorodibenzo-p-dioxin in rats. *Toxicol Appl Pharmacol.* 1982; 46:279-303.
34. National Toxicology Program. Carcinogenesis bioassay of 2, 3, 7, 8-tetrachlorodibenzo-p-dioxin in Osborne-Mendel rats and B6C3F1 mice. 1982. Washington, D.C.: Government Printing Office, NIH 82-1765.)
35. Menegon A, Board PG, et al. Parkinson's disease, pesticides and polymorphisms. *Lancet.* 1998; 352:1344-46.
36. Stephenson J. Exposure to home pesticides linked to Parkinson disease. *JAMA.* 2000; 283:3055-56.
37. Fingerhut, et al. Cancer mortality in workers exposed to dioxin. *NEJM.* 1991; 324:212-18.
38. Bailer JC. How dangerous is dioxin? *NEJM.* 1991; 324:260-262.
39. Handbook on Pest Management in Agriculture. 1991. Boca Raton, FL: CRC Press.

Chapter 11
Smoking

1. Glantz SA, Barnes DE, et al. Looking through a keyhole at the tobacco industry: the Brown and Williamson documents. *JAMA*. 1995; 274:219-224.
2. Mackay J. The global tobacco epidemic. *Public Health Rep*. 1998; 113:14-21.
3. Conference on Smoking and Health. *Lancet*. 1990; 28:1026.
4. Brown P. WHO agrees on measures to stop global spread of tobacco use. *BMJ*. 1999; 318:1437.
5. Yang G, Fan L, et al. Smoking in China: the 1996 National Prevalence Survey. *JAMA*. 1999; 282:1247-53.
6. Public Health Service. Smoking and health, a report of the surgeon general. U.S. Dept. of HEW. 1979.
7. Henningfield J, Fant R, et al. Tobacco dependence: Scientific and public health basis of treatment. *TEN*. 2000; 2:42-46.
8. Ambrosone CB, Freudenheim JL, et al. Cigarette smoking, N-acetyltransferase 2 genetic polymorphisms, and breast cancer risk. *JAMA;* 1996; 276:1494-1501.
9. Brinton LA, Schairer C, et al. Cigarette smoking and breast cancer. *Am J Epidemiol*. 1986; 123:614-622.
10. Brownson RC, Blackwell CW, et al. Risk of breast cancer in relation to cigarette smoking. *Arch Intern Med*. 1988; 148:140-144.
11. Chu SY, Stroup NE, et al. Cigarette smoking and the risk of breast cancer. *Am J Epidemiol*. 1990; 131:244-253.
12. Hiatt RA, Fireman BH. Smoking, menopause, and breast cancer. *JNCI*. 1986; 76:833-838.
13. Hiatt, et al. Breast cancer and serum cholesterol. *JNCI*. 1982; 68:885-889.
14. Meara J, McPherson K, Roberts M, et al. Alcohol, cigarette smoking and breast cancer. *Br J Cancer*.1989; 60:70-73.
15. Morabia A, Bernstein M, et al. Relation of breast cancer to passive and active exposure tobacco smoke. *Am J Epidemiol*. 1996; 143:918-928.
16. Palmer JR, Rosenberg L, et al. Breast cancer and cigarette smoking. *Am J Epidemiol*. 1991; 134:1-13.
17. Rohan TE, Baron JA. Cigarette smoking and breast cancer. *Am J Epidemiol*. 1989; 129:36-42.
18. Stockwell HG, Lyman GH. Cigarette smoking and the risk of female reproductive cancers. *Am J Obstet Gynecol*. 1987; 157:35-40.
19. Adami HO, et al. Cigarette smoking, alcohol and risk of breast cancer in young women. *Br J Cancer*. 1988; 58:832-37.
20. Field NA, Baptiste NS, et al. Cigarette smoking and breast cancer. *Int J Epidemiol*. 1992; 21:842-848.
21. London SJ, Colditz GA, et al. Prospective study of smoking and the risk of breast cancer. *JNCI*. 1989; 81:1625-1631.
22. Neugut A, et al. New warning for breast cancer patients who smoke. *Oncology Times*. 1993; 15:1.
23. Slattery M, et al. Cigarette smoking and exposure to passive smoke are risk factors for cervical cancer. *JAMA*. 1989; 261:1593-1598.
24. Trevathan E, et al. Cigarette smoking, dysplasia, carcinoma *in situ* of the uterine cervix. *JAMA*.1984; 250:499-502.
25. Hoff, et al. Relationship between tobacco smoking and colorectal polyps. *Scand J Gastroenterol*. 1987; 22: 13-16.
26. Kikendall, et al. Cigarettes and alcohol as risk factors for colonic adenomas. *Gastroenterology* 1989; 97:660-664.
27. Fenoglio, et al. Colorectal adenomas and cancer. *Cancer*. 1982; 50:2601-2608
28. Ricker, et al. Adenomatous lesions of the large bowel. *Cancer*. 1979; 43:1847-1857.
29. Zahm, et al. Tobacco smoking as a risk factor for colon polyps. *Am J Public Health*. 1991; 81:846-849.
30. Winn DM, Blot W, et al. Snuff dipping and oral cancer among women in the southern United States. *NEJM*. 1981; 304:745.19.
31. Pic A. Heavy smoking and exercise can trigger MI. *Int Med News*. 1981; 14:3.
32. Abbott, et al. Risk of stroke in male cigarette smokers. *NEJM*. 1986; 315:717-720.
33. Wolf, et al. Cigarette smoking as a risk factor for stroke. *JAMA*. 1988; 259:1025-1029.
34. Colditz, et al. Cigarette smoking and risk of stroke in middle-aged women. *NEJM*. 1988; 318:937-941.
35. Rogers, et al. Abstention from cigarette smoking improves cerebral perfusion among the elderly chronic smokers. *JAMA*. 1985; 253:2970-2974.
36. Baron JA. Smoking and estrogen-related disease. *Am J Epidemiol*. 1984; 119:9-22.

37. Baird, et al. Cigarette smoking associated with delayed conception. *JAMA.* 1985; 253:2979-2983.
38. Stjernfeldt, et al. Maternal smoking during pregnancy and risk of childhood cancer. *Lancet.* 1986; June 14:1350-1352.
39. Hopkin JM, Evans. Cigarette smoke induced DNA damage and lung cancer risks. *Nature.* 1980; 283:388.
40. Evans H, et al. Sperm abnormalities and cigarette smoking. *Lancet.* 1981; (March):627.
41. Hersey, et al. Effects of cigarette smoking on the immune system. *Med J Aust.* 1983; 2:425-9.
42. Burrows, et al. Interactions of smoking and immunologic factors in relation to airway obstruction. *Chest.* 1983; 84(6):657-61.
43. McSharry, et al. Effect of cigarette smoking on antibody response to inhaled antigens. *Clin Allergy.* 1985; 15:487-96.
44. Fielding and Phenow. Health effects of involuntary smoking. *NEJM.* 1988; 319:1452-1460.
45. Department of Health and Human Services. Health consequences of smoking: Chronic obstructive lung disease: A report of the surgeon general. Washington, D.C.: Government Printing Office. 1984; PHS: 84-50205.
46. Department of Health and Human Services. Health consequences of involuntary smoking: A report of the surgeon general. Washington, D.C.: GPO. 1987; Pub No.87-8398.
47. National Research Council, Committee on passive smoking. Environmental tobacco smoke: Measuring exposures and assessing health effects. Washington, D.C.: 1987; GPO.
48. Johnson K, Hu, Mao. The Canadian Cancer Registries Epidemiology Research Group. Passive and active smoking and breast cancer risk in Canada. *Cancer Causes Control.* 2000; 11:211-21.
49. Jee S, Ohrr H, Kim. Effects of husbands smoking on the incidence of cancer in Korean women. *Int J epidemiol.* 1999; 28:824-8.
50. Lash TL, et al. Active and passive cigarette smoking on the occurrence of breast cancer. *Am J Epidemiol.* 1999; 149:5-12.
51. Wells AJ. Breast cancer, cigarette smoking and passive smoking. *Am J Epidemiol.* 1991; 133:208-10.
52. Morabia A, Bernstein M, et al. Relation of breast cancer with passive and active exposure to tobacco smoke. *Am J Epidemiol.* 1996; 143:918-28.
53. Smith S, Deacon J, Chilvers. The UK National case control study. Alcohol, smoking, passive smoking, and caffeine in relation to breast cancer risk in young women. *Br J Cancer.* 1994; 70:112-9.
54. Sandler D, Everson, Wilcox. Passive smoking in adulthood and cancer risk. *Am J Epidemiol.* 1985; 121:37-48.
55. Sandler, Wilcox, Everson. Cumulative effects of lifetime passive smoking on cancer risk. *Lancet.* 1985; 1:312-5.
56. Hirayama T. Cancer mortality in nonsmoking women and smoking husbands in a large cohort study in Japan. *Prev Med.* 1984; 13:680-90.
57. Uberla. Lung cancer from passive smoking: Hypothesis or convincing evidence? *Ant Arch Occupa Environ Health.* 1987; 59:421-37.
58. Janerich D, et al. Lung cancer and exposure to tobacco smoke in the household. *NEJM.* 1990; 323(10):632-636.
59. Stjernfeldt, et al. Maternal smoking during pregnancy and risk of childhood cancer.MI 57.
60. Klonoff-Cohen H, Edelstein S, et al. The effect of passive smoking and tobacco exposure through breast milk on sudden infant death syndrome. *JAMA.* 1995; 273:795-798.
61. Slattery M, et al. Cigarette smoking and exposure to passive smoke are risk factors for cervical cancer. *JAMA.*1989; 261:1593-1598.
62. Kabat GC, et al. Bladder cancer in nonsmokers. *Cancer.* 1986; 57:362-367.
63. Hermanson B, et al. Beneficial six year outcome of smoking cessation in older men and women with coronary heart disease: Results from the CASS registry. *NEJM.* 1988; 319:1365-9.
64. LaCroix A, et al. Smoking and mortality of older men and women in three communities. *NEJM.* 1991; 324:1619-25.
65. Williamson D, et al. Smoking cessation and weight gain in a national cohort. *NEJM.* 1991; 324:739-45.
66. Sharfstein and Sharfstein. Campaign contributions from the AMA Political Action Committee to members of Congress. *NEJM.* 1994; 330:32-37.

Chapter 12
Alcohol and Caffeine

1. Smith-Warner S, et al. Alcohol and breast cancer in women: A pooled analysis. *JAMA.* 1998; 279:535-40.
2. Rosenberg L, Sloan D, et al. Breast cancer and alcoholic consumption. *Lancet.* 1982; 30:267.
3. Schatzkin, et al. 1987. Alcohol consumption and breast cancer in the epidemiologic follow-up study of the first NHANES. *NEJM.* 1987; 316:1169-1173.
4. Graham S. Alcohol and breast cancer. *NEJM.*1987; 316:1211-12.
5. Longnecker, et al. 1988. A meta-analysis of alcohol consumption in relation to risk of breast cancer. *JAMA.* 1988; 260:652-656.
6. Longnecker M. Alcoholic beverage consumption in relation to risk of breast cancer: Meta-analysis and review. *Cancer Causes and Control.* 1994; 5: 73-82.
7. Smith-Warner S A, Spiegelman D, et al. Alcohol and breast cancer in women: A pooled analysis of cohort studies. *JAMA.* 1998; 279: 535-540.
8. Editorial. Does alcohol cause breast cancer? *Lancet* June 8, 1985; 1311-12.
9. Webster, et al. Alcohol consumption and the risk of breast cancer. *Lancet* Sept 24, 1983:724-726.
10. Lindegard, et al. Alcohol and breast cancer. *NEJM* 317:1285-1286.
11. Willett, et al. Moderate alcohol consumption and the risk of breast cancer. *NEJM.* 1987; 316:1174-1180.
12. Ginsburg E, Mello N, et al. Effects of alcohol on estrogens in postmenopausal women. *JAMA.* 1996; 276:1747-51.
13. Friend T. Alcohol may speed up cancer. Society for Neuroscience meeting. *USA Today.* Oct. 1992; 28:1.
14. Stampfer, et al. A prospective study of moderate alcohol consumption and the risk of coronary heart disease and stroke in women. *NEJM.* 1988; 319:267-273.
15. Gill, et al. Stroke and alcohol consumption. *NEJM* 1986; 315:1041-1046.
16. Liu RS, Lemieux L, Shorvon SD. Association between brain size and abstinence from alcohol. *Lancet.* 2000; 355:1969-70.
17. Vatten LJ, et al. Coffee consumption and risk of breast cancer: A prospective study of 14,593 Norweigen women. *Br J Cancer.*1999; 62:267-70.
18. Posner J, et al. Association of coffee intake in women with breast cancer. *Surg.* 1986; 100:482-88.
19. Simon D, Yen D, Cole P. Coffee drinking and cancer of the lower urinary tract system. *JNCI.* 1975; 54(3):587.
20. Cnattingius S, Signorelli L, et al. Coffee intake and the risk of first trimester spontaneous abortion. *NEJM.* 2000; 343:1839-45.
21. Soyka LF. Effects of methylxanthines on the fetus. *Clinics in Perinatol.* 1979; 6:37.
22. Weathersbee P, Olsen L, Lodge. Caffeine and pregnancy. *Postgrad Med.* 1977; 62:64.
23. Mulvihill J. Caffeine as teratogen and mutagen. *Teratology* 1973; 8:69.
24. Weinstein, Mauer, Solomon. Effects of caffeine on chromosomes of human lymphocytes. *Mutat Res.* 1992; 16:391.
25. LaCroix A, et al. Coffee consumption and the incidence of coronary heart disease. *NEJM.* 1986; 315:977-982.
26. Barrett-Connor E, et al. Coffee-associated osteoporosis offset by daily milk consumption. *JAMA.* 1994; 271:280-283.

Chapter 13

Hormonal and Sexual-Social Factors

1. Adami, et al. The effect of female sex hormones on cancer survival. *JAMA.* 1990; 263:2189-93.
2. Kvale, et al. Menstrual factors and breast cancer risk. *Cancer.* 1988; 62:1625-31.
3. Marshall E. Search for a killer: focus on hormones. *Science.* 1993; 259:618-621.
4. Hughes and Jones. Intake of dietary fibre and the age of menarche. *Ann Human Biology.* 1985; 12:325-332.
5. Kalache, et al. Age at last full term pregnancy and risk of breast cancer. *Lancet.* 1993; 341:32-35.
6. Miller, et al. Multidisciplinary project on breast cancer: the epidemiology, etiology, and prevention of breast cancer. *Int J Cancer.* 1986; 37:174-177.
7. Kvale and Heuch. A prospective study of reproductive factors and breast cancer II: age at first and last birth. *Am J Epidemiol.* 1987; 126:842-850.
8. Brind J, Chinchilli VM, et al. Induced abortion as an independent risk factor for breast cancer: A comprehensive review and meta-analysis. *J Epidemiol Community Health.* 1996; 50:481-96.
9. Hsieh C, Wuu J, et al. Delivery of premature newborns and maternal breast cancer risk. *Lancet.* 1999; 353:1239.
10. Senghas R, Dolan M. Induced abortion and the risk of breast cancer. *NEJM.* 1997; 336:1834.

11. Krieger N. Exposure, susceptibility and breast cancer risk. *Breast Can Res Treat.* 1989; 1989; 13:205-223.
12. Somerville S. Connections. Is there a link between the permination of first pregnancy and breast cancer? Monograph. Life Dynamics. Lewisville, TX. 1994.
13. Pike, M., et al. Oral contraceptives and early abortion as risk factors for breast cancer in women. *Br J Cancer.* 1981; 43:72-76.
14. Brinton, et al. Reproductive factors in the etiology of breast cancer. *Brit J Cancer.* 1983; 47:757-782.
15. Parazzini, et al. Menstrual and reproductive factors and breast cancer in women with family history of the disease. *Int J Cancer.* 1991; 51:677-681.
16. Olsson, et al. Her-2/neu and INT2 proto-oncogene amplification in malignant breast tumors in relation to reproductive factors and exposure to exogenous hormones. *JNCI.* 1991; 83:1485-87.
17. Olsson, et al. Proliferation and DNA ploidy in malignant breast tumors in relation to early oral contraceptive use and early abortion. *Cancer.* 1991;67:1285-90.
18. Lindefors-Harris, et al. Risk of cancer of the breast after legal abortion during first trimester: a Swedish register study. *Brit Med J.* 1989; 299:1430-32.
19. Howe, et al. Early abortion and breast cancer risk among women under age 40. *Int J Epidem.* 1989; 18:300-304.
20. Russo, et al. Susceptibility of the mammary gland to carcinogenesis, II. Pregnancy interruption as a risk factor in tumor incidence. *Am J Pathol.* 1980; 100:497-509.
21. Brooks and Pauley. Breast cancer biology. In: Encyclopedia of Human Biology, ed. R. Dulbecco. 1990.
22. Swerdlow A, Stavola B, et al. Risks of breast and testicular cancers in young adult twins in England and Wales: evidence on prenatal and genetic aetiology. *Lancet.* 1997; 350:1723-28.
23. Trichopoulos D. Hypothesis: does breast cancer originate in utero? *Lancet.* 1990; 335:939-940.
24. Ekbom, et al. Evidence of prenatal influences on breast cancer risk. *Lancet.* 1992; 340:1015-18.
25. Brinton, et al. Epidemiology of minimal breast cancer. *JAMA.* 1992; 249:483-487.
26. Gammon and John. Recent etiologic hypothesis concerning breast cancer. *Epidemiol Rev.* 1993;15:163-168.
27. Yen S. Endocrinology of pregnancy. In: Maternal-Fetal Medicine, ed. Creasy and Resnic. Philadelphia: W.B. Saunders. pp. 375-403. 1989.
28. Newcomb, et al. Lactation and a reduced risk of premenopausal breast cancer. *NEJM.* 1993; 330:81-87.
29. McTiernan, et al. Evidence for a protective effect of lactation on risk of breast cancer in young women: results from a case-control study. *Am J Epidemiol.* 1986; 124:353-358.
30. Katsouyanni, et al. Diet and breast cancer: a case control study in Greece. *Int J Cancer.* 1986; 38:815-820.
31. Rosero-Bixby, et al. Reproductive history and breast cancer in a population of high fertility: Costa Rica. *Int J Cancer.* 1987; 40:747-754.
32. Yuan, et al. Risk factors for breast-/ cancer in Chinese women in Shanghai. *Cancer Res.* 1988; 48:1949-53.
33. Siskind, et al. Breast cancer and breast feeding: results from an Australian case-control study. *Am J Epidemiol.* 1992; 130:229-236.
34. Yoo, et al. Independent protective effect of lactation against breast cancer: a case-control study in Japan. *Am J Epidemiol.* 1992; 135:726-733.
35. United Kingdom National Case-Control Study Group. Breast feeding and risk of breast cancer in young women. *BMJ.* 1993; 307:17-20.
36. Henderson, et al. Endogenous hormones as a major factor in human cancer. Cancer Res. 1982; 42:3232-39.
37. Petrakis, et al. Influence of pregnancy and lactation on serum and breast fluid estrogen levels: implications for breast cancer risk. *Int J Cancer.* 1987; 40:587-591.
38. Ing, et al. Unilateral breast feeding and breast cancer. *Lancet.* 1977; (July 16):124-127.
39. Gemignani M, Petrek J. Pregnancy after breast cancer. *Cancer Control.* 1999; 6:272-76.
40. Kroman N, Jensen M, et al. Should women be advised against pregnancy after breast cancer treatment? *Lancet.* 1997; 350:319-22.
41. Donegan WL. Cancer and pregnancy. *CA Canc J Clin.* 1983; 33:194-214.
42. Orr JW, Shingleton. Cancer in pregnancy. Current problems in cancer. Yearbook Medical Publishers. 1983;8:3-50.

43. Danforth, D. How subsequent pregnancy affects outcome in women with a prior breast cancer. *Oncology*. 1991; 5:23-35.
44. Petrek, et al. Prognosis of pregnancy-associated breast cancer. *Cancer.* 1991; 67:869-872.
45. Lambe M, et al. Transient increase in the risk of breast cancer after giving birth. *NEJM*. 1994; 331:5-9.
46. Guinee VF, et al. Effect of pregnancy on prognosis for young women with breast cancer. *Lancet*. 1994; 343:1587-89.
47. Boyd NF, et al. Effect of low fat, high carbohydrate diet on symptoms of cyclical mastopathy. *Lancet*.1988; (July):128-129.
48. Henderson, et al. Endogenous hormones as a major factor in human cancer. *Cancer Res*. 1982; 42:3232-39.
49. Musey, et al. Long-term effect of a first pregnancy on the secretion of prolactin. *NEJM*. 1987; 316:229-234.
50. Herbst, et al. Adenocarcinoma of the vagina. *NEJM*. 1971; 284:878-81
51. Robboy SJ, et al. Increased incidence of cervical and vaginal dysplasia in 3980 diethylstilbesterol exposed young women. *JAMA*. 1984; 252:2979-90.
52. Greenberg, et al. Breast cancer in mothers given DES in pregnancy. *NEJM*. 1984; 311:1393-98.
53. Bibbo, et al. A twenty-five year follow up study of women exposed to DES during pregnancy. *NEJM*. 1978; 298:763-7.
54. Melnick, et al. Rates and risk of DES related clear cell adenocarcinoma of vagina and cervix. *NEJM*. 1987; 316:514-16.
55. Conley, et al. Seminoma and epididymal cysts in a young man with known DES exposure in utero. *JAMA*. 1983; 249:1325-26.
56. Loizzo, et al. Italian baby food containing DES: Three years later. *Lancet*. 1984;(May 5):1013-14.
57. Collaborative Group on Hormonal Factors in Breast Cancer. Breast cancer and hormonal contraceptives. *Lancet*. 1996; 347:1713-27.
58. Centers for Disease Control cancer and steroid hormone study: Long term oral contraceptive use and the risk of breast cancer. *JAMA*. 1983; 244:1591-95.
59. Rosenberg L, et al. Breast cancer and oral contraceptive use. *Am J Epidemiol*. 1984; 119:167-76.
60. Olsson, et al. Oral contraceptive use and breast cancer in young women in Sweden.Lancet. 1985; i:748-49.
61. Kalach, et al. Oral contraceptives and breast cancer. *Br J Hosp Med*. 1983; 30:278-83.
62. Royal College of General Practitioners. Breast cancer and oral contraceptives in the royal college of general practitioners study. *Br Med J*. 1981; 282:2089-93.
63. Hulka B, Stark A. Breast cancer: cause and prevention. *Lancet*. 1995; 346:883-87.
64. Grabick D, Hartmann L, et al. Risk of breast cancer with oral contraceptive use in women with a family history of breast cancer. *JAMA*. 2000; 284:1791-98.
65. Burke W. Oral contraceptives and breast cancer. *JAMA*. 2000; 284:1837-38.
66. Rookus M, et al. Oral contraceptives and risk of breast cancer in women aged 20-54 years. *Lancet* 1994; 344:844-51.
67. Pike MC, et al. Breast cancer in young women and use of oral contraceptives: Possible modifying effect of formulation and age at use. *Lancet*. 1983; (Oct 22):926-930.
68. McPherson, et al. Oral contraceptives and breast cancer. *Lancet*. 1983; ii:1414-15.
69. UK National Case Control Study Group. Oral contraceptive use and breast cancer risk in young women. *Lancet*. 1989; (May 6):973-82.
70. Vessey, et al. Neoplasia of the cervix uteri and contraception: A possible adverse effect of the pill. *Lancet*. 1983; (Oct 22): 930-34.
71. Neuberger, et al. Oral contraceptives and hepatocellular carcinoma. *Br Med J*. 1986; 292:1355-61.
72. Skegg D, Noonan E, et al. Depot medroxyprogesterone acetate and breast cancer. *JAMA*. 1995; 273:799-04.
73. WHO collaborative study of neoplasia and steroid contraceptives. Breast cancer, cervical cancer, and depot medroxy progesterone acetate. Lancet. 1984;(Nov. 24): 1207-08.
74. Gapstur S, Morrow, Sellers. Hormone replacement therapy and risk of breast cancer. *JAMA*. 1999; 281:2091-97.
75. Collaborative Group on Hormonal Factors in Breast Cancer. Breast cancer and hormone replacement therapy: collaborative reanalysis. *Lancet*. 1997; 350:1047-59.
76. Colditz G, Hankinson S, et al. The use of estrogens and progestins and the risk of breast cancer postmenopausal women. *NEJM*. 1995; 332:1589-93.
77. LeBlanc E, Viscoli, Henrich. Postmenopausal estrogen replacement therapy is associated with adverse breast cancer prognostic

indices. *J Women Health Gender Med.* 1999; 8:815-23.

78. Hulka B. Hormone-replacement therapy and the risk of breast cancer. *CA- Cancer J Clin.* 1990; 40:289-296.
79. Steinberg, et al. A meta-analysis of the effect of estrogen replacement therapy on the risk of breast cancer. *JAMA.* 1991; 265:1985-90.
80. Colditz G, Hankinson S, et al. The use of estrogens and progestins and the risk of breast cancer in postmenopausal women. *NEJM.*1995; 332:1589-93.
81. Epstein F. Estrogen and the risk of breast cancer. *NEJM.* 2001; 344:276-285.
82. Weiderpass E, Baron, et al. Low potency oestrogen and risk of endometrial cancer. *Lancet.* 1999; 353:1824-28.
83. Beresford S, Weiss, Voigt. Risk of endometrial cancer with use of oestrogen combined with progestagen in postmenopausal women. *Lancet.* 1997; 349:458-61.
84. Rodriguez C, Patel A, et al. Estrogen replacement therapy and ovarian cancer mortality in a large prospective study of US women. *JAMA.* 2001; 285:1460-65.
85. Orentreich N, Durr. Mammogenesis in transsexuals. *J Invest Dermatol.* 1982; 63:142.
86. Symmers WS. Carcinoma of the breast in transsexuals. *Br Med J.* 1968;1:83.
87. Simon J, Hsia J, Cauley J, et al. Postmenopausal Hormone Therapy and Risk of Stroke: The Heart and Estrogen-progestin Replacement Study (HERS). *Circulation.* 2001; 103: 638 – 642.
88. Mosca L, Collins P, Herrington D, et al. Hormone replacement therapy and cardiovascular disease: American Heart Association Statement. *Circulation* 2001; 104:499-03.
89. Commentary. Hormone therapy and heart disease after menopause. *Lancet.* 2001; 358:1196-97.
90. Girdler SS, O'Briant C, et al. A comparison of the effect of estrogen with or without progesterone on mood and physical symptoms in postmenopausal women. *J Women's Health Gender-Based Med.* 1999; 8(5):637-646.
91. Zweifel JE, O'Brien WH. A meta-analysis of the effect of hormone replacement therapy upon depressed mood. *Psychoneuroendocrinology.* 1997; 22:189-194.
92. Barrett-Conner, et al. Estrogen replacement therapy and cognitive function in older women. *JAMA.* 1993; 269:2637-41.
93. Geerlings M, Ruitenberg A, et al. Reproductive period and risk of dementia in postmenopausal women. *JAMA.* 2001; 285:1475-81.
94. LeBlanc E, Janowsky J, et al. Hormone replacement therapy and cognition. *JAMA.* 2001; 285:1489-99.
95. Mulnard R, et al. Estrogen replacement therapy for mild to moderate Alzheimer disease. *JAMA.* 2000; 283:1007-15.
96. Torgerson DJ, Bell-Syer, SE. Hormone replacement therapy and prevention of nonvertebral fractures: A meta-analysis of randomized trials. *JAMA.* 2001; 285:2891-97.
97. Spicer, et al. The question of estrogen replacement in patients with a prior diagnosis of breast cancer. *Oncology.* 1990; 4:49-54.
98. Hoffman D, et al. Breast cancer in hypothyroid women using thyroid supplements. *JAMA.* 1984; 251:616-619.

Chapter 14
Air and Water

1. Buell P. Relative impact of smoking and air pollution on lung cancer. *Arch Environ Health.* 1967; 15:291-297.
2. Cederlof R, et al. The relationship of smoking and social covariables to mortality and cancer mortality, a ten year follow up in Sweden. 1975; Stockholm: Depart of Environmental Hygiene, The Karolinska Institute.
3. Dean G. Lung cancer and bronchitis in Northern Ireland. *Br Med J.* 1966; 1:1506.
4. Lee ML, Novotny N, Bartle. Gas chromatography mass spectometric and nuclear magnetic resonance determination of polynuclear aromatic hydrocarbons in airborne particulates. *Anal Chem.* 1976; 48:1566.
5. Ware J. Particulate air pollution and mortality. *NEJM.* 2000; 343:1798-99.
6. Samet JM, Dominici F, et al. Fine particulate air pollution and mortality in 20 US cities. *NEJM.* 2000; 343:1742-9.
7. Dockery DW, et al. An association between air pollution and mortality in six U.S. cities. *NEJM* 1993; 329:1753-1759.
8. Hoffmann D, Schmeltz, Hecht, et al. Volatile carcinogens. Occurence, formation, and analysis. In: *Prevention and detection of cancer.* 1996. Part 1. Prevention. Vol. 2. Etiology, prevention methods, ed. H.E. Nieburgs. New York and Basel: Marcel Dekker, Inc., pps. 1943-59.
9. National Research Council. Vapor-phase organic pollutants. Committee on medical and biological effects of environmental pollutants. Washington, D.C.: National Academy of Sciences; 1976.

10. U.S. Department of Health and Human Services, National Institute for Occupational Safety and Health. 1988. Carcinogenic effects of exposure to diesel exhaust. Washington, D.C.: Government Printing Office. Bulletin No. 50. August.
11. Hocking M. Paper versus polystyrene: A complex choice. *Science.* 1991; 251:504-505.
12. Blumthaler and Ambach. How well do sunglasses protect against ultraviolet radiation? *Lancet.* 1991; 337:1284.
13. World Health Organization. Indoor air pollutants: Exposure and health effects assessment. 1983. Report No. 78. Nordlingen Copenhagen: WHO.
14. Nero AV. Indoor radon exposures from radon and its daughters. *Health Physics.* 1983; 45:277-88.
15. Abelson P. Uncertainties about health effects of radon. *Science* 1990; 250:353.
16. BEIR IV. Health risks of radon and other internally deposited alpha emitters. Wash DC: National Academy Press,1988.
17. Repace JL. Consistency of research data on passive smoking and lung cancer. *Lancet.* 1984; i:506.
18. US Environmental Protection Agency. Preliminary assessment of suspected carcinogens in drinking water. 1975. Washington, D.C.: Government Printing Office.
19. Harris RH, T Page. Carcinogenic hazards of organic chemicals in drinking water. In: Book A. Incidence of Cancer in Humans. 1975. ed. HH Hiatt, JD Watson, and JA Winsten. Cold Spring Harbor, NY: Cold Spring Harbor Laboratory.
20. Hogan MD et al. Association between chloroform and various site-specific cancer mortality rates. *J Environ Pathol Toxicol.* 1979; 2:873.
21. Cantor KP, et al. Associations of cancer mortality with halomethanes in drinking water. *JNCI.* 1978; 61:979.
22. National Research Council. 1978. Chloroform, carbon tetrachloride, and other halomethanes: An environmental assessment. Washington, D.C.: National Academy of Sciences.
23. Rafferty PJ. 1978. Public health aspects of drinking water quality in North Carolina. Master's thesis, Department of Environmental Sciences and Engineering, School of Public Health, University of North Carolina, Chapel Hill, NC.
24. Spivey GH, et al. 1977. Cancer and chlorinated drinking water. Final report. EPA No. CA-6-99-3349-J. Cincinnati, Ohio: U.S. EPA.
25. US Atomic Energy Commission. 1974. Plutonium and other transuranium elements; Sources, environmental distribution and biomedical effects. Wash DC: Govt Print Office.

Chapter 15

Electromagnetic Radiation

1. Land, et al. Breast cancer risk from low dose exposures to ionizing radiation. *JNCI.* 1980; 65:353-376.
2. Miller, et al. Mortality for breast cancer after radiation during fluoroscopic examinations in patients being treated for tuberculosis. *NEJM.* 1989; 321:1285-1289.
3. Feig SA. Radiation risks from mammography: Is it clinically significant? *AJR.* 1984; 143:469-475.
4. Hall FM. Screening mammography: potential problems on the horizon. *NEJM.* 1986; 314:53-55.
5. Paterson A, Frush D, Donnelly. Helical CT of the body are settings adjusted for pediatric patients? *AJR* 2001; 176: 297-301.
6. Donnelly LF, Emery K, et al. Minimizing radiation dose for pediatric body applications of single-detector helical CT at a large children's hospital. *AJR* 2001; 176: 303-306.
7. Roberts T. Women radiated for Hodgkin's have high breast cancer risk. *Radiology Today.* 1992; (Sept):12-13.
8. Li F, et al. Breast carcinoma after cancer therapy in childhood. *Cancer.* 1983; 51:521-523.
9. Boice JD, Harvey EB, et al. Cancer in the contralateral breast after radiation for breast cancer. *NEJM.* 1992; 326:781-785.
10. Storm H, O Jensen. Risk of contralateral breast cancer in Denmark. *Br J Cancer.* 1986; 54:483-492.
11. Storm H, Anderson H, et al. Adjuvant radiation therapy and risk of contralateral breast cancer. *JNCI.* 1992; 84:1245-1250.
12. Basco V, Coldman AJ. Radiation dose and second breast cancer. *Br J Cancer.* 1985; 52:319-325.
13. Bernstein J, Thompson WD, Risch N, et al. Risk factors predicting the incidence of second primary breast cancers. *Am J Epidemiol.* 1992; 136:925-936.
14. Fisher B, et al. Ten year results of a randomized clinical trial comparing radical mastectomy and total mastectomy with or without radiation. *NEJM.* 1985; 312:674-681.

15. McCredie J, et al. Consecutive primary carcinomas of the breast. *Cancer.* 1975; 35:1472-1477.
16. Schell S, et al. Bilateral breast cancer in patients with initial stage I and II. *Cancer.* 1982; 50:1191-1194.
17. Burns P. Bilateral breast cancer in northern Alberta. *Can Med Assoc Journal.* 1984; 130:881-886.
18. Horn P, W Thompson. Risk of contralateral breast cancer. *Cancer.* 1988; 62:412-424.
19. Parker R, et al. Contralateral breast cancers following treatment for initial breast cancer in women. *Am J Clin Oncol.*1989; 12:213-216.
20. Jacobson JA, Danforth, et al. Ten-year results of a comparison of conservation with mastectomy in the treatment for breast cancer. *NEJM.* 1995; 332:907-911.
21. Arriagada R, Le MG, et al. Conservative treatment vs mastectomy in early stage breast cancer. *J Clin Oncol.*1996; 14:1558-1564.
22. Sarrazin D, Le M, et al. Ten-year results of a randomized trial comparing conservative treatment to mastectomy. *Radiotherap Oncol.*1989; 14:177-184.
23. Zucali R, Luini, et al. Contralateral breast cancer after limited breast surgery plus radiotherapy of early mammary tumors. *Eur J Surg Oncol.* 1987; 13:413-417.
24. Neugut AI, Weinburg M, et al. Carcinogenic effects of radiotherapy for breast cancer. *Oncology.* 1999; 13:1245-1256.
25. Hildreth N, et al. The risk of breast cancer after irradiation of the thymus in infancy. *NEJM.* 1989; 321:1281-1284.
26. Modan B, et al. Increased risk of breast cancer after low dose radiation. *Lancet.* 1989; (March 25):629-631.
27. Land, et al. *JNCI.* 1993; (Oct. 20).
28. Bonnell JA. Effects of electric fields near power transmission plant. *J Roy Soc Med.* 1982; 75:933-44.
29. Pool R. Electromagnetic fields: The biological evidence. *JAMA.* 1990; 249:1378-1381.
30. Vena JE, et al. Use of electric blankets and risk of postmenopausal breast cancer. *Am J Epidemiol.*1992; 134:180-185.
31. Wertheimer, Leeper. Electrical wiring configurations in childhood cancer. *Am J Epidemiol.* 1979; 109:273-84.
32. Wertheimer, Leeper. Adult cancer related to electrical wires near the home. *Int J Epidemiol.* 1982; 11:354-55.
33. Gauger JR. Household appliance magnetic field survey. IEEE Trans PAS-104, No. 9. In: Epidemiological studies relating human health to electric and magnetic fields; criteria for evaluation, June 1988. Intl Electricity Res. Exchange.
34. Milham. Mortality from leukemia in workers exposed to electrical and magnetic fields. *NEJM.* 1982; 307:249.
35. Wright, et al. 1982. Leukemia in workers exposed to electrical and magnetic fields. *Lancet.* 1982; ii: 1160-61.
36. McDowall. Leukemia mortality in electrical workers in England and Wales. *Lancet.* 1983; 246.
37. Tynes, Anderson. Electromagnetic fields and male breast cancer. *Lancet.* 1990; 336:1596.
38. Demers PA, et al. Occupational exposure to electromagnetic fields and breast cancer in men. *Am J Epidemiol.* 1991; 134:340-347.
39. University of California News Service. 1988. 63:13.
40. Ozonoff DM. Fields of controversy. *Lancet.* 1997; 349:74.
41. Worries about radiation continue, as do studies. *The New York Times.* July 8, 1990.
42. Rothman KJ. Epidemiological evidence on health risks of cellular phones. *Lancet.* 2000; 356:1837-40.
43. Hyland GJ. Physics and biology of mobile telephony. *Lancet.* 2000; 356:1833-36.
44. Blettner M, Schlehofer B. Is there an increased risk of leukemia, brain tumors or breast cancer after exposure to high-frequency radiation? Review of methods and results of epidemiologic studies. *Abteilung Epidemiologie, Deutsches Krebsforschungszentrum. Med Klin* 1999; 94:150-8.
45. Galeev AL. Effects of the microwave radiation from the cellular phones on humans and animals. Russian Acad. Sci., Moscow, Russia. *Ross Fiziol Zhlm IM Sechenova.* 1998; 84:1293-302.
46. Juutilainen J, de Seze R. Biological effects of amplitude-modulated radiofrequency radiation. *Scand J Work Environ Health.* 1998; 24(4):245-54.
47. Senior K. Mobile phones: are they safe? *Lancet.* 2000. 355:1793.
48. *Immunol Lett.* 1986. 13:295-299.

Chapter 16
Sedentary Lifestyle

1. Olivera S, Christos P. The epidemiology of physical activity and cancer. *Ann NY Acad Sci.* 1997; 833:79-80.

2. Hoffman-Goetz L, Apter D, et al. Possible mechanisms mediating an association between physical activity and breast cancer. *Cancer.* 1998; 83:621-628.
3. Nieman DC, Henson DA. Role of endurance exercise in immune senescence. *Med Sci Sports Exerc.* 1994; 26:172-81.
4. Tomasi, et al. Immune parameters in athletes before and after strenuous exercise. *J Clin Immunol.* 1982; 2:173-178.
5. Soppi, et al. Effect of strenuous physical stress on circulating lymphocyte number and function before and after training. *J Clin Lab Immunol.* 1982; 8:43-46.
6. Robertson, et al. The effect of strenuous physical exercise on circulating blood lymphocytes and serum cortisol levels. *J Clin Lab Immunol* 1981; 5:53-57.
7. Hanson, et al. Immunological responses to training in conditioned runners. *Clin Soc.* 1981; 60:225-228.
8. Green, et al.. Immune function in marathon runners. *Ann Allergy.* 1983; 47:73-75.
9. Busse WW, et al. The effect of exercise on the granulocyte response to isoproterenol in the trained athlete and unconditioned individual. *J Allergy Clin Immunol* . 1980; 65:358-364.
10. Eskola, et al. Effect of sport stress on lymphocytes and antibody formation. *Clin Exp Immunol.* 1978; 32:339-345.
11. Yu, et al. Effect of corticosteroid on exercise induced lymphocytosis. *Clin Exp Immunol.* 1977; 28:326-331.
12. Hedfors, et al. Variations of blood lymphocytes during work studied by cell surface markers, DNA synthesis and cytotoxicity. *Clin Exp Immunol.* 1976; 24:328-335.
13. Cannon and Kluger. Endogenous pyrogen activity in human plasma after exercise. *Science.* 1983; 220:617-619.
14. Dinarello and Wolff. Molecular basis of fever in humans. *Am J Med.* 1982; 72:799-819.
15. Gershbein LL, et al. An influence of stress on lesion growth and on survival of animals bearing parental and intracerebral leukemia. *Oncology* 1974; 30:429.
16. DeRosa G, NR Suarez. Effect of exercise on tumor growth and body composition of the host. *Fed Am Soc Exp Biol.* 1980; 1118.
17. Albanes D, Blair A, et al. Physical activity and risk of breast cancer in NHANES I population. *Am J Pub Health.* 1989; 79:744-750.
18. Bernstein L, Henderson BE, et al. Physical exercise and reduced risk of breast cancer in young women. *JNCI.* 1994; 86:1403-1408.
19. D'Avanzo B, Nanni O, et al. Physical activity and breast cancer risk. *Cancer Epidemiol Biomarkers Prev.* 1996; 5:155-160.
20. Fredenreich CM, Rohan TE. Physical activity and risk of breast cancer. *Eur J Cancer Prev.* 1995; 4:145-151.
21. Frisch RE, Wyshak, et al.. Lower prevalence of breast cancer in cancers of the reproductive system among former college athletes compared to non-athletes. *Br J Cancer* 1985; 52:885-891.
22. McTiernan A. Exercise and breast cancer – time to get moving. *NEJM.* 1997; 336:1311-1312.
23. Mittendorf R, Longnecker MP, et al. Strenuous physical activity in young adulthood and risk of breast cancer. *Cancer Causes Control.* 1995; 6:347-353.
24. Thune I, Brenn T, Lund E, Gaard M. Physical activity and the risk of breast cancer. *NEJM.* 1997; 336:1269-1275.
25. Vena JE, Graham S, et al. Occupational exercise and risk of cancer. *Am J Clin Nutr.* 1987; 45:318-327.
26. Vihko VJ, Apter DL, et al. Risk of breast cancer among female teachers of physical education and languages. *Acta Oncol.* 1992; 31:201-204.
27. Zheng W, Shu XO, et al. Occupational physical activity and the incidence of cancer of the breast, corpus uteri, and ovary in Shanghai. *Cancer.* 1993; 71:3620-3624.
28. Gammon MD, Britton JB, et al. Does physical activity reduce the risk of breast cancer? Review of the epidemiological evidence. *Menopause.* 1996; 3:172-180.
29. Rockhill B, Willett WC, Hunter DJ, et al. A prospective study of recreational physical activity and breast cancer risk. *Arch Intern Med.* 1999; 159:2290-2296.
30. Segal R, Evans W, Johnson D, et al. Structured exercise improves physical functioning in women with Stages I and II breast cancer: Results of a randomized controlled trial. *J Clin Oncol.* 2001; 19:657-665.
31. Garabrant, D.H., et al. Job activity and colon cancer risk. *Am J Epidemiol.* 1984; 119(6):1005-1014.
32. Vena, J.E., et al. Lifetime occupational exercise and colon cancer. *Am J Epidemiol.* 1985; 122(3):357-365.
33. Gerhardsson, M., et al. Sedentary jobs and colon cancer. Am J Epidemiol. 1986; 123(5):775-780.

34. Manson JE, Hu FB, Rich-Edwards JW, et al. A prospective study of walking as compared with vigorous exercise in the prevention of coronary heart disease in women. *NEJM*. 1999; 341:650-658.
35. Duncan JJ, Gordon NF, Scott CB. Women walking for health and fitness. How much is enough? *JAMA*. 1991; 266:3295-99.
36. Dunn AL, Marcus BH, et al. Comparison of lifestyle and structured intervention to increase physical activity and cardiorespiratory fitness: a randomized trial. *JAMA*. 1999; 281:327-34.
37. Andersen RE, Wadden TA, Bartlett SJ, et al. Effects of lifestyle activity vs structured aerobic exercise in obese women: a randomized trial. *JAMA*. 1999; 281:335-340.
38. Mittleman M, Maclure M, et al. Triggering of acute myocardial infarction by heavy physical exertion. *NEJM*. 1993; 329:1677-83.
39. Willich S, Lewis M, et al. Physical exertion as a trigger of acute myocardial infarction. *NEJM*. 1993; 329:1684-90.
40. Erikssen G, Liestol K, et al. Changes in physical fitness and changes in mortality. *Lancet*. 1998; 352:759-62.
41. Somers VK, et al. Effects of endurance training on baroreflex sensitivity and blood pressure in borderline hypertension. *Lancet*. 1991; 337:1363-68.
42. Louis Harris and Associates, Inc. Perrier survey of fitness in America. 1978. Study No. S 2813. New York, NY.
43. Paffenbarger R, et al. Physical activity, all cause mortality, and longevity of college alumni. *NEJM*. 1986; 314:605-613.
44. Harris SS, et al. Physical activity counseling for healthy adults as a primary preventive intervention in the clinical setting report for the U.S. Preventive Services Task Force. *JAMA*. 1989; 261:3590-3598.
45. Medical News and Perspectives. Exercise, health links need hard proof, say researchers studying mechanisms. *JAMA*. 1991; 265:2928.
46. Horton E. Exercise and decreased risk of NIDDM. *NEJM*. 1991; 325(3):196-97.
47. Helmrich S, et al. Physical activity and reduced occurrence of non-insulin-dependent diabetes mellitus. *NEJM*. 1991; 325:147-52.
48. Petty BG, et al. Physical activity and longevity of college alumni, letter. *NEJM* 1986; 315(6):399.
49. Winningham ML, et al. Exercise for cancer patients: Guidelines and precautions. *Physician and Sports Medicine*. 1986; 14(10):125-134.

Chapter 17
Stress

1. LeShan LL. Psychological states as factors in the development of malignant disease: A critical review. *JNCI*. 1959; 22:1-18.
2. Angeletti R, Hickey W. A neuroendocrine marker in tissues of the immune system. *Science*. 1985; 230:89-90.
3. Bulloch K. Neuralmodulation of Immunity.1985. New York: Raven Press, 111.
4. Riley V. Psychoneuroendocrine influences on immunocompetence and neoplasia. *Science*.1985; 212:1100-09.
5. Berczi I. The stress concept and neuroimmunoregulation in modern biology. *Ann N Y Acad Sci*. 1998; 85:3-12.
6. Cohen F, Kearney KA, et al. Differential immune system changes with acute and persistent stress for optimists vs pessimists. *Brain Behav Immun*. 1999; Jun;13:155-74.
7. Davis SL. Environmental modulation of the immune system via the endocrine system. *Domest Anim Endocrinol*. 1998;15:283-9.
8. Hiramoto RN, Solvason HB, et al. Psychoneuroendocrine immunology: perception of stress can alter body temperature and natural killer cell activity. *Int J Neurosci* 1999; 98:95-129.
9. Kemeny ME, Gruenewald TL Psychoneuroimmunology update. *Semin Gastrointest*. 1999;10:20-9.
10. Miller AH. Neuroendocrine and immune system interactions in stress and depression. *Psychiatr Clin North Am*. 1998; 21:443-63.
11. Nieman DC. Nutrition, exercise, and immune system function. *Clin Sports Med* 1999; 18:537-48.
12. Peters ML, Godaert GL, et al. Immune responses to experimental stress: effects of mental effort and uncontrollability. *Psychosom Med*. 1999;61:513-24.
13. R~aberg L, Grahn M, et al. On the adaptive significance of stress-induced immunosuppression. *Proc R Soc Lond B Biol Sci*. 1998; 265:1637-41.
14. Rozlog LA, Kiecolt-Glaser JK, et al.Stress and immunity: implications for viral disease and wound healing. *J Periodontol*. 1999; 70:786-92.

15. Bartrop R, et al. Depressed lymphocyte function after bereavement. *Lancet.* 1977; i:834-836.
16. Schleifer SJ, et al. Suppression of lymphocyte stimulation following bereavement. *JAMA.* 1983; 250:374-377.
17. Kronfol Z, et al. Impaired lymphocyte function in depressive illness. *Life Science.* 1983; 33:241-247.
18. Schleifer SJ, et al. Lymphocyte function in major depressive disorder. *Arch J Psychiatry.*1984; 41:484-486.
19. Schleifer SJ, et al. Lymphocyte function in ambulatory depressed patients, hospitalized schizophrenic patients, and patients hospitalized for herniorrhaphy. *Arch Jen Psychiatry.* 1985; 42:129-133.
20. Locke S, et al. Life change, stress, psychiatric symptoms, and natural killer cell activity. *Psychosomatic Med.*1984; 46:441-53.
21. Heisel JS, et al. Natural killer cell activity and MMPI scores of a cohort of college students. *Am J Psychiatry.* 1984; 143:1382-86.
22. Jemmott JB, et al. Academic stress, power motivation and decrease in secretion rate of salivary secretory immunoglobulin A. *Lancet.* 1983; ii:1400-02.
23. Ader R, N Cohen. Behaviorally conditioned immunosuppressant. *Psychosomatic Medicine* 1985; 37:333-340.
24. Black S, et al. Inhibition of mantoux reaction by direct suggestion under hypnosis. *Br Med J.* 1963; 1:1649-1652.
25. Smith GR, et al. Psychological modulation of human immune response to varicella zoster. *Arch Intern Med.*1985; 145:2110-12.
26. Horne RL, RS Picard. Psychosocial risk factors for lung cancer. *Psychosomatic Medicine.* 1979; 41:503-514.
27. Jacobs TJ, E Charles. Life events and the occurrence of cancer in children. *Psychosomatic Medicine.* 1980; 42:11-24.
28. Bloom BL, et al. Marital disruption as a stressor: A review and analysis. *Psychological Bulletin.* 1978; 85:867-894.
29. Fox BH. Premorbid psychological factors as related to cancer incidence. *J Behavioral Medicine.* 1978; 1:45-133.
30. Bloom BL, et al. Marital disruption as a stressor: A review and analysis. *Psychological Bulletin.* 1978; 85:867-894.
31. LeShan LL. An emotion and life history pattern associated with neoplastic disease. *Ann NY Acad Sci.*1966; 125:780-793.
32. Ernster BL, et al. Cancer incidence by marital status: U.S. third national cancer survey. *JNCI.* 1979; 63:567-585.
33. Mastrovito RC, et al. Personality characteristics of women with gynecological cancer. *Cancer Detection and Prevention.* 1979; 2:281-287.
34. Stavraky KC, et al. Psychological factors in the outcome of human cancer. *J Psychosomatiegc Res.* 1968; 12:251-259.
35. Bacon CL, et al. A psychosomatic survey of cancer of the breast. *Psychosomatic Medicine.* 1952; 14:453 560.
36. Greer S, T Morris. Psychological attributes of women who develop breast cancer: A controlled study. *J Psychosomatic Res.* 1975; 19:147-153.
37. Horne RL, RS Picard. Psychosocial risk factors for lung cancer. *Psychosomatic Medicine.* 1979; 41:503-514.
38. Paykel ES. Recent life events in the development of depressive disorders. In: *The Psychobiology of the Depressive Disorders.* 1979; ed. R.A. Depue. New York: Academic Press.
39. Schmale A, et al. The psychological setting of the uterine cervical cancer. *Ann NY Acad Sci.* 1966; 125:807-813.
40. Editorial. Stress and colorectal cancer. *Epidemiol.* 1993; Sept 37.
41. Rogentine G, et al. Psychological factors in prognosis of malignant melanoma. *Psychosomatic Med.* 1979; 41:647-655.
42. Newcomer JW, Selke G, Melson AK, et al. Decreased memory performance in healthy humans induced by stress-level cortisol treatment. *Arch Gen Psychiatry.* 1999;56:527-533
43. Kiecolt-Glaser J, Marucha PT et al. Slowing of wound healing by psychological stress. *Lancet.* 1995; 346:1194-96.
44. Hansen D, Lou, Olsen. Serious life events and congential malformations: a national study with complete follow-up. *Lancet.* 2000; 356:875-80.
45. Cox DJ, Gonder-Frederick LA. The role of stress in diabetes mellitus. In *Stress, coping and disease,* Hillsdale, NJ: Erlbaum. 1991:119-134.
46. Halford WK, Cuddihy, Mortimer. Psychological stress and blood glucose regulation in Type I diabetic patients. *Health Psychology* 1990;9:516-528.
47. Bieliauskas LA. *Stress and its relationship to health and illness.* Boulder, CO: Westview. 1982.

48. Morris T, et al. Patterns of expression of age and their psychological correlates in women with breast cancer. *J Psychosom Res.* 1981; 25:111-117.
49. Grassi L, et al. Eventi stressanti supporto sociale e caratteristiche psicologiche in pazienti affecte da carcinoma della mammella. *Revista di Psichiatria.* 1986; 21:315-328.
50. Watson M, et al. Emotional control and automatic arousal in breast cancer patients. *J Psychosom Res.* 1984; 28:467-474.
51. Gross J. Emotional suppression in cancer onset and progression. *Soc Sci Med.*1989; 12:1239-1248.
52. Jasmin, et al. Evidence for a link between certain psychological factors and the risk of breast cancer in a case controlled study. *Ann Oncol.* 1990; 1:22-29.
53. Watson M, et al. Relationships between emotional control, adjustment to cancer, and depression and anxiety in breast cancer patients. *Psycholog Med.* 1991; 21:51-57.
54. Fallowfield LJ, Hall A, et al. Psychosocial outcomes of different treatment policies in women with early breast cancer. *BMJ.* 1990; 301:575-80.
55. Mulder CL, VanDer Pompe, et al. Do psychosocial factors influence the course of breast cancer? A review. *Psycho-Oncology.* 1992; 1:155-67.
56. Spiegel D, Bloom JR, et al. Effect of psychosocial treatment on survival of patients with metastatic breast cancer. *Lancet.* 1989; I:888-91.
57. Fawzy FI, Fawzy NW, et al. Effects of an early structured psychiatric intervention, coping, on recurrence and survival 6 years later. *Arch Gen Psychiatry.* 1993; 50:681-89.
58. House J, et al. Social relationships and health. *Science.* 1988; 241:540-545.
59. Spiegel E, et al. Effect of psychosocial treatment on survival of patients with metastatic breast cancer. *Lancet* 1989; ii:888-891.
60. Greer S, Morris T, Pettingale KW, et al. Psychosocial response to breast cancer and 15-year outcome. *Lancet.* 1990; 335:49-50.
61. Levy S, et al. Immunological and psychosocial predictors of disease recurrence in patients with early stage breast cancer. *Behavioral Medicine.* 1991; Summer. pp. 67-75.
62. Derogatis L, et al. Psychological coping mechanisms and survival time in metastatic breast cancer. *JAMA.* 1979; 242:1504-1508.
63. Greer S, et al. Psychological response to breast cancer and 15-year outcome. *Lancet.* 1990; 335:49-50.
64. Maunsell E. Better survival in patients with confidants. *Oncology News International.* 1993; December:16.
65. Phillips et al. Psychology and survival. *Lancet.* 1993; 342:1142-45.
66. Urbani D. Can regular sex ward off colds and flu? *New Scientist.* April 19, 1999. Study by Drs. Charnetski and Brennan at Wilkes University. The effect of sexual behavior on the immune system.
67. Nunn C, Gittleman, Antonovics. Promiscuity and the primate immune system. *Science.* 2000; 290:1168-1170.
68. Kinsey AC, Pomeroy WB, et al. Sexual behavior in the human female. Philadelphia, Saunders. 1953.
69. Wellings K, Field J, et al. Sexual behaviour in Britain. Harmondsworth: Penquin B. 1994.

Chapter 18
Lack of Spirituality

1. Van Biema D. Does heaven exist? *Time.* March 1, 1997: 70-8.
2. Kaplan M. Ambushed by spirituality. *Time.* June 24, 1996:62.
3. McNichol T. The new faith in medicine. *USA Today.* April 7, 1996:4.
4. Matthews DA. Prayer and spirituality. *Rheum Dis Clin North Am.* 2000; 26:177-87.
5. Koenig HG, et al. The relationship between religious activities and blood pressure in older adults. *Intl J Psych In Medicine.* 1998; 28:189-213.
6. Baider L, Russak SM, et al. The role of religious and spiritual beliefs in coping with malignant melanoma: An Israeli sample. *Psycho-Oncology.* 1999; 8: 27-35.
7. Gioiella ME, Berkman B, Robinson M. Spirituality and quality of life in gynecology patients. *Cancer Pract.* 1998; 6:333-8.
8. Holland JC, Passik S, et al. The role of religious and spiritual beliefs in coping with malignant melanoma. *Psycho-Oncology* 1999; 8:14-26.
9. Mytko JJ, Knight SJ. Body, mind, and spirit: towards the integration of religiousity and spirituality in cancer quality of life research. *Psychooncology.* 1999; 8:439-50.
10. Roberts JA, Brown, Elkins, Larson. Factors influencing views of patients with gynecological cancer about end-of-life decisions. *Am J Obstet Gyn.* 1997; 176:166-172.

11. Taylor EJ, Outlaw FH, Bernardo TR, Roy A. Spiritual conflicts associated with praying about cancer. *Psychooncology.* 1999; 8:386-94.
12. Bliss JR, McSherry E, Fassett J. NIH Conference on Spirituality and Health Care. 1995.
13. Byrd RC. Positive therapeutic effects of intercessory prayer in a coronary care unit population. *Southern Med Journal.* 1988; 81:826-829.
14. Harris RC, et. al. The role of religion in heart transplant recipients long-term health and well-being. *J Religion and Health.* 1995; 34:17-32.
15. Harris WS, et al. A randomized controlled trial of the effects of remote intercessory prayer on outcomes in patients admitted to the coronary care unit. *Arch Int Med.* 1999; 159;2273-78.
16. McSherry E, Ciulla, et al. *Social Compass.* 1987; 35:515-37.
17. Azhar MZ, Varma SL, Dharap. Acta Psychiatrica Scandinavica. 1994; 90:1-3.
18. Ardelt M. Wisdom and life satisfaction in old age. *J Gerontology, Psychological Sciences.* 1997; 52:15-27.
19. Chu CC, Klein HE. *JAMA.* 1985; 77:793-796.
20. Kendler KS, Gardner CO, Prescott. Religion, psychopathology, and substance use and abuse: A multimeasure, genetic-epidemiologic study. *Am J Psychiatry.* 1997; 154:322-329.
21. Koenig HG, Larson DB, Weaver AJ. Research on religion and mental illness. In: Spirituality and Religion in Recovery from Mental Illness, ed., Roger Fallott. New Directions for Mental Health Services 1998.
22. Koenig HG, George LK, Peterson. Religiosity and remission of depression in medically ill older adults. *Am J Psychiatry.* 1998; 155:536-542.
23. Koenig HG, Pargament KI, Nielson J. *J Nervous and Mental Diseases.* 1998; 186:513-521.
24. McCullough ME, Larson DB. Religion and depression: a review of the literature. *Twin Research.* 1999; 2:126-136.
25. McCullough ME. Research on religion-accommodative counseling: review and meta-analysis. *J Counseling Psychology.* 1999; 46:1-7.
26. Miller L, et al. Religiosity and depression: Ten-year follow-up of depressed mothers and offspring. *J Am Acad Child Adolescent Psychiatry.* 1997; 36:1416-25.
27. Myers DG, Diener E. Who is happy? *Psychological Science.* 1995; 6:10-19.
28. Pfeiefer S, Waelty. Psychopathology and religious commitment: A controlled study. *Psychopathology.* 1995; 28:70-77.
29. Pressman P, Lyons JS, et al. *Am J Psychiatry.* 1990; 147:758-59.
30. Propst LR, et al. *J Consulting and Clin Psychology.* 1992; 60:94-103.
31. Strawbridge WJ. et al. Religiosity buffers effects of some stressors on depression but exacerbates others. *J Gerontology, Social Sciences.* 1995; 53:5115-26.
32. Weaver AJ, et al. An analysis of research on religious and spiritual variables in three major mental health nursing journals. *Issues in Mental Health Nursing.* 1998; 19:263-276.
33. Weaver AJ, Samford, Larson JA, et al. A systematic review of research on religion in four major psychiatric journals: 1991-1995. *J of Nervous and Mental Disease.* 1998; 186:187-189.
34. Weaver AJ, Kline AE, et al. Is religion taboo in psychology? A systematic analysis of research on religion in seven major American psychological association journals: 1991-1994. *J of Psychology and Christianity.* 1998;17:220-32.
35. Koenig HK, Cohen HJ, et al. Attendance at religious services, Interleukin-6, and other biological parameters of immune function in older adults. *Intl J Psychiatry in Medicine.* 1997; 27:233-250.
36. Bradley DE. Religious involvement and social resources: Evidence from the data set "Americans' Changing Lives." *Journal for the Scientific Study of Religion.* 1995; 34:259-267.
37. Daaleman, TP, Frey B. Prevalence and patterns of physician referral to clergy and pastoral care providers. *Archives of Family Med* 1998; 7: 548-553.
38. Florell JL Bulletin of the American Protestant Hospital Association. 1997; 37:29-36.
39. Fryback PB, Reinert BR. Spirituality and people with potentially fatal diagnosis. *Nurs Forum.* 1999; 34:13-22.
40. Goldman N, Korenman S, Weinstein R. Marital status and health among the elderly. *Social Science and Medicine.* 1995; 40: 1717-30.
41. Hill PC, Butter EM. The role of religion in promoting physical health. *J Psychology and Christianity.* 1995; 14:141-155.
42. Hummer RA, Rogers RG, Nam CB. Religious involvement and U.S. adult mortality. *Demography.* 1999; 36: 1-13

43. Kaldjian LC, et al. End-of-life decisions in HIV-positive patients: The role of spiritual beliefs. *AIDS*.1998; 12:103-107.
44. Kark JD, et al. *Am J Public Health*. 1996; 86:341-346.
45. Koenig HG, Pargament KL, Nielson J. Religious coping and health status in medically ill hospitalized older adults. *J of Nervous and Mental Disease* 1998; 186:513-521.
46. Koenig HG, et al. *J Gerontology*. 2000; 7:321-328.
47. Koenig HG, Larson DB. Use of hospital services, religious attendance, and religious affiliation. *Southern Medical Journal*. 1998; 91:925-932.
48. Koenig HG. *Intl J Geriatric Psychiatry*. 1998; 13:213-224.
49. Levin JS, Lyons JS, Larson DB. Prayer and health during pregnancy: Findings from the Galveston Low Birthweight Survey. *Southern Med J* 1993; 86:1022-27.
50. McBride JL, Arthur G, et al. The relationship between a patient's spirituality and health experiences. *Family Medicine* 1998; 30:122-126.
51. McDowell D, Galanter M, et al. Spirituality and the treatment of the dually diagnosed: An investigation of patient and staff attitudes. *J Addictive Diseases*. 1996; 15:55-68.
52. Oman D, Reed D. Religion and mortality among the community-dwelling elderly. *Am J Public Health*. 1998; 88:1469-75.
53. Oxman TE, Freeman DH, Manheimer ED. Lack of social participation or religious strength or comfort as risk factors for death after cardiac surgery in the elderly. *Psychosomatic Medicine*. 1995; 57:5-15.
54. Smith BW. Coping as a predictor of outcomes following the 1993 Midwest flood. *J Social Behavior Personality*. 1996; 11: 225-39.
55. Strawbridge W, et al. *Am J Public Health*. 1997; 87:957-961.
56. Bjarnason T. Parents, religion and perceived social coherence: A Durkheimian framework of adolescent anomic. *J of Scientific Study of Religion*. 1998; 37:742-54.
57. Daaleman TP, Frey B. Spiritual and religious beliefs and practices of family physicians: A National Survey. *J Family Practice*. 1999; 48: 98-104.
58. Ebrahim S, Wannamethee, et al. Marital status, change in marital status, and mortality in middle-aged British men. *Am J of Epidemiology*. 1995; 142: 834 842.
59. Idler EL, Kasl SV. *J Gerontology*. 1997; 52B: S307-S316.
60. Koenig HG, Larson DB, Hays JC, et al. Religion and the survival of 1010 hospitalized veterans. *J Religion and Health*. 1999; 37: 15-29.
61. Levin JS, Chatters LM. Religion, health, and psychological well-being in older adults: Findings from three national surveys. *J of Aging and Health*. 1998; 10: 504-531.
62. Liu QA, Ryan, et al. The influence of local church participation on rural community attachment. *Rural Sociology*. 1998; 63:432-450.
63. Nathanson IG. Divorce and women's spirituality." *J of Divorce and Remarriage*. 1995; 22:179-188.
64. Wilson J, Musick M. Personal autonomy in religion and marriage: Is there a link? *Review of Religious Res*. 1995; 37:3-18.
65. Koenig HG, et al. *J Gerontology*. 1998; 53(A).
66. Miller WR. Researching the spiritual dimensions of alcohol and other drug problems. *Addiction*. 1998; 93:979-90.

Chapter 19

Genetics and Breast Implants

1. Lichtenstein P, Holm N, et al. Environmental and heritable factors in the causation of cancer. *NEJM*. 2000; 343:78-85.
2. Easton DF, et al. Genetic linkage analysis in familial breast and ovarian cancer: results from 214 families. *Am J Hum Genet*. 1993; 52:678-701.
3. Ferguson-Smith, et al. Genomic imprinting and cancer. *Cancer Survive*. 1990; 9:487-503.
4. Reik W. 1989. Genomic imprinting and genetic disorders in man. *Trends Genet*. 1989; 5:331-336.
5. Karp J, et al. Oncology. *JAMA*. 1993; 270:237-239.
6. Hall J, et al. Linkage of early onset familial breast cancer to chromosome 17q21. *Science*. 1990; 250:1684.
7. Coles C, et al. Evidence implicating at least two genes on chromosome 17p in a breast cancer. *Lancet*. 1990; 336:761-763.
8. Weber B. Susceptibility genes for breast cancer. *NEJM*. 1994; 331:1523-1524.
9. Narod, et al. Familial breast, ovarian cancer locus on chromosome 17q12-23. *Lancet*. 1991; 338:82.
10. Arason A, et al. Linkage analysis of chromosome 17q markers and breast-ovarian cancer in Icelandic families and possible relationship to prostatic cancer. *Am J Hum Genet*. 1993; 52:711.

11. Ford D, et al. The risks of cancer in BRCA1 mutation carriers. *Am J Hum Genetics.* 1994; 53:298.
12. Ford D, et al. Risks of cancer in BRCA1 - mutation carriers. *Lancet.* 1994; 343:692-695.
13. Emery J, Murphy M, Lucasseh A. Heritary cancer – evidence for current recommended management. *Lancet Onc.* 2000; May:9-16.
14. Schrag D, Kuntz K, et al. Decision analysis – effects of prophylactic mastectomy or oopherectomy on life expectancy among women with BRAC1 or BRCA2 mutation. *NEJM.* 1997; 336:1465-71.
15. Verhog L, Brekelmans C, et al. Survival and tumour characteristics of breast cancer patients with germline mutations of BRCA1. *Lancet.* 1998; 351:316-21.
16. Culotta E, Koshland. p53 sweeps through cancer research. *Science.* 1994; 262:1958-61.
17. Hollstein M, et al. 1991. p53 mutations in human cancers. *Science.* 1991; 253:49-52.
18. Harris C. p53: at the crossroads of molecular carcinogenesis and risk assessment. *Science.* 1993; 262:1980-81.
19. Li F, Fraumeni J. Soft tissue sarcomas, breast cancer, and other neoplasms: a familial syndrome? *Ann Intern Med.* 1969; 71:747-751.
20. Skolnick M, et al. Inheritance of proliferative breast disease in breast cancer kindreds. *Science.* 1990; 250:1715-20.
21. Smith H, et al. Allelic loss correlated with primary breast cancer. *PNAS.* 1991; 88:3847-51.
22. Nelson N. Institute of Medicine finds no link between breast implants and disease. *JNCI.* 1999; 91:1191.
23. Berkel H, Birdsell D, et al. Breast augmentation: A risk factor for breast cancer? *NEJM.* 1992; 326:1649-53.
24. Deapen DM, Brody G. Augmentation mammoplasty and breast cancer: A 5 year update of the Los Angeles study. *Plas Reconstr Surg.* 1992; 89:660-65.
25. Bryant H, Brasher P. Breast implants and breast cancer – reanalysis of a linkage study. *NEJM.* 1995; 332:1535-39.
26. Petit J, Le M, et al. Can breast reconstruction with gel-filled silicone implants increase the risk of death and second primary cancer in patients treated by mastectomy for breast cancer? *Plast Reconstr Surg.* 1994; 94:115-19.
27. McLaughlin JK, Fraumeni J, et al. Breast implants, cancer, and systemic sclerosis. *JNCI.* 1994; 86:1424.
28. Gerszten K, Gerszten P. Silicone breast implants: An oncologic perspective. *Oncology.* 1998; 12:1427-1443.
29. Oppenheimer B, Oppenheimer E, et al. Further studies of polymers as carcinogenic agents in animals. *Cancer Res.* 1995; 15:333-40.
30. Fisher JC. The silicone controversy – when will science prevail? *NEJM.* 1992; 326:1696-98.
31. Janowsky E, Kupper L, Hulka B. Meta-analyses of the relation between silicone breast implants and the risk of connective tissue diseases. *NEJM.* 2000; 342:781-790.
32. Karlson EW, Tanasijevic M, et al. Monoclonal gammopathy of undetermined significance and exposure to breast implants. *Arch Intern Med* 2001 Mar 26;161:864-867.
33. Speizer FE, Schur PHAngell M. Shattuck lecture – evaluating the health risks of breast implants. *NEJM.* 1996; 334:1513-18.
34. Gabriel S, Woods, et al. Complications leading to surgery after breast implantation. *NEJM.* 1997; 336:677-82.
35. Sanchez-Guerrero J, Colditz G, et al. Silicone breast implants and the risk of connective tissue diseases and symptoms. *NEJM.* 1995; 332:1666-70.
36. Giltay E, Moens H, et al. Silicone breast prostheses and rheumatic symptoms: A retrospective follow up study. *Ann Rheum Dis.* 1994; 53:194-96.
37. Strom B, Reidenberg M, et al. Breast silicone implants and risk of lupus. *J Clin Epidemiol.* 1994; 47:1211-14.
38. Dugowson C, Daling, et al. Silicone breast implants and risk for rheumatoid arthritis. *Arthritis Rheum.* 1992; 35:S66.
39. Hochberg M, Perlmutter D, et al. Association of augmentation mammoplasty with systemic sclerosis: Results from a multicenter study. *Arthritis Rheum.* 1994; 37:S369.
40. Hennekens C, Lee I, et al. Self-reported breast implants and connective tissue diseases in female health professionals. *JAMA.* 1996; 275:616-21.
41. Weisman M, Vecchione T, et al. Connective tissue disease following breast augmentation: A preliminary test of the human adjuvant disease hypothesis. *Plast Reconstru Surg.* 1988; 82:626-30.
42. Cook L, Daling J, et al. Characteristics of women with and without breast augmentation. *JAMA.* 1997; 277:1612-17.

43. Council on Scientific Affairs, AMA. Silicone gel breast implants. *JAMA.* 1993; 270:2602-06.

Chapter 20
Breast Cancer Detection

1. Thomas DB, DL Gao, SG Self, et al. Randomized trial of breast self-examination in Shanghai: methodology and preliminary results. *JNCI.* 1997; 89: 355-365.
2. Semiglazov VF, Moiseenko VM, Manikhas AG, et al. Interim results of a prospective randomized study of self-examination for early detection of breast cancer (Russia, St. Petersburg, WHO). *Vopr Onkol* 1999;45(3):265-71.
3. Holmberg L, Ekbom A, Calle E, et al. Breast cancer mortality in relation to self-reported use of breast self-examination. A cohort study of 450,000 women. *Breast Cancer Res Treat.* 1997; 43:137-40.
4. Semiglazov, et al. Current evaluation of the contribution of self-examination to secondary prevention of breast cancer. *Eur J Epidemiol.* 1987; 3:78-83.
5. Phillips, et al. Breast self-examination: Clinical results from prospective study. *Br J Cancer.* 1984; 50:7-12.
6. Morrison AS. Is self-examination effective in screening for breast cancer? *JNCI.* 1991; 83:226-227.
7. Baxter N, with Canadian Task Force on Preventive Health Care. Preventive health care, 2001 update: Should women be routinely taught breast self-examination to screen for breast cancer? *CMAJ* 2001; 164:1837-46.
8. Mant, et al. Breast self-examination and breast cancer at diagnosis. *Br J Cancer.* 1987; 55:207-211.
9. Frank and Mai. Breast self-examination in young women: More harm than good? *Lancet.* 1985; (Sept 21):654-658.
10. Mittra I, Baum M, et al. Is clinical breast examination an acceptable alternative to mammographic screening? *BMJ.* 2000; 321:1071-73.
11. Fletcher, et al. Physicians' abilities to detect lumps in silicone breast models. *JAMA.* 1985; 253:2224-28.
12. Breslow, et al. Final report of the NCI ad hoc working groups on mammography in screening for breast cancer and summary report. *JNCI.* 1977; 59:467-541
13. Bailar JC. Mammography: A contrary view. *Ann Intern Med.* 1976; 84:77-84.
14. Mittra I. Breast screening: the case for physical examination without mammography. *Lancet.* 1994; 343:342-344.
15. Seidman, et al. Survival experience in the Breast Cancer Detection Demonstration Project. *Cancer.* 1987; 37:258-290.
16. Sener, et al. Potential accuracy of Xeroradiographic examination of the breast with respect to menopausal status and location of pathological findings. *Breast.* 1977; 3:39-47.
17. Hermansen, et al. Diagnostic reliability of combined physical examination, mammography, and fine needle puncture in breast tumors. *Cancer.* 1987; 60:1866-71.
18. Ries LAG, Kosary CL, et al. SEER cancer statistics review, 1973-1996. Bethesda, MD. National Cancer Institute. 1999.
19. Testimony of Samuel Broder, M.D., Director of National Cancer Institute, National Institutes of Health, Dept. HHS, before Subcommittee on Aging, Senate Committee on Labor and Human Resources, March 9, 1994.
20. Marwick C. NCI Board votes to keep mammography guidelines. *JAMA.* 1993; 270:2783.
21. Eastman P. ACS vigorously defends mammography screening for women in their forties. *Oncology Times.* January 1994:28-30.
22. Shapiro S. The call for change in breast cancer screening guidelines. *Am J Public Health.* 1994. 84:10-12.
23. Guidelines for Screening Mammography. *Oncology Bulletin* February 1994:7.
24. National Institutes of Health Consensus Conference Statement. January 21-23, 1997.
25. Shapiro S, et al. Periodic breast cancer screening in reducing mortality from breast cancer. *JAMA.* 1971; 215:1777-85.
26. Beahrs O, et al. Report of the working group to review the National Cancer Institute - American Cancer Society Breast Cancer Detection Demonstration Projects. *JNCI.* 1979; 62:640-709.
27. UICC Multidisciplinary Project on Breast Cancer. UICC *Tech Rep Ser.* 1982:69.
28. Tabar L, et al. Screening for breast cancer - the Swedish trial. *Radiology.* 1981; 138:219-222.
29. Miller A, et al. The National Study of Breast Cancer Screening. Protocol for a Canadian randomized controlled trial of screening for breast cancer in women. *Clin Invest Med.* 1981; 4.277-258.
30. Roberts, M., et al. The Edinburgh randomized trial of screening for breast cancer. Br J Cancer. 1984; 50:77-84.

31. UK Trial of Early Detection of Breast Cancer Group. Trial of early detection of breast cancer. *Br J Cancer*. 1981; 44:618-27.
32. Verbeek A, et al. Reduction of breast cancer mortality through mass screening with modern mammography. *Lancet*. 1984; (June):1222-24.
33. Collette J, et al. Evaluation of screening for breast cancer in a non-randomized study by means of a case control study. *Lancet*. 1984; i:1224-26.
34. Palli, et al. A case controlled study of the efficacy of a non-randomized breast cancer screening program in Florence, Italy. *Int J Cancer*. 1986; 38:501-504.
35. Shapiro S, et al. Ten to fourteen year effects of breast cancer screening on mortality. *JNCI*. 1982; 69:349-355.
36. Gad A, et al. Screening for breast cancer in Europe: achievements, problems, and future. *Rec Results Cancer Res*.1984; 90:179-194.
37. Eddy D, et al. The value of mammography screening in women under age 50 years. *JAMA*. 1988; 259:1512-19.
38. Bailar John C. Mammography before age 50 years? *JAMA*. 1988; 259:1548-49.
39. Miller A, et al. Report on a workshop of the UICC project on evaluation of screening for cancer. *Int J Cancer*. 1990; 46:761-769.
40. Baines CJ, et al. Canadian National Breast Screening Study: Assessment of technical quality by external review. *A J R*. 1990; 153:23-32.
41. Baines CJ. Evaluation of mammography and physical exam has independent screening modalities in the Canadian National Breast Screening Study. In: Practical Modalities of an Efficient Screening for Breast Cancer in the European Community, ed. G. Ziant. Amsterdam: Elsevier. 1989; pp. 3-9.
42. Kopans DB. The Canadian Screening Program: A different perspective. *A J R*. 1990; 155:748-749.
43. Miller AB. Breast screening in women under 50. *Lancet*. 1991; 338:113.
44. Elwood, et al. The effectiveness of breast cancer screening in young women. *Curr Clin Trials*. 1993; 2:227.
45. Tabar L, et al. The Swedish two county trial of mammographic screening for breast cancer. *J Epidemiol Commun Health*. 1989; 43:107-114.
46. Tabar L, et al. Update of the Swedish two-county program of mammographic screening for breast cancer. *Radiol Clin N Am*. 1992; 30:187-210.
47. Alexander F, Anderson T, et al. 14 years of follow-up from the Edinburgh randomized trail of breast cancer screening. *Lancet*. 1999; 353:1903-08.
48. UK Trial of Early Detection of Breast Cancer group. 16 year mortality from breast cancer in the UK Trial of Early Detection of Breast Cancer. *Lancet*. 1999; 353:1909-14.
49. Frisell J, et al. Randomized study of mammography screening: Preliminary report on mortality in the Stockholm trial. *Breast Cancer Res Treat*. 1991; 18:49-56.
50. Kerilkowske K, et al. Efficacy of screening mammography. *JAMA*. 1995; 273:149-154.
51. Thomas BA. Population breast cancer screening: theory, practice, and service implications. *Lancet*. 1995; 345:205-206.
52. Kattlove H, et al. Benefits and costs of screening and treatment for early breast cancer. *JAMA*. 1995; 273:142-148.
53. Kerlikowske K, et al. Positive, predictive value of screening mammography by age and family history of breast cancer. *JAMA*. 1993; 270:2444-50.
54. Spratt, et al. Geometry, growth rates, and duration of cancer and carcinoma *in situ* of the breast before detection by screening. *Cancer Res*. 1986; 46:970-974.
55. Nystrom L, et al. Breast screening with mammography: Overview of Swedish trials. *Lancet*.1993; 341:973-78.
56. Elmore J, Barton M, et al. Ten-year risk of false positive screening mammograms and clinical breast examinations. *NEJM*. 1998; 338:1089-96.
57. Devitt JE. False alarms of breast cancer. *Lancet*. 1989; (November 25): 1257-58.
58. Slazmann P, Kerlikowske K, Phillips. Cost effectiveness of extending screening mammography guidelines to include women 40-49 years of age. *Ann Intern Med*. 1997; 127:955-65.
59. Lee JM. Screening and informed consent. *NEJM*. 1993; 328:438-439.
60. Gotzsche P, Olsen O. Is screening for breast with mammography justifiable? *Lancet*. 2000; 355:129-34.
61. Antman K, Shea S. Screening mammography under age 50. *JAMA*. 1999; 281:1470-72.
62. Wright C, Mueller B. Screening mammography and public health policy: need for perspective. *Lancet*. 1995; 346:29-32.
63. Miller A, To T, Baines C, Wall C. Canadian National breast screeing study-2: 13-

year results of a randomized trial in women aged 50-59 years. *JNCI.* 2000;92:1490-9.

64. Kerlikowske K, Salzmann P, et al. Continuing screening mammography in women aged 70 to 79 years. *JAMA.* 1999; 282:2156-63.
65. Leibman J, et al. Modified mammography detects breast cancer in women with breast implants. *Oncology.* 1989; 3:89.
66. Leibman J, et al. Imaging of the augmented breast. *Oncology.* 1990; 4:71.
67. Watmough DJ. X-ray mammography and breast compression. *Lancet.* 1992 340:122.
68. Smatchio K, et al. Ultrasonic treatment of tumours: absence of metastases following treatment of a hamster fibrosarcoma. *Ultrasound Med Biol.* 1979; 5:45-49.
69. Egan RL. Mammographic patterns and breast cancer risk. *JAMA.* 1980; 244:287.
70. Andersson I, et al. Mammographic screening and mortality from breast cancer: the Malmo mammographic screening trial. *BMJ.* 1988; 297:943-948.
71. Clark D, Chambers IR, et al. Pressure measurements during automatic breast compression in mammography. *J Biomed Eng* 1990;12:444-6.
72. Boyd NF, Jensen HM, et al. Mammographic densities and the prevalence and incidence of histological types of benign breast disease. Reference Pathologists of the Canadian National Breast Screening Study. *Eur J Cancer Prev* 2000;9:15-24.
73. Knight JA, Martin LJ, et al. Macronutrient intake and change in mammographic density at menopause: results from a randomized trial. *Cancer Epidemiol Biomarkers Prev* 1999;8:123-8.
74. Boyd NF, Lockwood GA, et al. Mammographic densities and risk of breast cancer among subjects with a family history of this disease. *JNCI* 1999;91:1404-8.
75. Rutter CM, Mendelson M, et al. Changes in breast density associated with initiation, discontinuation, and continuing use of hormone replacement therapy. *JAMA.* 2001; 285:171-76.
76. Sterns EE, Zee, SenGupta, Saunders FW. Thermography. Its relation to pathologic characteristics, vascularity, proliferation rate, and survival. *Cancer* 1996 Apr 1;77:1324-8.
77. Jones BF. A reappraisal of the use of infrared thermal image analysis in medicine. *IEEE Trans Med Imaging* 1998; 17:1019-27.
78. Brawley O. NCI abandons mammographic guidelines. *Oncology.* March 1994:9.

Chapter 21
Cancer Angiogenesis

1. Folkman J. Tumor angiogenesis: therapeutic implications. *NEJM.* 1971; 285:1182.
2. Folkman J. et al. Isolation of a tumor factor responsible for angiogenesis. *J Exp Med.*1971; 133:286-7.
3. Folkman J. The vascularization of tumors. *Scientific American.*1976; 234:59-68.
4. Liotta L, Stetler-Stevenson W. Tumor invasion and metastasis: an imbalance of positive and negative regulation. *Canc Research.* 1991; 51:5054S-59S.
5. Ingber D E. Extracellular matrix as a solid-state regulator in angiogenesis: identification of new targets for anti-cancer therapy. *Seminars in Cancer Biol.* 1992; 3:57-63.
6. Liotta L, et al. Quantitative relationships of intravascular tumor cells, tumor vessels, and pulmonary metastases following tumor implantation. *Cancer Res.* 1974; 34:997.
7. Fidler I J, Hart I. Biologic diversity in metastatic neoplasms origins and implications. *Science.* 1982; 217:998-1001.
8. Weidner N, et al. Tumor angiogenesis and metastasis correlation in invasive breast carcinoma. *NEJM.* 1991;324:1.
9. Toi M, et al. Tumor angiogenesis is an independent prognostic indicator in primary breast carcinoma. *Int J Cancer*. 1993;55:371.
10. Srivastava A, et al. The prognostic significance of tumor vascularity in intermediate thickness skin melanoma. *Am J Pathol.*1988; 133:419.
11. Macchiarini P, et al. Relation of neovascularization to metastasis on non small cell lung cancer. *Lancet.*1992; 340:145.
12. Weidner N, et al. Tumor angiogenesis correlates with metastasis in invasive prostate carcinoma. *Am J Pathol* 1993; 143:401.
13. Bouch N. Understanding tumor angiogenesis. *Contemporary Onc.* 1994. April:14-23.
14. Pili R, et al. Altered angiogenesis underlying age-dependent changes in tumor growth. *JNCI.* 1994; 86:1303 14.
15. Guo J, Stolina M, et al. Stimulatory effects of B7-related protein-1 on cellular and humoral and humoral immune responses in mice. *J Immunol* 2001; 166: 5578-84.
16. Folkman J, Klagsbrun M. Angiogenic factors. *Science.*1987; 235:445-446.
17. Jackson D. et al. Stimulation and inhibition of angiogenesis by placental proliferin and proliferin related protein. *Science.* 1994; 266:1581-84.

Chapter 22

Establishing the Diagnosis and Stage

1. Haagensen CD. In: Diseases of the Breast. Philadelphia: W.B. Saunders Company. 1986; p. 253.
2. Ciatto S, et al. The value of routine cytological examination of breast cyst fluids. *Acta Cytol.* 1987; 31:301-304.
3. Wolberg WH, et al. Fine needle aspiration for breast mass diagnosis. *Arch Surg.* 1989; 124:814-18.
4. Miller TR, et al. Cancer Detection and Prevention. 1992.
5. Herman JB. Mammary cancer subsequent to aspiration of cyst in the breast. *Ann Surg.* 1971; 173:40.
6. Harrington, Lesnick. The association between gross cysts of the breast and breast cancer. *Breast.* 1981; 7:13.
7. Rosemond G, et al. Needle aspiration of breast cysts. *Surg Gynecol Obstet.* 1969; 128:351-354.
8. Schwartz GF, Feig SA. Management of patients with non-palpable breast lesions. *Oncology.* 1991; 5:39-44.
9. Schwartz GF. The role of excision and surveillance alone in subclinical DCIS of the breast. *Oncology.* 1994; 8:21-35.
10. Freund, et al. Breast cancer arising in surgical scars. *J Surg Oncology.* 1976; 8:477-80.
11. Ramirez AJ, Westcombe AM, et al. Factors predicting delayed presentation of symptomatic breast cancer: a systematic review. *Lancet.* 1999; 353:1127-31.
12. Richards MA, Westcombe AM, et al. Influence of delay on survival in patients with breast cancer: a systematic review. *Lancet.* 1999; 353:1119-26.
13. Richards MA, et al. The influence on survival of delay in presentation and treatment of symptomatic breast cancer. *BJ Cancer.* 1999; 79:858-64.
14. Brenner R, Sickles EA. Acceptability of periodic follow-up as an alternative to biopsy for mammographically detected lesions interpreted as probably benign. *Radiology.* 1989; 171:645-46.
15. Silverstein M, Lagios M, et al. The influence of margin width on local control of ductal carcinoma in situ of the breast. *NEJM.* 1999; 340:1455-61.
16. Meyer J, et al.Biopsy of occult breast lesions. *JAMA.* 1990; 253:2341-43.

Chapter 23

Localized Treatment Options for Breast Cancer

1. Cody H. Sentinel lymph node mapping in breast cancer. *Oncology.* 1999; 13:25-43.
2. Rovere GQ, Bird PA. Sentinel lymph node biopsy in breast cancer. *Lancet.* 1998; 352:421-22.
3. Harris P, et al. Current status of conservative surgery and radiotherapy as primary local treatment for early carcinoma of the breast. *Breast Cancer Res Treat.* 1985; 5:24-5.
4. Winchester D, Cox J. Standards for diagnosis and management of invasive breast carcinoma. *CA Cancer J Clin* 1998; 48:83-107.
5. Fisher B, et al. Ten-year results of a randomized clinical trial comparing radical mastectomy and total mastectomy with or without radiation. *NEJM.* 1985; 312:674-681.
6. Early Breast Cancer Trialist' Collaborative Group. Effects of radiotherapy and surgery in early breast cancer. *NEJM.* 1995; 333:1444-55.
7. Marks L, Prosnitz L. Lumpectomy with and without radiation for early-stage breast cancer and DCIS. *Oncology.*1997; 11:1361-72.
8. Fisher B, et al. Eight-year results of a randomized clinical trial comparing total mastectomy and lumpectomy with or without irradiation in the treatment of breast cancer. *NEJM.* 1989; 320:822-28.
9. Veronesi U, et al. Breast conservation is the treatment of choice in small breast cancer: long term results of a randomized trial. *Eur J Cancer.*1990; 26:668-70.
10. Sarrazin D, et al. Ten year results of a randomized trial comparing a conservative treatment to mastectomy in early breast cancer. *Radiother Oncol.* 1989; 14:177-184.
11. Straus K, et al. Results of the National Cancer Institute Early Breast Cancer Trial. *JNCI Monograph* 1992; No.11. Wash, D.C.: Govt Printing Office, pp. 27-32.
12. Spitalier J, et al. Breast conserving surgery with radiation therapy for operable mammary carcinoma: a 25-year experience. *World J Surg.* 1986; 10:1014-20.
13. Fourquet A, et al. Prognostic factors of breast recurrence in conservative management of early breast cancer: A 25 year follow-up. *Int J Radiat Oncol Biol Phys.* 1987; 17:719-25.
14. NIH Consensus Conference. Treatment of early stage breast cancer. *JAMA.* 1991; 256:391-395.
15. Veronesi U, et al. Quadrantectomy versus lumpectomy for small size breast cancer. *Eur J Cancer.* 1990; 26:671-673.

16. Fisher B, et al. Significance of ipsilateral breast tumor recurrence after lumpectomy. *Lancet.* 1991; 338:327-31.
17. Weidner N, et al. Tumor angiogenesis and metastases - correlation in invasive breast carcinoma. *NEJM.* 1991; 324:1-8.
18. McGuire WL. The optimal timing of mastectomy: low tide or high tide? *Ann Intern Med.* 1991; 115:401-403.
19. Farrow DC, et al. Geographic variation in the treatment of localized breast cancer. *NEJM.* 1992; 326:1097-1101.
20. Nattinger AB, et al. Geographic variation in the use of breast conserving treatment for breast cancer. *NEJM.* 1992; 326:1102-1107.
21. Silliman RA, et al. Age as predictor of diagnostic and initial treatment intensity in newly diagnosed breast cancer patients. *J Gerontol.* 1989; 44:M46-M50.
22. Physicians often fail to recognize post-mastectomy pain syndrome. *Oncology News International.* Nov 1993: 20.

Chapter 24
Conventional Systemic Treatment for Breast Cancer

1. Kennedy BJ. Hormone therapy for advanced breast cancer. *Cancer.* 1965; 18:1551-57.
2. Legha SS, et al. Hormonal therapy of breast cancer: New approaches and concepts. *Ann Intern Med.* 1978; 88:69-77.
3. Murphy B, Muss H. Hormonal therapy of breast cancer: State of the art. *Oncology.* 1997;11:7-13.
4. Taylor SG, Gelman R, et al. Combination chemotherapy compared to tamoxifen as initial therapy for stage IV breast cancer in elderly women. *Ann Intern Med.* 1986; 104:455-61.
5. Anonymous. A randomized trial in post-menopausal patients with advanced breast cancer comparing endocrine and cytotoxic therapy. The Australian and New Zealand Breast Cancer Trials group. *J Clin Oncology.* 1986; 4:186-93.
6. Early Breast Cancer Trialists' Collaborative Group. Systemic treatment of early breast cancer by hormonal, cytotoxic, or immune therapy. *Lancet.* 1992; 339:1-15; and 71-85.
7. Early Breast Cancer Trialists' Collaborative Group. Ovarian ablation in early breast cancer: overview of the randomized trials. *Lancet.* 1996; 348:1189-96.
8. Early Breast Cancer Trialists' Collaborative Group. Tamoxifen for early breast cancer: an overview of the randomized trials. *Lancet.* 1998; 351:1451-67.
9. Early Breast Cancer Trialists' Collaborative Group. Ovarian ablation for early breast cancer. *Cochrane Database Syst Rev* 2000;(2):CD000485
10. Hortobagyi G. Treatment of breast cancer. *NEJM.*1998; 339:974-84.
11. Barley V. Time for reappraisal of ovarian ablation in early breast cancer. *Lancet.* 1996; 348:1184.
12. Goldhirsh A, et al. Effect of systemic adjuvant treatment on first sites of breast cancer relapse. *Lancet.* 1994; 343:377-81.
13. Pritchard K. Adjuvant systemic therapy for breast cancer: a tale of relapse and survival. *Lancet.* 1994; 343:370-71.
14. Scottish Cancer Trials Breast Group and ICRF Breast Unit. Ovarian ablation versus CMF in premenopausal women with stage II breast cancer: the Scottish Trial. *Lancet.* 1993; 341:1293-98.
15. Ejlertsen B, Dombernowski, et al. Comparable effect of ovarian ablaton and CMF in premenopausal ER+ patients. *Proc Am Soc Clin Oncol.* 1999; 18:Abstract 248.
16. Jakesz R, et al. Comparison of adjuvant therapy with tamoxifen and goserelin vs. CMF in premenopausal stage I and II ER+ patients: Austrian Group. *Proc Am Soc Clin Oncol.* 1999; 18:Abstract 250.
17. Gelber R, et al. Adjuvant chemotherapy plus tamoxifen compared to tamoxifen alone – meta analysis. *Lancet.* 1996; 347:1066-71.
18. McCarthy N, Swain S. Update on adjuvant chemotherapy for early breast cancer. *Oncology.* 2000;14:1267-87.
19. Dodwell DJ. Cytotoxic drugs: A search for dose response. *Lancet.* 1993; 341:614-16.
20. Stewart, et al. Dose response in the treatment of breast cancer. *Lancet.* 1994; 343:402-04.
21. Rodenhuis S, Richel D, et al. Randomized trial of high-dose chemotherapy and haemopoietic progenitor-cell support in operable breast cancer with extensive nodal involvement. *Lancet.* 1998; 352:515-21.
22. Antman K, Heitjan D, Hortobagyi G. High dose chemotherapy for breast cancer. *JAMA.* 1999; 282:1701-03.
23. Nissen-Meyer R, et al. Short perioperative versus long-term adjuvant chemotherapy. *Recent Results Can Res.* 1988, 98:91-98.
24. CRC Adjuvant Breast Trial Working Party. Cyclophosphamide and tamoxifen as

adjuvant therapies in the management of breast cancer. *Br J Cancer.* 1988; 57:604-07.

25. The Ludwig Breast Cancer Study Group. Prolonged disease-free survival after one course of perioperative adjuvant chemotherapy for node negative breast cancer. *NEJM.* 1989; 320:491-96.
26. Hrushesky WJ. The clinical application of chronobiology to oncology. Am J Anat. 1983; 168:519-42.
27. Haus E, et al. Chronobiology in hematology and immunology. *Am J Anat.* 1983, 168:467-517.
28. Rivard GE, et al. Maintenance chemotherapy for childhood acute lymphoblastic leukemia: better in the evening. *Lancet.* 1985 (Dec 7): 1264-66.
29. Dodwell D. Adjuvant chemotherapy for early breast cancer: doubts and decisions. *Lancet.* 1998; 351:1506-07.
30. Glick JH. Adjuvant therapy of node negative breast cancer: another point of view. *JNCI.* 1988; 80:1076.
31. The Ludwig Cancer Study Group. Prolonged disease-free interval after one course of perioperative adjunctive chemotherapy for node negative breast cancer. *NEJM.* 1989; 320:491-96.
32. Fisher B, et al. A randomized trial evaluating sequential methotrexate and fluorouracil in the treatment of patients with node negative breast cancer who have estrogen receptor negative tumors. *NEJM.* 1989; 320:473-78.
33. Fisher B, et al. A randomized trial evaluating tamoxifen in the treatment of patients with node negative breast cancer who have estrogen receptor positive tumors. *NEJM.* 1989; 320:479-84.
34. Mansour EG, et al. Efficacy of adjuvant chemotherapy in high risk node negative breast cancer. *NEJM.* 1989; 320:485-90.
35. McGuire WL. Adjuvant therapy of node negative breast cancer. *NEJM.* 1989; 320:525-27.
36. NIH Consensus Conference. Treatment of early stage breast cancer. JAMA. 1991; 265:391-95.
37. McGuire WL, et al. How to use prognostic factors in axillary node negative breast cancer patients. *JNCI.*1990; 82:1006-15.
38. McGuire WL, Clark. Prognostic factors and treatment decisions in axillary node negative breast cancer. *NEJM.* 1992; 326:1756-61.
39. Hillner and Smith. Efficacy and cost effectiveness of adjuvant chemotherapy in women with node negative breast cancer. *NEJM.* 1991; 324:160-168.
40. Kramer BS. Breast cancer-control: weighing cost versus effect. *Contemp Oncology.* 1991; Nov-Dec:43-50.
41. Bagenal FS, et al. Survival of patients with breast cancer attending Bristol Cancer Help Center. *Lancet.*1990; 336:606-10.
42. Stadtmauer E, O'Neill, et al. Conventional dose chemotherapy compared with high dose chemotherapy plus autologous hematopoietic stem cell transplantation for metastatic breast cancer. *NEJM.* 2000; 342:1069-76.
43. Basade MM, Gulati S. High-dose chemotherapy in metastatic breast cancer. *Lancet.* 1998; 351:386-87.
44. Bergh J. Where next with stem cell supported high-dose therapy for breast cancer? *Lancet.* 2000; 355:944-45.
45. Stephenson J. Bone marrow/stem cells: No edge in breast cancer. *JAMA.* 1999; 281:1576-78.
46. Rose LJ. The problem of evidence: Law and medicine look at autologous bone marrow transplant. *Managed Care & Cancer.* 1999; Nov/Dec: 14-19.
47. Editorial. Chaos surrounds high-dose chemotherapy for breast cancer. *Lancet.* 1999; 353:1633.
48. McCarthy M. Unproven breast-cancer therapy widely used in USA. *Lancet.* 1996; 347:1617.
49. Slamon D, et al. Use of chemotherapy plus a monoclonal antibody against Her2 for metastatic breast cancer that overexpresses Her2. *NEJM.* 2001; 344:783-92.
50. Kimmick G, Muss H. Systemic therapy for older women with breast cancer. *Oncology.* 2001; 15:280-299.
51. Muss H. How to treat the older woman with breast cancer. *Contemporary Oncology.* 1993; (May):27-38.
52. Goldhirsch A, et al. Treatment of breast cancer in elderly patients. *Lancet.* 1990;336:564-65.
53. Christman K, et al. Chemotherapy of metastatic breast cancer in the elderly. *JAMA.* 1992; 268:57-62.
54. Burstein H, Winer E. Primary care for survivors of breast cacner. *NEJM.* 2000; 343:1086-94.
55. American Society of Clinical Oncology. Recommended breast cancer surveillance guidelines. *J Clin Oncol.* 1997; 15:2149-56.

56. Holland JF. Karnofsky Memorial Lecture: Breaking the cure barrier. *J Clin Oncol.* 1983; 1:74-90.

57. Legha SS, et al. Complete remissions in metastatic breast cancer treated with combination drug therapy. *Ann Intern Med.* 1979; 91:847-52.

58. Blumenschein, et al. Seven year follow-up of stage IV patients entering complete remission from FAC presented at the Third European Oncology Res Treat Conf, April 19, 1983. Amsterdam, the Netherlands.

59. Lippman M, et al. Diagnosis and Management of Breast Cancer. Philadelphia, PA: W.B. Saunders Company, 1988; pp. 375-406.

60. Zwaveling, et al. An evaluation of routine follow-up for detection of breast cancer recurrences. *J Surg Oncol.* 1987; 34:194-97.

61. Broyn and Froyen. Evaluation of routine follow-up after surgery for breast cancer. *ACTA Chir Scand.* 1982; 148:401-04.

62. The GIVIO Investigators. Impact of follow-up testing on survival and health-related quality of life in breast cancer patients. *JAMA.* 1994;271:1587-92.

63. Rosselli M, et al. Intensive diagnostic follow-up after treatment of primary breast cancer. *JAMA.* 1994; 271:1593-97.

64. Fisher B, et al. Endometrial cancer in tamoxifen-treated breast cancer patients: Findings from NSABP B-14. *JNCI.* 1994; 86:527-537.

65. Barakat R. The effect of tamoxifen on the endometrium. *Oncology.* 1995; 9:129-139.

66. Bergman L, Beelen M, et al. Risk and prognosis of endometrial cancer after tamoxifen for breast cancer. *Lancet.* 2000; 356:881-87.

67. Barakat R, et al. Effect of adjuvant tamoxifen on the endometrium in women with breast cancer: Prospective study using endometrial biopsy. *J Clin Oncol.* 2000; 18:3459-63.

68. Gerber B, et al. Effects of adjuvant tamoxifen on the endometrium in postmenopausal women with breast cancer: A prospective study using transvaginal ultrasound. *J Clin Oncol.* 2000; 18:3464-70.

69. Adler A, et al. Immunocompetence, immunosuppression, and human breast cancer. *Cancer.* 1980; 45:2061-83.

70. Mandeville R, et al. Biological markers and breast cancer. Depressed immunocompetence. *Cancer.* 1982, 50:1280-88.

71. Greenspan EM. Prior tuberculosis in long term survivors of breast and ovarian cancer from a New York oncology practice (1954-1974). *Mt Sinai J Med.* 1985; 52:465-68.

72. Cassileth, B., et al. Survival and quality of life among patients receiving unproven as compared with conventional cancer therapy. *NEJM.* 1991; 324:1180-85.

73. Dodwell D. Adjuvant chemotherapy for early breast cancer: doubts and decisions. *Lancet.* 1998; 351:1506-07.

74. Rajagopal S, Goodman, Tannock. Adjuvant chemotherapy for breast cancer: discordance between physicians' perception of benefit and the results of clinical trials. *Lancet.* 1998;351:1506-07.

75. Richards M, Ramirez A, et al. Offering choice of treatment to patients with cancers: a review. *Eur J Cancer.* 1995; 31A:112-16.

76. Editorial. Breast Cancer: have we lost our way? *Lancet.* 1993; 341:343-44.

77. Lancet Conference Summary. The challenge of breast cancer. *Lancet.* 1994; 343:1085-86.

Chapter 25
Male Breast Cancer

1. Adami HO, et al. The survival pattern in male breast cancer: an analysis of 1429 patients from the Nordic countries. *Cancer.* 1989; 64:1177-82.

2. Bagley CS, et al. Adjuvant chemotherapy in males with cancer of the breast. *Am J Clin Oncol.* 1987; 10:55-60.

3. Eldar S, et al. Radiation carcinogenesis in the male breast. *Eur J Surg Oncol.* 1989; 15:274-78.

4. Orentreich, et al. Mammogenesis in transsexuals. *J Invest Dermatol.* 1974; 63:142.

5. Symmers WC. Carcinoma of the breast in transsexuals. *Br Med J.* 1968; 1:83.

6. Treves and Holleb. Cancer of the male breast. *Cancer.* 1955; 8:1239.

7. Fodor. Breast cancer in a patient with gynecomastia. *Plast Reconstruct Surg.* 1989; 84:976-79.

8. Lin RS. Epidemiological findings in male breast cancer. *Proc Am Assoc Cancer Res.* 1980; 21:72.

9. Fisher B, et al. Eight year results of a randomized clinical trial comparing total mastectomy and lumpectomy with or without irradiation in the treatment of breast cancer. *NEJM.* 1989; 320:822-28.

10. Veronesi U, et al. Comparison of Halsted mastectomy with quadrantectomy, axillary dissection, and radiotherapy in early breast

cancer: Long-term results. *Eur J Cancer Clin Oncol.* 1986; 22:1085-89.
11. Friedman M, et al. Estrogen receptors in male breast cancer: clinical and pathological correlations. *Cancer.* 1981 47:134-37.
12. Gupta N, et al. Estrogen receptors in male breast cancer. *Cancer.* 1980; 46:1781-84.
13. Everson R, et al. Clinical correlations of steroid receptors and male breast cancer. *Cancer Res.* 1980; 40:991-97.
14. Donegan W, et al. Carcinoma of the male breast. A 30 year review of 28 cases. *Arch Surg.* 1973; 106:273-279.
15. Horn B, Roof Y. Male breast cancer. *Oncology.* 1976; 33:188-91.
16. Ribeiro G. Tamoxifen in the treatment of male breast carcinoma. *Clin Radiol.* 1983; 34:625-28.
17. Donegan W. Cancer of the breast in men. *CA Cancer J Clin.* 1991; 41:339-54
18. Kinne D. Management of male breast cancer. *Oncology.* 1991; March:45-48.

Chapter 26
Quality of Life and Ethics

1. *Cancer Treat Rep.* 1985. 69:1155-57.
2. Hurny C, et al. Quality of life studies in international groups. *Eur J Cancer.* 1992; 28:118-24.
3. Kurtzman S, et al. Rehabilitation of the cancer patient. *Am J Surg.* 1988; 155:791-803.
4. Bullard DG, et al. Sexual health care and cancer. *Front Radiat Ther Oncol.* 1980; 14:55-58.
5. Silberfarb PM, et al. Psychosocial aspects of neoplastic disease. Functional status of breast cancer patients. *Am J Psychiatry.* 1980; 137:450-455.
6. Jamison KR, et al. Psychosocial aspects of mastectomy. *Am J Psychiatry.* 1978; 135:432-36.
7. Battersby C, et al. Mastectomy in a large public hospital. *Aust N Z J Surg.* 1978; 48:401-04.
8. Taylor SE, et al. Attributions, beliefs about control and adjustment to breast cancer. *J Person Soc Psychol.* 1984; 46:489-502.
9. Steinberg MD, et al. Psychological outcome of lumpectomy versus mastectomy in the treatment of breast cancer. *Am J Psychiatry.* 1985; 142:34-39.
10. Margolis G, et al. Psychological effects of breast conserving cancer treatment and mastectomy. *Psychosom Med.* 1990; 31:33-39.
11. Psychological Aspects of Breast Cancer Study Group: Psychological response to mastectomy. *Cancer.* 1987; 59:189-96.
12. Vinokur AD, et al. Physical and psychosocial functioning in adjustment to breast cancer. *Cancer.* 1989; 63:394-405.
13. Dean C, et al. Affects of immediate breast reconstruction on psychosocial morbidity after mastectomy. *Lancet.* 1983; 1:459-62.
14. Noone RB, et al. Patient acceptance of immediate reconstruction following mastectomy. *Plast Reconstruct Surg.* 1982; 69:632-40.
15. Schain W, et al. The sooner the better: a study of women undergoing immediate versus delayed breast reconstruction. *Am J Psychiatry.* 1985; 142:40-46.
16. Masters and Johnson. Human Sexual Response. 1966; Boston: Little, Brown.
17. Schover LR. The impact of breast cancer on sexuality, body image, and intimate relationships. *CA Cancer J Clin.* 1991; 41:112-120.
18. Steinhauser K, Christakis N, et al. Factors considered important at the end of life by patients, family, physicians, and other care providers. *JAMA.* 2000; 284:2476-82.
19. President's Commission for the Study of Ethical Problems in Medicine. *Making Health Care Decisions.* 1982; **2**: 245-246.
20. Arato v. Avedon. 5 Cal 4th 1172, 23 Cal Rptr. 1993. 2D. 131, 858P. 2D 598.
21. Smith TJ. Editorial. *JAMA.* 1998; 279:1746-48.
22. Moertel CG. Off-label drug use for cancer therapy and National Health Care Priorities. *JAMA.* 1991; 266:3031-32.

Chapter 27
Untreated Breast Cancer: Its Natural History

1. Bloom HJ, et al. Natural history of untreated breast cancer (1805-1933). Comparison of untreated and treated cases according to histological grade of malignancy. *Br Med J.* 1962; ii:213-221.
2. Buchanan JB, et al. Tumor growth, doubling times, and inability of the radiologist to diagnosis certain cancers. *Radiol Clin N Am.* 1983; 21:115-26.
3. Haagensen CD, et al. Breast Carcinoma-Risk and Detection. 1981. Philadelphia: W.B. Saunders.
4. Fournier D, et al. Growth rate of 147 mammary carcinomas. *Cancer.* 1980; 45:2198-07.

5. Kramer WM, Rush. Mammary duct proliferation in the elderly. *Cancer.* 1973; 31:130-137.
6. Nielsen M, et al. Precancerous and cancerous breast lesions during lifetime and at autopsy. *Cancer.*1984; 54:612-615.
7. Baum M. The curability of breast cancer. *Br Med J.* 1976; i:439-442.
8. Fox MS. On diagnosis and treatment of breast cancer. *JAMA.* 1979; 241:489-494.
9. Brinkley D, Haybittle. Long term survival of women with breast cancer. *Lancet.* 1984; i:1118.
10. Le MG, et al. Long term survival of women with breast cancer. *Lancet.* 1984; ii:922.
11. Rutqvist LF, Wallgren. Long term survival of 458 young breast cancer patients. *Cancer.* 1985; 55:658-65.
12. Skrabanek P. False premises and false promises of breast cancer screening. *Lancet.* 1985; (August):316-19.
13. Jackson A. On carcinoma of the breast and its treatment. *Med Pre.* 1988; i:552-553
14. Lewison EF, Montague, eds. Diagnosis and Treatment of Breast Cancer. 1981. Baltimore: Williams and Wilkins, pg. 3.
15. Fisher B. Laboratory and clinical research in breast cancer: a personal adventure: the David A. Karnofsky Memorial Lecture. *Cancer Res.* 1980; 40:3863-74.
16. Fisher ER. Pathobiological considerations in the treatment of breast cancer. In: Controversies in Breast Disease, ed. Grundfest-Broniatowski and Esselstyn. 1988; New York: Marcel Dekker, pp. 151-180.
17. Dunken W, Kerr. The curability of breast cancer. *Br Med J.* 1976; ii:781-783

Chapter 28
The Simone Ten Point Plan

1. Enas, AE. Triglycerides and small, dense low-density lipoprotein. *JAMA.* 1998; 280:1990.

Glossary of Medical Terms

Adjuvant treatment. Treatment given in addition to the primary treatment.

Aspiration. Removal of liquids or solids from a lump using a needle and syringe.

Autosomal dominant trait. A single gene, acting alone, to produce an outcome.

Axilla. Armpit.

Benign. A noncancer, nonmalignant growth.

Biopsy. The gross and microscopic examination of tissues removed from the body to make a medical diagnosis; excisional biopsy is the removal of the entire breast lump, whereas incisional biopsy is the removal of a small piece of the breast mass.

Brachytherapy. See Implant radiation.

Cancer. A malignant uncontrollable growth that invades surrounding tissues and spreads to other organs as well.

Carcinoma. A cancer that begins in the lining or coverings of organs.

Chemotherapy. Chemical drugs used to treat an illness.

Computed tomography (CT). A computerized X-ray study that details the cross-sectional anatomy of a part of a body.

Cyst. A sac in an organ filled with fluid, gas, or semisolids.

Diagnostic mammography. An X-ray of the breast done for a woman who has symptoms. See also Mammogram; Screening mammography.

Duct. Tubes in breast from lobes to the nipple through which milk is delivered.

Estrogen. A hormone produced mainly in the ovaries responsible for the development of female characteristics and the menstrual cycle.

External radiation. Radiation from a machine outside the body delivered to a site in the body. See also Implant radiation; Radiation therapy.

Genotype. The hereditary make-up of someone as determined by genes.

Gynecologist. Physician who treats diseases of the female organs.

Hormone therapy. Adding or removing hormones to treat cancer.

Hormones. Steroid chemicals produced by various organs for different purposes.

Implant radiation (also known as brachytherapy). A radioactive substance is placed directly into the tissue in the body that needs treatment. See also External radiation; Radiation therapy.

Lobe. A section of the breast.

Lobule. A division of the lobe in the breast.

Local-regional therapy. Treatment directed to the tumor bed and its adjacent surrounding tissues.

Lumpectomy. Removal of only the breast lump; excisional biopsy is sometimes used synonymously.
Lymph nodes. Oval or round bodies located along the lymphatic vessels that remove bacteria or foreign particles from the lymph. Cancers can spread to lymph nodes causing the lymph nodes' size to increase.
Lymphedema. Fluid that sometimes collects in the tissues of extremities as a result of removing lymph vessels or lymph nodes.
Malignant. A cancerous tumor that is growing and spreading.
Mammogram. See Diagnostic or Screening mammography.
Mastectomy. Surgical removal of the breast.
Mendelian inheritance. Classical genetics that has two genes operating to produce a single outcome.
Menopause. The time when menstrual cycles stop permanently.
Metastasis. The spread of cancer from the primary organ, like breast, to another more distant organ, like bone.
Oncologist. Physician who treats cancer.
Palpation. Examining organ by feeling to detect abnormalities.
Pathologist. Physician who reads prepared microscopic slides containing biopsied tissue in order to determine a diagnosis.
Pathology. The study and classification of tissue specimens with the use of a microscope.
Progesterone. A female hormone secreted by the ovaries.
Prosthesis. The artificial replacement of a body part, as with a breast that is worn underneath clothing.
Radiation therapy. Treatment of cancer using high energy radiation from X-ray or other sources. See also External or Implant radiation.
Screening. Tests used to find disease when a person has no symptoms of an illness.
Screening mammography. An X-ray of the breast done for a woman with no symptoms. See also Diagnostic mammography; Mammogram.
Staging. Determining where the cancer is located in the body.
Systemic therapy. Treatment that travels to all parts of the body, usually by way of the bloodstream.
Tumor. The Latin word that means growth or swelling; today's usage refers to an abnormal growth of tissue; it does not imply, however, that the mass is a cancer.
Tumor marker. Something detectable in the body that may suggest a cancer is growing.
Ultrasound. A diagnostic test that bounces sound waves off body tissues, a process that can differentiate solid from liquid. This is most useful to distinguish the contents of a mass in a breast. A solid mass needs further in vestigation, but a liquid-filled mass may not.

Sources of Information

National Cancer Institute (NCI), Cancer Information Service – call 800-4-CANCER for your questions and booklets on topics.

NCI Comprehensive and Clinical Cancer Centers around the country – call 301-496-4000 to find the Center near you.

National Cancer Institute Building 31, Room 10A24
9000 Rockville Pike Bethesda, MD 20892

NABCO – National Alliance of Breast Cancer Organizations

9 East 37th Street, 10 Floor New York, NY 10016
212-889-0606 888-806-2226 www.nabco.org

The American Society of Plastic and Reconstructive Surgeons

444 East Algonquin Road Arlington Heights, IL 60005
847-228-9900 800-635-0635

The Health Insurance Association of America (HIAA) will answer your questions concerning insurance coverage.

Fulfillment Department PO Box 41455
Washington, DC 20018 202-866-6244

The YWCA Encore Program – support for breast cancer patients.

National Headquarters 726 Broadway
New York, NY 10003 212-614-2827

PDQ (Physicians Data Query) – NCI database provides prognostic, stage, treatment information, and protocol summaries. A computer modem is needed. For information, call the NCI at 310- 496-7403.

National Organizations

4-Cancer 800-4-CANCER A service of the National Cancer Institute. Supplies information about cancer prevention, symptoms, kinds of cancer, clinical trials, second opinions, and referrals to support groups.

Share 212-382-2111 Provides emotional support and information. Will place callers' names on mailing list for educational seminars.

Y-Me 800-221-2141 All counselors are breast-cancer survivors. Provides information on early detection, accredited mammography facilities and cancer centers, and referrals to physicians and support groups.

About the Author (DrSimone.com)

During your life, there are people you would like to meet....and there are people you should meet. Meet now Charles B. Simone, Masters of Medical Sciences, Medical Doctor, **Internist** (trained at the Cleveland Clinic 1975-1977), **Medical Oncologist** (National Cancer Institute 1977-1982), **Tumor Immunologist** (National Cancer Institute 1977-1982), and **Radiation Oncologist** (Univ of Pennsylvania 1982-1985).

While thoroughly engrossed in basic science at the NCI, Dr Simone found new direction as a result of his patients. Vice President Humphrey died not of his cancer but of malnutrition and a young man with cancer was dying because he lacked certain vitamins. Newly interested in nutrition and cancer his research led to the landmark book, *Cancer and Nutrition* (1981) thrusting him into the alternative medicine arena. In 1992 he was asked to help organize the Office of Alternative Medicine, National Institutes of Health. He later received FDA approval to investigate the use of shark cartilage to treat advanced cancers.

In 1993 he was called upon to write the language that led to the compromise in the US Congress ensuring that all Americans have free access to information and food supplements – the Dietary, Health and Education Act of 1994 (DSHEA). Then he helped win landmark cases against the Food and Drug Administration [*Pearson v. Shalala*] in which the FDA was found to violate the First and Fifth Amendment rights of American citizens. For all this patriotic work in behalf of the American people, he was bestowed the first **Bulwark of Liberty Award** in May 2001 by the American Preventive Medical Association and the Foundation for Alternative Medicine.

He has authored more than 60 peer-reviewed articles and many books: Cancer and Nutrition, How to Save Yourself from a Terrorist Attack, Prostate Health, KidStart, others.

Dr. Simone consults for heads of state of the US and other countries, celebrities, and advises many governments. He testifies for the US Congress regarding health, cancer, disease prevention, children's health programs, FDA reform, alternative medicine, and the dissemination of truth to patients. He appears on 60 MINUTES, Prime Time Live, MS NBC, Fox, and others.

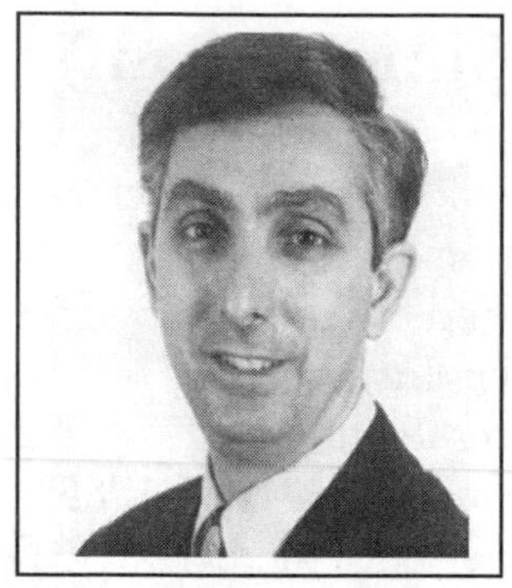

"What is needed is some person, some institution, some inescapable "force" that captures the imagination of our citizens and demonstrates that cancer and other diseases will be eliminated only when each of us comes to understand that this can only occur as part of a lifelong process of sanity, balance, moderation, and self-respect."

About Charles B. Simone, M.D. ....

"Nancy joins me in sending you our best wishes for the success of your vital work."
Ronald Reagan, President

"Dr. Charles B. Simone, an expert in the field of cancer research and treatment, is an individual for whom I have the highest respect."
Peter W. Rodino, Jr., Former Chairman, Judiciary

"If everyone would follow Dr. Simone's plan, we would make major strides toward putting the cancer doctors out of work."
Robert A. Good, MD, PhD, Frm Chairman, Memorial Cancer, NYC

"I congratulate Dr. Simone on innovative work."
Dr. Linus Pauling, two-time Nobel Laureate

"Valuable and timely. Should prove beneficial to the public."
George E. Stringfellow, American Cancer Society

"Thank you for having the courage to come forward. Your testimony is a powerful indicator of the great need for change in America's system of health care and the importance of an individual's freedom of choice when treating illness."
Dan Burton, Chairman Committee Government Reform and Oversight

"Thank you for all your work on behalf of alternative therapies."
Tom Harkin, US Senator

"Excellent work." **Dr. Denis Burkitt**

"Your work will reduce cancer." **William Bennett, Frm Sec Education**

Index